NEW EDITION

THE

36-HOUR

DAY

*a family guide to caring at home for
people with Alzheimer's disease and
other confusional illnesses*

Nancy L. Mace and Peter V. Rabins, MD
with Beverly A. Castleton,
Evelyn McEwen and Barbara Meredith

CO-PUBLISHED WITH AGE CONCERN

Hodder & Stoughton

A MEMBER OF THE HODDER HEADLINE GROUP

This book is dedicated to everyone
who gives a '36-hour day' to the care
of a person with a dementing illness.

British Library Cataloguing in Publication Data

Mace, Nancy L.
   36 Hour Day. – 2Rev.ed
   I. Title
   649.8

ISBN 0-340-56382-6

Original USA edition
Copyright © 1981 by The Johns Hopkins University Press
UK edition (with adaptations) first published 1985, fourth impression 1988,
fifth impression 1990

Second UK edition 1992
Impression number 10 9 8 7 6 5 4 3 2
Year   1999 1998 1997 1996 1995

Whilst the advice and information in this book is believed to be true
and accurate at the date of going to press, neither the author nor the
publisher can accept any legal responsibility or liability for any errors
or omissions that may be made.

Typeset by Rowland Phototypesetting Limited, Bury St Edmunds, Suffolk
Printed in Great Britain for Hodder & Stoughton Education, a
division of Hodder Headline Plc, 338 Euston Road, London NWI 3BH
by Atheneum Press Limited.

Authors' Details

In the USA

Nancy L Mace, MA, is a consultant to the Office of Technology Assessment, US Congress, and to the Alzheimer's Association. She was formerly an Assistant in Psychiatry and Co-ordinator of the T Rowe and Eleanor Price Teaching Service of the Department of Psychiatry and Behavioral Sciences of the Johns Hopkins University School of Medicine.

Peter V Rabins, MD, MPH, is Associate Professor of Psychiatry, Director of the Psychogeriatric Unit, and Director of the T Rowe and Eleanor Price Teaching Service of the Department of Psychiatry and Behavioral Sciences of the Johns Hopkins University School of Medicine.

In the UK

Beverly Ann Castleton, MA, MB, BChir, FRCP, is a Consultant Physician in the Care of the Elderly and Young Physically Disabled at St Peter's Hospital, Chertsey and Weybourne Trust, Surrey.

Evelyn McEwen, MA Cantab, MSc, is Divisional Director Services, at Age Concern England.

Barbara Meredith, BA, MSc, is Information and Policy Officer for Health and Personal Social Services, Age Concern England.

Contents

Foreword to the first edition

A great many people are involved in the care of elderly patients with dementia, from the doctor and nurse who manage the illness but who can remain detached from the problem, to the sufferer and the care-giving relation, from whom the problem never goes away. The doctor is preoccupied with whether or not he has made the correct diagnosis, undertaken the necessary investigations and prescribed the safest and most effective treatment. The nurse worries how the patient eats, drinks, and sleeps; when and how she uses the toilet; whether she is going to wander away. Meanwhile the patient may be preoccupied with her bowels or with waiting for her long-deceased husband to return from work to eat the meal she has prepared for him. The patient's daughter (and I make no apology for casting both patient and carer in the feminine role, because this is as it is in the majority of cases) is preoccupied with how much longer the patient will exhaust and torment her with outrageous behaviour, and how much longer she will be able to bear it; with what is going to happen next; with what caused it all; with whether she will suffer from the same thing herself in her own old age.

The doctor, nurse, social worker and health visitor endeavour to become aware of the preoccupations of patients, colleagues and relatives, just as relatives want to know what is pre-occupying the doctors. But in many cases the gap remains unbridged. And indeed it is a formidable task to understand, let alone to explain how an intelligent and considerate person, in charge of her own life and sensitive to the needs of others, becomes an irresponsible, dangerous, unfeeling automaton. Also, what happens to a devoted carer who finds herself trapped within four walls with a crazed, unpredictable caricature of a person once loved, now pitied for what she has lost and resented for what she has done to others.

If it is possible for a book to explain these horrifying and bewildering processes in terms that a lay person can understand, this one does so. Its striking title, *The 36-Hour Day*, emphasises that the true victim of this disease is the carer; her many tasks mean that she has not enough hours in the day for the patient's needs let alone for her own. The professional skill of doctors and nurses can do much to mitigate the manifestations of the disease, and even in a few cases to eradicate it. But their work finishes and they go home at night to tranquillity, while the carer battles on bewildered and unenlightened.,

This book has now been made available to British readers on the initiative of Age Concern England. The considerable work of 'translating' the terminology and the references to services to fit the British scene has been skilfully executed by Dr Beverly Castleton, with the assistance of the staff of Age Concern England. It is to be hoped that at least one of the 36 hours of the carer's day, and one of the 24 hours of the 'professional's' day, can be set aside for reading this book and referring to it, because it contains much wisdom, sound sense, good advice and practical assistance which can help carers and professionals to understand one another's preoccupations. A more tolerable life for the carer entails better care for the patient and less pressure on doctors and nurses. We should all be grateful for this book.

Professor Bernard Isaacs
Department of Geriatric Medicine
University of Birmingham

Preface to the first edition

Although this book was written for the families of people with dementing illnesses, we recognise that other people, including those suffering from these conditions, may read this book. We welcome this. We hope that the use of such words as *patient* and *brain-injured person* will not discourage those who have these illnesses. These words were chosen because we want to emphasise that the people who suffer from these conditions are ill, not 'just old'. We hope the tone of the book conveys that we think of you as individuals and people and never as objects.

This book is not intended to provide medical or legal advice. The services of a competent professional should be obtained when legal, medical, or other specific advice is needed.

At present not all professionals are knowledgeable about dementia. We frequently refer to trained personnel who can help you, but we recognise that you may have difficulty finding the help you need. You, the care giver, will need to utilise both professional resources and your own good judgement. This book cannot address the particulars of your situation, but is intended only as a general guide.

In addition we recognise that criteria for allocating services are often locally determined and the provision and availability of such services as home care assistants, meals-on-wheels, day centres, district nursing and community psychiatric nursing vary from area to area. Charging policies may also differ from one local authority to another.

We use examples of family situations to illustrate our discussion. These examples are not descriptions of real families or patients. They are based upon experiences, feelings, and solutions that families and patients have discussed with us. Names and other identifying information have been changed.

Both men and women suffer from these diseases. To simplify reading, we will use the masculine pronouns *he* and *his* and the feminine pronouns *she* and *her* in alternate chapters.

Acknowledgements

So many people have given of their time, experience, and wisdom that it is not possible to name them all. We wish to thank all those known and anonymous who have contributed ideas and information.

The influence of the teachers and colleagues who shaped our ideas in the first edition remains. Paul R McHugh, MD, Director of the Department of Psychiatry and Behavioral Science at the Johns Hopkins University School of Medicine, who encouraged us to write the first edition, continues to be a dynamic influence in our approach to these issues.

In the nine years following the publication of the first edition of The 36-Hour Day, hundreds of family care-givers and professionals have shared their ideas and solutions to problems. We have used many of these ideas in the revised edition. Many people have mentioned areas that needed further elaboration in the revised edition. A few people who suffer from a dementing illness have read and shared their comments. Our friends and colleagues, translators of foreign editions, physicians, dentists, and others have answered our questions and offered suggestions. Over time we have considered this information and tested it against the experience of care-givers and professionals. This process of learning, growth, testing, and reshaping created the revised edition. It would be impossible to list every name and would violate the privacy of many. Nevertheless, we are indebted to the generosity of this worldwide community.

The Alzheimer's Association has distributed countless copies of the first edition and its board members and staff have contributed to the revised edition. Kathryn Ling, Tom Kirk, Joan Dashiell, and Nancy Lombardo, PhD, made generous contributions of time to this edition.

David Chavkin reviewed the accuracy of sections on nursing home reform legislation, Medicare, and Medicaid. Staff members at the National Senior Law Center also advised us on legal issues. The staff of the National Citizens Coalition for Nursing Home Reform, particularly Barbara Frank, Ruth Nee, MSW, Sarah Burger, MSW, and Elma Holder, MSPH, reviewed the sections on nursing homes and nursing home law. Gene Vandekieft assisted us in understanding insurance issues. Katie Maslow, MSW, of the Office of Technology Assessment, US Congress, and Lisa Gwyther, MSW, of Duke University, long supporters of the first edition, shared expertise in many areas. Jean Marks, MSW, and her staff in the New York City chapter of the Alzheimer's Association shared their experiences of confused people living alone and of minority families. Ray Rasco also shared his knowledge of confused people who live alone. The Internal Revenue Service Information Department and John Kenneally provided information about tax law. Thomas Milleson, DDS, and Richard Dixon, DDS, gave us guidance in dental care. Carter Williams, MSW, and Mildred Simmons helped us understand the role of physical restraints. Mary Barringer, RN, and Jean Marks helped us with incontinent care. Thomas Price, MD, gave us information about multi-infarct dementia. Glenn Kirkland, MS, reviewed the entire manuscript and gave us extensive valuable comment; he also researched the 'gadgets' that might be useful to families.

A good editor is vital to a good book, and The 36-Hour Day has had the good fortune to have two good editors dedicated to its success. Anders Richter, editor to the first edition, facilitated many of the foreign language editions. It was he who initiated the writing of the revised edition. Wendy Harris has carried on the tradition of energy, skill, and dedication in the editorial management of The 36-Hour Day. We are indebted to both of these fine editors.

Acknowledgements for the UK edition

I have to echo the thoughts of Nancy Mace and Peter Rabins that so many people have helped by giving of their time and expertise to advise on the content of this second edition that it is not possible to name them all. They have my sincere thanks.

Certain colleagues do require to be mentioned by name. I would like to thank Professor Tom Arie, Professor of Psychiatry, Department of Health Care of the Elderly, Nottingham, for his advice and encouragement during the writing of the 1st Edition. Mary Baker, Welfare Director of the Parkinson's Disease Society, shared with me her extensive knowledge of the needs of carers and patients suffering from debilitating chronic neurological states, and advised on parts of the text. Gill Williams provided invaluable help in writing the section on incontinence problems. Hilary Young and Pat Kilminster provided material on occupational therapy. Monica Unwin and Clive Evers of the Alzheimer's Disease Society have provided considerable information which has made a most helpful contribution towards the text of the second edition.

Finally a special thank-you goes to my long-suffering secretary, Sheila Van Piggelen, for her support and enthusiasm in chasing sources of information.

                                                            Beverly Castleton

I would like to thank my former colleague at Age Concern, Chris Cloke for work in the first edition and my colleagues now for their unfailing willingness to answer questions of detail in many parts of the book. In particular I would like to thank Vinnette Marshall for managing the project for us so effectively.

                                                            Evelyn McEwen

1 Dementia

For two or three years, Mary had known that her memory was failing. First she had trouble remembering the names of her friends' children, and one year she completely forgot about the strawberry jam she had made. She compensated by writing things down. After all, she told herself, she was getting older. But then she would find herself groping for a word she had always known, and she worried that she was becoming senile.

Recently, when she was talking with a group of friends, Mary would realise that she had forgotten more than just an occasional name – she had lost the thread of the conversation altogether. She compensated for this too: she always made an appropriate answer, even if she secretly felt confused. No one noticed, except perhaps her daughter-in-law, who said to her best friend, 'I think Mother's memory is going.' It worried Mary – sometimes depressed her – but she always denied that anything was wrong. There was no one to whom she could say, 'I am losing my mind. It is literally slipping away as I watch.' Besides, she didn't want to think about it, didn't want to think about getting old, and, most importantly, she didn't want to be treated as if she were senile. She was still enjoying life and able to manage.

Then, in the winter, Mary became ill. At first she thought it was only a cold. She saw a doctor, who gave her some pills, and asked her what she expected at her age, which annoyed her. She rapidly became worse. She went to bed, afraid, weak and very, very tired. Mary's daughter-in-law received a telephone call from Mary's neighbour. Together they found the old woman semiconscious, feverish, and mumbling incoherently.

During the first few days in the hospital, Mary had only an intermittent, foggy notion of what was happening. The doctors told her family that she had pneumonia, and that her kidneys were working poorly. All the resources of a modern hospital were mobilised to fight the infection.

Mary was in a strange place, and nothing was familiar. People, all strangers, came and went. They told her where she was, but she forgot. In strange surroundings, she could no longer compensate for her forgetfulness, and the delirium caused by the acute illness aggravated her confusion. She thought her husband came to see her: a handsome young man in his war uniform. Then, when her son came, she was surprised that they would come together. Her son kept saying, 'But Mum, Dad has been dead for twenty years.' But she knew he wasn't, because he had just been there. Then, when she complained to her daughter-in-law that she never came, she thought the girl lied when she said, 'But mother, I was just here this morning.' In truth, she could not remember the morning.

People came and poked and pushed, and shoved things in and out and over her. They stuck needles into her and they wanted her to breathe through a mask over her mouth and nose. She did not understand and they could not explain that the inhalations she received through the mask would improve her breathing. The *mask became part of her nightmare. She could not remember where she was. When she had to go to the toilet, they put cotsides on her bed and refused to let her go, so that she cried and wet herself.*

Gradually, Mary got better. The infection cleared and the dizziness passed. Only during the acute phase of her illness did she imagine things, but after the fever and infection had passed, the confusion and forgetfulness seemed more severe than before. Although the illness had probably not affected the gradual course of her memory loss, it had weakened her considerably and taken her out of the familiar setting in which she had been able to function. Most significantly, the illness had focused attention on the seriousness of her situation. Now her family realised she could no longer live alone.

The people around Mary talked and talked. No doubt they explained their plans, but she forgot. When she was finally released from the hospital, they took her to her son's home. They were happy about something that day, and led her into a room. Here at last were some of her things, but not all. She thought perhaps the rest of her things had been stolen while she was sick. They kept saying they had told her where her things were, but she couldn't remember what they said.

This is where they said she lived now, in her son's home – except that long ago she had made up her mind that she would never live with her children. She wanted to live at home. At home she could find things. At home she could manage – she believed – as she always had. At home, perhaps, she could discover what had become of a lifetime of possessions. This was not her home: her independence was gone, her things were gone, and Mary felt an enormous sense of loss. Mary could not remember her son's loving explanation – that she couldn't manage alone and that bringing her to live in his home was the best arrangement he could work out for her.

Often, Mary was afraid, a nameless, shapeless fear. Her impaired mind could not put a name or an explanation to her fear. People came, memories came, and then they slipped away. She could not tell what was reality and what was a memory of people past. The bathroom was not where it was yesterday. Dressing became an insurmountable ordeal. Her hands forgot how to button buttons. Belts hung inexplicably about her, and she could not think how to manage them or why they hung there.

Mary gradually lost the ability to make sense out of what her eyes and ears told her. Noises and confusion made her feel panicky. She couldn't understand, they couldn't explain, and often panic overwhelmed her. She worried about her things: a chair, and the china that had belonged to her mother. They said they had told her over and over again, but she could not remember where her things had gone. Perhaps someone had stolen them. She had lost so much. What things she still had, she hid, but then she forgot where she hid them.

'I cannot get her to have a bath,' her daughter-in-law said in despair. 'She smells. How can I send her to the day centre if she won't have a bath?' For Mary, the bath became an experience of terror. It was a mystery. From day to day she could not remember how to manage the water: sometimes it all ran away, sometimes it kept rising and rising, so that she could not stop it. The bath

involved remembering so many things. It meant remembering how to undress, how to find the bathroom, how to wash. Mary's fingers had forgotten how to undo a zip; her feet had forgotten how to step into the bath. There were so many things for an injured mind to think about that panic overcame her.

How do any of us react to trouble? We might try to get away from the situation for a while, and think it out. One person may go out for a beer; another may weed the garden or go for a walk. Sometimes we react with anger. We fight back against those who cause, or at least participate in, our situation. Or we become discouraged for a while, until nature heals us or the trouble goes away.

Mary's old ways of coping with trouble remained. Often when she felt nervous, she thought of going for a walk. She would pause on the doorstep, look out, drift out, and walk away – away from the trouble. Yet the trouble remained and now it was worse, for Mary would be lost, nothing would be familiar: the house had disappeared, the street was not the one she knew – or was it one from her childhood, or where they lived when the boys were growing up? The terror would wash over her, clutching at her heart. Mary would walk faster.

Sometimes Mary would react with anger. It was an anger she herself did not understand. But her things were gone, her life seemed gone. The compartments of her mind sprang open and fell shut, or vanished altogether. Who would not be angry? Someone had taken her things, the treasures of a lifetime. Was it her daughter-in-law, or her own mother-in-law, or a sister resented in childhood? She accused her daughter-in-law, but quickly forgot the suspicion. Her daughter-in-law, coping with an overwhelming situation, was unable to forget.

Many of us remember the day we began secondary school. We lay awake the night before, afraid of getting lost and not finding the classrooms the next day in a strange building. Every day was like that for Mary. Her family began sending her to a day centre. Every day a driver came to pick her up, and every day her daughter-in-law came to get her, but from day to day Mary could not remember that she would be taken home. The rooms were not dependable. Sometimes Mary could not find them. Sometimes she went in the men's toilet. Sometimes she did not know whether they would come to get her in the evening.

Many of Mary's social skills remained, so she was able to chat and laugh with the other people in the day centre. As Mary relaxed in the centre, she enjoyed the time she spent there with other people, although she could never remember what she did there well enough to tell her daughter-in-law.

Mary loved music; music seemed to be imbedded in a part of her mind that she retained long after much else was lost. She loved to sing old, familiar songs. She loved to sing at the day centre. Even though her daughter-in-law could not sing well, Mary did not remember that, and the two women discovered that they enjoyed singing together.

The time finally came when the physical and emotional burden of caring for Mary became too much for her family and she went to live in a care home. After the initial days of confusion and panic passed, Mary felt secure in her small, sunny bedroom. She could not remember the schedule for the day, but the reliability of the routine comforted her. Some days it seemed as if she were still at the day centre, sometimes she was not sure. She was glad the toilet was close by, where she could see it and did not have to remember where it was.

Mary was glad when her family came to visit. Sometimes she remembered their names, more often she did not. She never remembered that they had come last week and so she regularly scolded them for abandoning her. They could never think of much to say, but they put their arms around her frail body, held her hand, and sat silently or sang old songs. She was glad when they didn't try to remind her of what she had just said, or that they had come last week, or ask her if she remembered this person or that one. She liked it best when they just held her and loved her.

Someone in your family has been diagnosed as having a dementia. This could be Alzheimer's disease, multi-infarct dementia, or one of several other diseases. Perhaps you are not sure yet which condition it is. Whatever the name of the disease, a person close to you has lost some of his intellectual ability – the ability to think and remember. He may become increasingly forgetful. His personality may appear to change, or he may become depressed, moody, or withdrawn.

Many, although not all, of the disorders that cause these symptoms in adults are chronic and irreversible. When a diagnosis of an irreversible dementia is made, the patient and his family face the task of learning to live with this illness. Whether you decide to care for the person at home or to have him cared for in a care home or hospital, you will find yourself facing new problems and coping with your feelings about having someone close to you develop an incapacitating illness.

This book is designed to help you with that adjustment and with the tasks of day-to-day management of a chronically ill family member. We have found that there are questions many families ask. This material can help you begin to find answers, but it is not a substitute for the help of your doctor and other professionals.

What is dementia?

You may have discovered that many names have been given to the symptoms of memory loss, and loss of thinking and reasoning capacity in adults. This is the result of different descriptions and definitions recorded in older medical books. Commonly used terms include 'organic brain syndrome', 'senility', 'hardening of the arteries', or 'chronic brain syndrome'. Your doctor may mention 'Alzheimer's disease', 'multi-infarct disease', 'senile dementia', or 'presenile dementia'. In this book we will refer to these conditions as *dementia*.

Doctors use the word *dementia* in a specific way. It means a loss or impairment of mental powers. It comes from two Latin words, which mean *away* and *mind*. *Dementia* does not mean insane. It has been chosen by the medical profession as the least offensive and most accurate term to describe this group of illnesses. *Dementia* describes a group of symptoms and is not the name of a disease or diseases that cause the symptoms.

There are two major conditions that result in the symptoms of mental confusion, memory loss, disorientation, intellectual impairment, or similar problems. These two conditions may look similar to the casual observer and can be confused. (They will be discussed in more detail in Chapter 17.)

The first condition, *delirium*, comprises a group of symptoms in which the person is less alert than normal. He is often drowsy, but may fluctuate between drowsiness and restlessness. Like the impaired person, he is also confused, disoriented, or forgetful. These conditions have also been called 'acute confusional states' or 'reversible confusional states'. Delirium can be caused by illnesses such as pneumonia or kidney infection, malnutrition, or reactions to medications.

With the second condition, *dementia*, there is impaired intellectual functioning in a person who is clearly awake. The symptoms of dementia can be caused by several different diseases. Some of these diseases are treatable, others are not. Thyroid disease, for example, may cause a dementia that can be reversed with correction of the thyroid abnormality. In Chapter 17 we have summarised some of the diseases that can cause dementia.

Alzheimer's disease appears to be the most frequent cause of irreversible dementia in adults. The intellectual impairment progresses gradually from forgetfulness to total disability. Structural changes in the brain are visible in post-mortems of people who suffered from Alzheimer's disease. The cause of the illness is not known, and, at present, doctors know of no way to stop or cure it. However, much can be done to make the patient comfortable and help the family feel in control of the situation.

Multi-infarct dementia is believed to be the second most common cause of irreversible dementia. This is a series of strokes within the brain. Sometimes the strokes may be so tiny that neither you nor the afflicted person is aware of any change, but together they can destroy enough bits of brain tissue to affect memory and other intellectual functions. This condition used to be called 'hardening of the arteries', but post-mortem studies have shown that it is stroke damage rather than inadequate circulation that causes the problem. In some cases, treatment can reduce the possibility of further damage.

Alzheimer's disease and multi-infarct dementia sometimes occur together. The diagnosis and characteristics of these diseases are discussed in detail in Chapter 17.

People who have a dementing illness may also have other illnesses, and their dementia may make them more vulnerable to other health problems. Other illnesses or reactions to medications often cause delirium in people with dementing illnesses. The delirium can make the person's mental functions and behaviour worse. It is vital to his general health, and to make his care easier, to detect and treat other illnesses promptly. It is important to find a GP who is sympathetic and who will respond quickly to this need.

Depression is common in older people, and can be the cause of memory loss, confusion, or other changes in mental function. Dementia caused by depression is reversible. The depressed person's memory frequently gets better when the depression is treated. Although depression can also occur in a person with an irreversible dementia, depression should always be treated.

Several other uncommon conditions cause dementia. These will be discussed in Chapter 17.

The dementing diseases know no social or racial lines: the rich and the poor, the wise and the simple alike become victims. There is no reason to be ashamed or embarrassed because a family member has a dementing illness. Many brilliant and famous people have suffered from dementing illnesses. Although dementias associated with the final stage of syphilis were common in the past, these are very rare today.

The only other known link between dementia and venereal disease is that associated with Acquired Immune Deficiency Syndrome (AIDS). As yet, this disease rarely affects the elderly population.

Severe memory loss is *never* a normal part of growing older. According to the best studies available, 5 per cent of older people suffer from a severe intellectual impairment and a similar number may suffer from milder impairments. The diseases become more prevalent in people who survive into their eighties and nineties, but about 80 per cent of those who live into very old age never experience a significant memory loss or other symptoms of dementia. A slight forgetfulness is common as we age, but usually it is not enough to interfere with our lives. Most of us know elderly people who are active and in full command of their intellect in their seventies, eighties or nineties. Margaret Mead, Pablo Picasso, Arturo Toscanini and Duke Ellington were all still active in their careers when they died: all were past 75; Picasso was 91.

As more people in our population live into later life, it becomes crucial that we learn more about dementia. The total number of significantly affected sufferers in the United Kingdom is estimated to be about ¾ of a million.

The person with a dementing illness

The person suffering from a dementing illness has difficulty remembering things, although he may be skilful at concealing this. His ability to understand, reason and use good judgement may be impaired. The onset and the course of the condition depend upon which disease caused the condition and upon other factors, some of which are unknown to researchers. Sometimes the onset of the trouble is sudden: looking back, you may say, 'After a certain time, Dad was never himself.' Sometimes the onset is gradual: family members may not notice at first that something is wrong. Sometimes the afflicted person himself may be the first to notice. The person with a mild dementia is often able to describe his problem clearly: 'Things just go out of my mind. I start to explain and then I just can't find the words.'

People respond to their problems in different ways. Some people become skilful at concealing the difficulty. Some keep lists to jog their memory. Some vehemently deny that anything is wrong or blame their problems on others. Some people become depressed or irritable when they realise that their memory is failing. Others remain outwardly cheerful. Usually, the person with a mild to moderate dementia is able to continue to do most of the things he has always done. Like a person with any other disease, he is able to participate in his treatment, in family decisions, and in planning for the future.

Early memory problems are sometimes mistaken for stress, depression, or even mental illness. This misdiagnosis creates an added burden for the person and the family.

A wife recalls the onset of her husband's dementing illness, not in terms of his forgetfulness, but in terms of his mood and attitude:

'I didn't know anything was wrong. I didn't want to see it. Charles was quieter than usual; he seemed depressed, but he blamed it on people at work. Then his boss told him he was being transferred – a demotion, really – to a smaller branch office. They didn't tell me anything. They suggested we take a holiday. So we did. We went to Scotland. But Charles didn't get any better. He was depressed and irritable. After he took the new job, he couldn't manage that either; he blamed it on the younger men. He was so irritable, I wondered what was wrong between us after so many years. We went to a marriage guidance counsellor and that only made things worse. I knew he was forgetful, but I thought that it was caused by stress.'

Her husband said at the time, 'I knew something was wrong. I could feel myself getting uptight over little things. People thought I knew things about the plant that I – I couldn't remember. The counsellor said it was stress. I thought it was something else, something terrible. I was scared.'

Some people experience changes in personality. Many of the qualities that a person has always had may remain: he may always have been sweet and lovable and may remain so, or he may always have been a difficult person to live with and may become more so. Other people may change dramatically, from amiable to demanding, or from energetic to apathetic. They may become passive, dependent and listless, or they may become restless, easily upset and irritable. Sometimes they become demanding, fearful, or depressed.

> *A daughter says, 'Mother was always the cheerful, outgoing person in the family. We knew she was becoming forgetful, but the worst thing is that she doesn't want to do anything anymore. She doesn't do her hair, she doesn't keep the house tidy, she absolutely won't go out.'*

Often, little things enormously upset people with memory problems. Tasks that were previously simple may now be too difficult to undertake, and a person may react to this by becoming upset, angry, or depressed.

> *From another family: 'The worst thing about Dad is his temper. He used to be easy-going. Now he is always shouting over the least little thing. Last night he told our ten year old son that Alaska is not a state of the USA. He was shouting and arguing and stalked out of the room. Then, when I asked him to have a bath, we had a real fight. He insisted he had already had a bath.'*

It is important for those around him to remember that much of the person's behaviour is beyond his control: for example, he may not be able to keep his anger in check or to stop pacing the floor. The changes that occur are not the result of an unpleasant personality grown old; they are the result of damage to the brain and are usually beyond the control of the patient.

In those illnesses in which the dementia is progressive, the person's memory will gradually become worse, and his troubles cannot be concealed. He may become unable to recall what day it is or where he is. He may be unable to do simple tasks such as dressing, and may not be able to put words together coherently. As the dementia progresses, it becomes clear that the damage to the brain affects many functions, including memory, motor functions (co-ordination, writing, walking) and speaking. The person may have difficulty finding the right names for familiar things, and he may become clumsy or walk with a shuffle. The sick person's abilities may fluctuate from day to day, or even from hour to hour. This makes it harder for families to know what to expect.

Some people with dementing illnesses have hallucinations (hearing, seeing, or smelling things that are not real). This experience is real to the person experiencing it and can be frightening for family members. Some people become suspicious of others; they may hide things or accuse people of stealing from them. Often, they simply mislay things and, in their confusion, think someone has stolen them.

> *A son recalls: 'Mum is so paranoid. She hides her purse. She hides her money, she hides her jewellery. Then she accuses my wife of stealing it. Now she is accusing us of stealing the silverware. The hard part is that she doesn't seem to be ill. It's hard to believe she isn't doing this deliberately.'*

In the final stages of a progressive dementing illness, so much of the brain has been affected that the person is often confined to bed, unable to control urination and unable to express himself. In the last stages of the illness, the patient may require skilled nursing care.

It is important to remember that not all these symptoms may be apparent in one person. Your family member may never experience some of these symptoms or may experience others we have not mentioned. The course and prognosis of the disease will vary according to the specific disorder and the individual person.

Where do you go from here?

You know or suspect that someone close to you has a dementing illness. Where do you go from here? You will need to take stock of your current situation, and then identify what needs to be done to help the impaired person and to make the burdens on yourself bearable. There are many questions you must ask. This book will help you find some answers.

The first thing you need to know is the cause of the disease and its prognosis. Each disease that causes dementia is different. You may have been given different diagnoses and different explanations of the disease, or you may not know what is wrong with the person. However, you must have a diagnosis and some information about the course of the disease before you or the doctor can respond appropriately to day-to-day problems or plan for the future. It is usually better to know what to expect. Your understanding of the illness can help to dispel fears and worries and will enable you to plan how best you can help the person with a dementing disease. Chapter 2 describes how a diagnostic assessment is done.

Even when the disease itself cannot be halted, *much can be done to improve the quality of life for the afflicted person and for the family*. Chapters 3 to 9 list many of the problems that families face in caring for a person with a dementing illness and offer suggestions for managing them.

Dementing illnesses vary according to specific diseases and to the individuals concerned. You may never face many of the problems discussed in these chapters. You may find it helpful to glance through them and read only those sections that apply to you.

The key to coping is common sense and ingenuity. Sometimes a family is too close to the problem to see clearly a way of managing. At other times no one is more ingenious at solving a difficult problem than the family members themselves. Many of the ideas offered here were developed by family members who have called or written to us to share them with others. These ideas will point you in the right direction.

At some stage you may find that you will need additional help in caring for an impaired person. Chapter 10 discusses the kinds of help that may be available and how to locate them.

You and the impaired person are part of a family that needs to work together to cope with an illness. Chapter 11 focuses on families and the problems that can arise within them. Chapter 12 discusses your feelings and the effects the illness may have on you. Caring for yourself is important both for you and the confused person who is dependent on you, and this topic is discussed in Chapter 13.

Chapter 14 is written for young people who know someone with a dementing illness. Perhaps, as a parent, you will want to read this chapter too and plan a time to discuss it with your son or daughter. The entire book is written in such a way that a young person will be able to understand any other sections he or she may want to read.

Chapter 15 deals with legal and financial matters. Although it may be painful to plan ahead, it is most important to do so. Perhaps now is the time to deal with certain matters you may have been avoiding.

A time may come when the impaired person cannot live alone. Chapter 16 discusses residential nursing homes and other living arrangements. The availability of good care homes is very variable throughout the UK. The funding arrangements for care in the statutory and private sectors are undergoing considerable review in the wake of the NHS and Community Care Act passed in 1990. We urge you to read Chapter 16 on the care accommodation which might be available and to plan ahead, even if you do not intend at this stage to use these forms of care. We would also advise you to seek professional help and advice on what the changes in the system may mean to you. Possible sources of such help are listed in that chapter.

Chapter 17 describes the diseases that cause dementia and explains how they differ from other brain disorders. However, it is written to give you a general understanding of terms and conditions, not as a tool for diagnosis.

Chapter 18 briefly reviews the research into Alzheimer's disease and multi-infarct dementia. The reading list in Appendix I refers you to other, more detailed information on research.

You may want to use this handbook to inform others about the diseases that cause dementia. The dementing illnesses affect large numbers of people, but their effects on families and their potential management are sometimes poorly understood by professionals and by the general community. Education does not always have to come from the professional person. You, the family, can effectively inform others. Share what you know about dementia with your GP, nursing home staff and others. Basic education on a personal level will help to bring dementia out into the open and into the light of research. This will result in improved care, improved emotional and financial support, and research to seek cures or preventive measures. Use what you know and use this handbook. You will increase the understanding of those around you, and you will reach families who have been struggling in isolation.

Caring for a person with a dementing illness is not easy. We hope the information in this book will help you, but we know that simple solutions are not yet at hand.

Often the text of this book discusses problems. However, it is important to remember that confused people and their families do still experience joy and happiness. Since dementing illnesses develop slowly, they often leave intact the impaired person's ability to enjoy life and to enjoy other people. When things go badly, remind yourself that no matter how bad the person's memory is, or how strange his behaviour, he is still a unique and special human being. We can continue to love a person even after he has changed drastically, and even when we are deeply troubled by his present state.

2 Getting medical help for the impaired person

This book is written for you, the family. It is based on the assumption that you and the sick person are receiving professional medical care. The family and the medical professionals are partners in the care of the impaired person. Neither should be providing care alone. This book is not meant to be a substitute for professional skills. However, we recognise that, at the time of writing, families may have difficulty finding the kind of medical care they need. Misconceptions about dementia do exist among professionals. Not all doctors or other professionals have the time, interest or skills to diagnose or care for a person with a dementing illness. As the public learns more about the dementing illnesses, this will become a thing of the past.

What should you expect from your doctor and other professionals? The first thing is an accurate diagnosis. Once a diagnosis has been made, you will need the continuing help of a doctor, and perhaps other professionals, to manage the dementing illness, to treat concurrent illnesses, and to help you find the resources you need. This chapter is written as a guide to help you find the best possible medical care in your community.

In the course of a dementing illness, you may need the special skills of a doctor, psychologist, social worker, nurse, occupational therapist or physiotherapist. Each is a highly trained professional whose skills complement those of the others. They can work together, first to assess the impaired person and then to help you with continuing care. They may use the skills of other professionals as well.

The assessment of the person with a suspected dementia

It is important that a thorough assessment be made when a person suffers from difficulty in thinking, remembering, or learning, or shows changes in personality. A complete assessment tells you and the doctors several things:

1   the exact nature of the person's illness;
2   whether or not the condition can be reversed or treated;
3   the nature and extent of the disability;
4   the areas in which the person can still function successfully;
5   whether the person has other health problems that need treatment and that might be making her mental problems worse;

6   the social and psychological needs and resources of the sick person
    and the family or care-giver; and
7   the changes you can expect in the future.

Procedures vary depending on your GP or which hospital consultant
is approached. However, a good assessment includes a medical and
neurological examination, an assessment of the person's social support,
and an evaluation of her remaining abilities.

The assessment may begin with a careful examination by a consultant.
He will take a *detailed history* from someone who knows the person well
and from the patient if possible. This tells the doctor how the person
has changed, tells him what symptoms the person has had, and gives
him information about other medical conditions. The doctor will also
give the person a *physical examination*, which may reveal other health
problems. A *neurological examination* (including, among other tests, asking
the person to balance with her eyes closed and tapping her ankles or
knees with a rubber hammer) may reveal changes in the functioning of
the nerve cells of the brain or spine.

The doctor will also carry out a *mental state examination*, in which he
asks the person questions about the time, date and place where she is.
Other questions test her ability to remember, to concentrate, to do
abstract reasoning, to do simple calculations and to copy simple designs.
Each of these reveals problems of function in different parts of the brain.
When the doctor carries out this examination, he will take into consideration the person's education and the fact that the person may be nervous.

The doctor will order *laboratory tests*, including a number of blood tests.
The *FBC* (full blood count) detects anaemia and evidence of infection,
either of which malfunctions can cause or complicate a dementing illness.
Blood chemistry tests check for liver and kidney problems, diabetes and a
number of other conditions. *Vitamin B12 level tests and folate level tests* check
for vitamin deficiencies, which might cause dementia. *Thyroid studies*
assess the function of the thyroid gland. Thyroid problems are among
the more common reversible causes of dementia. The *VDRL test* can
indicate a syphilis infection (syphilis was a common cause of dementia
before the discovery of penicillin), but a positive VDRL test does not
necessarily indicate that the person has ever had syphilis. The blood
tests usually involve inserting one needle, which is no more unpleasant
than a pin prick.

A *lumbar puncture* (*LP*) is performed in order to rule out an infection
in the central nervous system (for example, tuberculosis) and it may also
be used to reveal other abnormalities. It is usually done after a local
anaesthetic has been injected into the back and has few complications.
However, this particular investigation is rarely carried out as often there
is no reason to suspect these conditions.

An *EEG* (*electroencephalograph*) records the electrical activity present in
the brain, and involves attaching little wires to the head with a paste-like

material. It is painless, but may confuse the forgetful person. It aids in the diagnosis of delirium and can also offer evidence of abnormal brain functioning, but occasionally it records a 'normal' result in a demented person.

A *CAT scan* (*computerised axial tomogram*) is a sophisticated X-ray that produces a picture of the brain. (Ordinary skull X-rays show primarily the bones, and do not show the brain itself.) Changes compatible with Alzheimer's disease may be visible on a CAT scan, but such a diagnosis should not be made on the basis of a CAT scan alone. The CAT scan can detect evidence of stroke, multi-infarct dementia, tumours, changes in the flow of the fluid that surrounds the brain, and collections of blood which can put pressure on the brain.

The scan involves lying on a table and placing one's head in an object that looks like a very large hair dryer. It is painless, but may confuse an already impaired person. If so, a mild sedative can be prescribed to help the person relax. It is not performed on all patients, but is ordered when the doctor considers it to be necessary to aid diagnosis.

A new diagnostic tool, *MRI* or *NMR* (*magnetic resonance imaging* or *nuclear magnetic resonance* scanner), provides the physician with a picture similar to that of a CAT scan, but it uses magnetic energy rather than X-rays to produce an image. At present, MRI is not being used to evaluate all patients with dementia, but only those who are very young or whose condition raises certain diagnostic questions (such as whether they have had a small stroke). CAT scanning is more widely available, is less expensive and often provides more straightforward information.

The detailed history, physical and neurological examinations, and laboratory tests will identify or rule out each of the known causes of dementia. In addition to the medical assessment, other evaluations are carried out in order to understand the patient's abilities and to help you plan for the future.

A *psychiatric and psychosocial evaluation* is based on interviews with the patient and her family. This provides the basis for the development of a specific plan for the care of the individual. It may be done by the doctor, nurse and/or the social worker who works with the doctor. It includes helping the family assess their own emotional, physical and financial resources, the home in which the person lives, the community resources, and the patient's ability to accept or participate in plans.

It is important for the physician to determine whether the patient is depressed. Depression can cause symptoms similar to dementia and it can make an existing dementia worse. Whenever there is a question about depression, a psychiatrist experienced in caring for older people should see the patient. Depression is quite common and usually responds well to treatment.

An *occupational therapy assessment* helps to determine how much the person is able to do for herself and what can be done to help her compensate for her limitations and how she can be assisted to continue with any interests. It is carried out by an occupational therapist. These therapists are important members of the team. Their skills are sometimes over-looked because in the past they were consulted only in cases where there was the potential for physical rehabilitation. However, they are also able to identify what the person can still do, and to devise ways to help the person remain as independent as possible. Part of this assessment is an *ADL* (*activities of daily living*) *assessment*. The person is observed in a controlled situation to see if she can manage money, prepare a simple meal, dress herself and perform other routine tasks. It is noted whether she can carry out part of these tasks. Occupational therapists are familiar with a variety of appliances that can help some people.

Neuropsychological testing (also called *cerebral function testing* or *psychometric testing*) may be done to determine in which areas of mental function the person is impaired and in which she is still independent. This testing takes several hours. The tests assess such aspects as memory, reasoning, co-ordination, writing, and the ability to express oneself and understand instructions. The testing psychologist or occupational therapist will be experienced in making people feel relaxed and will take into consider-ation differences in education and interests.

The final part of the assessment is your *discussion* with the doctor and perhaps with other members of the assessment team. At this stage, the doctor will explain his findings to you and to the patient if she is able to understand at least part of what is happening.

The doctor should give you a specific diagnosis (he may explain that he cannot be certain) and a general idea of the person's prognosis (again, he may not be able to tell you exactly what to expect). The findings of other tests, such as the ADL, the psychological tests and the detailed history, will also be explained to you. You should be able to ask questions and come away with an understanding of the findings of the assessment. The doctor may make recommendations, about the use of medication or health services, or he may refer you to a social worker who can advise you about health and social services. You, he and the afflicted person may identify specific problems and set up a plan to cope with them.

A complete assessment may take more than one day. It may be neces-sary, or you may ask to arrange to spread the evaluation over more than one day so that the patient will not get too tired. It usually takes several days for the laboratories to report their findings to the doctor and for him to put all the information together into a report.

Assessments may be done on either an inpatient or on an outpatient basis. In some districts, assessments take place in specialist memory clinics. Several factors, including especially the general health of the patient, affect the decision to do an inpatient or an outpatient assessment.

Sometimes family members, and occasionally professionals, advise against 'putting a confused person through the "ordeal" of an assess-ment'. We feel that every person with memory and thinking problems should be fully assessed. An assessment is not an unpleasant ordeal. Staff accustomed to working with demented people are usually gentle and kind. It is important that they make the patient as comfortable as possible so that they will be able to measure her best performance.

As we have said, there are many reasons why a person might develop the symptoms of dementia. Some of these are treatable. If a treatable problem is not found because an assessment is not done, the afflicted person and her family may suffer unnecessarily for years. Certain diseases can be treated if they are found promptly, but can cause irreversible damage if they are neglected.

Even if a person is found to have an irreversible dementia, the assessment will give you information about how best to care for the impaired person and how best to manage her symptoms. It gives you a basis on which to plan for the future, and, also, it is important that you know that you have done all that you can for her.

How an assessment is arranged

In some areas, it has in the past been difficult to find a doctor interested in carrying out a thorough assessment of a person with a suspected dementia. This is changing. Your GP may do the assessment, or he may refer you to a hospital specialist who may be a neurologist, a psychiatrist, a psychogeriatrician or a geriatrician.

How do you decide whether an accurate diagnosis has been made for someone in your family? In the final analysis, you must settle on a doctor whom you trust and who you feel has done all he can, and then rely on his judgement. This is much easier when you understand something about the terminology, the diagnostic procedures and the dementia. If you have been given differing diagnoses, discuss the matter frankly with your doctor. It is important that you feel certain that an accurate diagnosis has been made. Occasionally a physician will make a diagnosis of Alzheimer's disease without undertaking a complete evaluation. It is not possible to make an accurate diagnosis without a complete assessment involving tests that rule out other conditions. If this happens to you, we suggest you consider obtaining a second opinion.

You may hear about people with similar symptoms who are 'miraculously' restored to health, or you may come across such statements as 'senility can be cured'. Considerable confusion has arisen over this issue because some of the causes of dementia are reversible, and because dementia and delirium (see Chapter 17) are sometimes confused. There are some unscrupulous individuals who offer bogus 'cures' for these tragic illnesses. An accurate diagnosis and a doctor you trust will reassure you that all that can be done is being done. You can also be kept informed about the progress of legitimate research through the Alzheimer's Disease Society and from the major research institutes.

Medical treatment and management of dementia

Dementing illnesses are diseases that require continuing medical attention. The availability of professional services varies. You, the care-giver, will provide much of the co-ordination of care. However, there are times when you will also need the help of professionals.

The doctor

You will need a doctor who will prescribe and adjust medication, answer your questions, and treat other concurrent illnesses. The doctor who provides continuing care will not usually be the specialist providing the initial assessment of the patient. He may be your family doctor or a member of a geriatric or psychogeriatric unit, such as a clinical assistant in charge of a day hospital. This doctor can refer the patient to a neurologist, psychiatrist or geriatrician if necessary. The doctor who provides continuing care must:

1　be willing and able to spend the necessary time with you and the sick person;
2　be knowledgeable about dementing illnesses and the special susceptibility of impaired patients to other diseases, medication and delirium;
3　be easily accessible;
4　be able to make referrals to occupational therapists, physiotherapists, social workers and other professionals.

Many GPs are able and willing to provide such care, but unfortunately there will be doctors who do not meet these criteria. Some doctors have large practices and may not have the time to focus on your problems. It is impossible for any one person to keep up with all the advances in medicine, so some doctors may not be skilled in the specialised care of a person with dementia. Finally, some doctors are uncomfortable caring for people with chronic incurable diseases. However, no physician should give you a diagnosis without following through with referrals to professionals who can give the help and follow-up you need. You may have to talk to more than one doctor before you find one who is right for you. Discuss your needs and expectations honestly with him, and talk over how you can best work with him. Doctors have been trained to keep patients' problems confidential. Because of this, some doctors are reluctant to talk to other members of the family or will talk only to the patient's spouse. However, there may be good reasons why you need to know about the patient. Physicians who work with many families of demented patients find that conferring with the whole family is important. Discuss this problem frankly with the doctor and ask him to be as open as he can with the whole family.

Changing your GP

If you are not happy with your GP, there may be another doctor within the practice whom you could see. You are also at liberty to change to a doctor in another practice who is willing to take on you or your relative. Doctors do not have to accept all the people who apply to join their lists of patients. All you have to do is to go to the new doctor's surgery and ask to be registered. You do not have to give a reason to your previous doctor about why you wish to change to another practice. Your local Family Health Services Authority will have a list of GPs and if you cannot find one who is willing to take you on, it will allocate you to a GP in the area.

The nurse and paramedics

In addition to the knowledge and experience of a doctor, you may need the skills of a nurse. Health visitors, district nurses, practice nurses and community psychiatric nurses (CPN), together with GPs, are part of the Primary Health Care Team working from the surgery or health centre. In most areas now, the community nursing team includes CPNs who can usually take referrals from a GP. In some districts, the CPNs are hospital based and may only take referrals from psychiatrists and psychogeriatricians.

The nurse may be the person whom you can reach most easily and who can co-ordinate the work that you, the doctor and others undertake to provide the best possible care. She may be the person who understands the difficulties of caring for a patient at home. She can observe the patient for changes in her health status which need to be reported to the doctor, and she can give you support and counselling. After talking with you, she can identify and help to solve many of the problems you face. She can teach you how to provide practical care for the person (coping with catastrophic reactions, giving baths, helping with eating problems, managing a wheelchair). She can teach you how and when to give medicine, and how to know whether it is working correctly. The nurse comes to your home to assess the patient and to offer suggestions for simplifying the patient's environment and minimising the effort you need to expend.

The district nurse may also be helpful to you if the patient is frail and needs considerable help with dressing, bathing and transferring, or if she is bedbound. There may well be a local Twilight Nursing Service, often used as a 'putting to bed' service, and this can be invaluable when caring for the impaired person. A Terminal Care Service for those dying at home may also be available.

The nurse will be able to give advice on coping with incontinence, and will have access to a supply of nursing aids such as commodes, incontinence appliances and disposable pads which she can arrange to have delivered to your home. There may be specialist advice available in your district from a continence adviser and a stoma care therapist.

The community occupational therapist may be asked to advise on how to maintain the activities of daily living and on specific aids to assist this, and can organise stair rails, toilet rails and raised toilet seats to be fitted. She can also supply feeding aids. The community physiotherapist may also be available to help.

There are private nursing agencies which can provide services not available locally under the NHS, but this is, of course, an expensive alternative.

The social worker

Social workers have a unique combination of skills: they should know the resources and services available in your community, and be skilled in assessing your situation and needs, and matching these with available services. They are professionals whose skills in helping you find resources can be invaluable. They can also provide practical counselling, and help you and your family think through plans and solve disagreements over care.

Your GP will be able to refer you to a community social worker, or, if the sick person is in hospital, the hospital social worker may be able to help you.

There will be a Social Services Department in your area which is part of a local authority. To locate such departments, look in your local telephone directory or call in at your local Citizens Advice Bureau. Anyone with a problem or query can seek help from the Social Services

Department without necessarily having to be referred by a doctor.
The duty social worker will probably be able to give you immediate
advice or will refer you to the appropriate agency to deal with your
problem.

3 Characteristic problems of dementia

In Chapters 3 to 9 we discuss many of the problems that families may encounter in caring for a person with a dementing illness. Although as yet nothing can be done to cure some dementing illnesses, it is important to remember that *much can be done to make life easier for you and the person with a dementing illness*. The suggestions we offer come from our clinical experience and from the experiences that family members have shared with us.

Each individual and each family is different. You may never experience many of the problems we discuss in these chapters. The problems you will face are influenced by the nature of the specific disease, by your personality, by the ill person's personality, and, often, by other factors, such as where you live. We do not want you to consider that what follows is a catalogue of situations lying ahead of you. It is, however, a comprehensive list of possible difficulties you may encounter, to be used as a reference guide when a specific problem arises.

The brain, behaviour and personality: why people with dementia do the things they do

The very nature of brain injuries can make them difficult to live with. The brain is a vast, complex, mysterious organ. It it the source of our thoughts, our emotions and our personality. Injury to the brain can cause changes in emotions, personality and the ability to reason. Most dementing illnesses do their damage gradually, so the effects are not seen suddenly, unlike the effects of a major stroke or head injury. Consequently, the behaviour of a person with a dementing illness often seems puzzling in contrast to behaviours due to other illnesses. It is not always evident that many of the visible symptoms (changes in personality, for example) are the result of a disease, because the patient often looks well.

You may wonder which behaviours are caused by the disease and which are deliberate or wilful, and family members may disagree over this. In the following chapters, we discuss some of the behaviour problems you may face and suggest ways you can respond. Understanding that the damage to the brain causes these behaviours will help you to cope with them.

The brain is an incredibly complex organ composed of billions of microscopic neurones, or brain cells. All the brain's tasks – thinking, talking, dreaming, walking, listening to music and thousands of others

– are carried out when these cells communicate with one another. This communication is accomplished by a chemical, manufactured inside the cell, that jumps the tiny gap from one cell to the neighbouring cell. Because it is known that some of these chemicals are in short supply in the brains of people with Alzheimer's disease, scientists are studying the chemicals in an effort to alleviate the symptoms of the disease.

Different parts of the brain carry out different tasks. When a person has a stroke and cannot speak, we know that the stroke occurred in the speech centre of the brain and destroyed cells that are necessary for the person to talk. A stroke often causes extensive damage, but only to a few areas of the brain. In dementia, damage is done in many areas and affects many aspects of mental function. While a stroke does all its damage at once, Alzheimer's disease gradually does more and more damage. This means that different cognitive abilities are damaged *unevenly*, and the patient will be able to do some things but not others. For example, he may be able to remember things from long ago but not from yesterday.

Our brains carry out thousands of tasks and we are usually not aware of most of them. We assume that other people's brains, like ours, are working as they should – but with a person who has dementia we cannot make this assumption. When the person does something odd or inexplicable, it is usually because some part of the brain has failed to do its job. In addition to controlling memory and language, the brain enables us to move our various body parts, filters out the things we don't want to pay attention to, gives feedback on the things we do, enables us to recognise familiar objects, and co-ordinates all the activities it is carrying out. *When the brain damage is uneven, the person may do things that don't make sense to us.*

> *John Barstow can remember he was angry with his wife, but he cannot remember her explanation of why she did what she did. In fact, he may not even remember what she did that made him angry.*

Researchers believe that our brain stores and processes memories of emotions differently from memories of fact. It is possible for the dementia to damage one without damaging the other as much. Old social skills and the ability to make customary social remarks are often retained longer than insight and judgement. Thus a person may sound fine to the doctor but in fact be unable to responsibly care for himself.

It may be that damaged nerve cells, like a loose light bulb, connect sometimes and fail other times. This may be why a person can do something one day and not another. Even when we do something that seems simple, the brain must carry out many tasks. *If the dementia prevents the brain from performing any one of the steps in a task, the task will not get done.*

'I asked my sister to make us both a cup of tea, but she ignored me. Then half an hour later, she went to the kitchen and made herself a cup of tea.'

Obviously, the sister was still able to carry out this task, but probably was not able to understand or act on language even though she heard the request.

Behaviour problems are caused by the damage to the brain and are not something the person can control or prevent. Behaviour that upsets you is almost never deliberate and almost never intended to 'get your goat'. Because the brain itself is damaged, the person has a severely limited ability to learn things or understand explanations. It is futile to expect the person to remember or learn, and frustrating to both of you to try to teach him. The person does not want to act like this and *is trying as hard as he can.*

Mrs Robinson helped out in her older daughter's kitchen, but when she visited her younger daughter she only sat and criticised. The younger daughter felt that Mrs Robinson had always preferred the older sister and that her refusal to help was a less than subtle reminder of her preference. In fact, the mother had been familiar with the older sister's kitchen before she became forgetful, but could no longer learn new information, even things as simple as where the dishes were kept in her younger daughter's unfamiliar kitchen.

A person's feelings also affect his behaviour. The person with dementia probably feels lost, worried, anxious, vulnerable and helpless much of the time. He may *also* be aware that he fails at tasks and feel that he is making a fool of himself. Imagine what it must feel like to want to say something nice to your care-giver but all that comes out are swear words. Think how frightening it must be if a familiar home and familiar people now seem strange and unfamiliar. If we can find ways to make a person with dementia feel more secure and comfortable, behaviour problems may decline.

Other little things also affect behaviour. When a person is not feeling well, he will be less able to think. In Chapter 6 we discuss how *illness, pain, and medication* can make a person's thinking – and behaviour – worse.

When you speak to a person, he must hear you: the first step in the processes of communication is *sensory input. The ability to repeat immediately what is heard may be retained, but the next step, to store what was said, at least temporarily, is often lost in people with dementia. If the person cannot temporarily store what you said, he cannot respond.* Often a person can store only part of what was said and will act only on that part. If you say 'The grand-children are coming to dinner, so you must have a bath', he may retain only 'have a bath' and act accordingly. If he retains nothing of what you said, he may be angry when you lead him to the bathroom. As well as retaining what was heard, the person must comprehend what the words mean and evaluate what was said. Many things may go wrong in this process and may result in a reply that seems inappropriate to you. The person will act on what he *thinks* he heard. But he can act only on what his ears heard, his brain registered, his dictionary understood and his mind processed. If his brain scrambles the message, he will respond in a way that is appropriate to what he understood, and if, in his confusion, he thinks that you are a stranger or that he is a young man and you are his mother, his response will be based on faulty understanding of the situation. A person who was usually placid may respond calmly, a person who was usually irritable may respond with anger, but whatever the response, it will be appropriate to the message *received*, not necessarily the message you gave.

The final step in communication is the person's answer. Things can go wrong here, too. What comes out may not be what the confused person intended. This too can sound like an intentional evasion, insult, or foolish answer.

There is much that we do not know about this process. Neuropsychologists study the mind and try to understand these complex cognitive processes. Often a neuropsychologist can work out why a particular person acts as he does, and sometimes can devise a way round the disability. Although there is still an enormous amount to learn about how this process works, when people with a dementing illness say or do things that don't make sense or that seem nasty or deliberate, it is almost certainly the brain damage at work. *The person you are caring for is often miserable and is doing the best he can.* In the rest of this book we will show you many ways you can help.

Because the brain is so complex, even the best experts are often at a loss. In addition, most families do not have access to a neuropsychologist. Do the best you can, regard problems as the brain damage at work, not as something you did or something the confused person intended. Affection, reassurance and calm are best, even when things make no sense.

Care-giving: some general suggestions

Be informed.   The more you know about the nature of dementing illness, the more effective you will be in devising strategies to manage behaviour problems.

Share your concerns.   When a person is only mildly to moderately impaired, he can take part in managing his problem. You may be able to share with each other your grief and worries. Together you may be able to devise memory aids that will help him remain independent. Mildly impaired people may benefit from counselling that can help them accept and adjust to their limitations.

Try to solve your most frustrating problems one at a time. Families tell us that the day-to-day problems often seem to be the most insurmountable. Getting mother to have her bath or getting supper prepared, eaten and cleaned up can become daily ordeals. *If you are at the end of your tether, single out one thing that you can change to make life easier, and work on that.* Sometimes changing small things makes a big difference.

Get enough rest.   One of the dilemmas families often face is that the care-giver may not get enough rest, or may not have the opportunity to get away from his care-giving responsibilities. This can make the care-giver less patient and less able to tolerate irritating behaviour. If things are getting out of hand, ask yourself if this is what is happening to you. If so, you may want to focus on finding ways to get more rest or more frequent breaks from your care-giving responsibilities. We recognise that this is difficult to arrange. We discuss this in Chapter 10.

Use your common sense and imagination – they are your best tools.   Adaptation is the key to success. If a thing cannot be done one way, ask yourself if it must be done at all. For example, if a person can eat successfully with his fingers but cannot use a fork and spoon appropriately, don't fight the problem; serve as many finger foods as possible. Accept changes. If the person insists on sleeping with his hat on, this is not harmful; go along with it.

Maintain a sense of humour – it will get you through many crises.   The ill person is still a person. He needs and enjoys a good laugh too. Sharing your experiences with other families will help you. Surprisingly, these groups of families often find their shared experiences both sad and funny.

Try to establish an environment that allows as much freedom as possible, but also offers the structure that confused people often need.   Establish a regular, predictable, simple routine for meals, medication, exercising, bedtime and other activities. Do things the same way and at the same time each day. If you establish regular routines, the person may gradually learn what to expect. Change routines only when they aren't working. Keep the person's surroundings reliable and simple. Leave furniture in the same place. Put away clutter.

Remember to talk to the confused person.   Speak calmly and gently. Make a point of telling him what you are doing and why. Let him have a part in deciding things as much as possible. Avoid talking *about* the patient in his presence, and remind others about this also.

Have an identity bracelet made for the confused person. Include on it the nature of his disease (for example, 'memory impaired') and your telephone number. This is one of the single most important things you can do. Many confused people get lost or wander away at one time or another and an identity bracelet can save you hours of frantic worry.

Keep the impaired person active but not upset. Families often ask if retraining, reality orientation, reminiscence therapy or keeping active will slow down or stop the course of the disease. Likewise, they may ask if being idle hastens the course of the disease. Some people with dementing illnesses become depressed, listless, or apathetic. Families often wonder whether encouraging such a person to do things will help him to function better.

The relationship of activity to the course of dementing illness is not clear. Research continues in this area. Activity helps to maintain physical well-being and may help to prevent other illnesses and infections. Being active helps the ill person to continue to feel that he is involved in the family and that his life has meaning.

It is clear that people with dementing illnesses cannot learn as well as before because brain tissue has been damaged or destroyed. It would be unrealistic to expect them to learn new skills. However, some individuals can learn simple tasks or facts if they are repeated often enough. Some impaired people who feel lost in a new place eventually 'learn' their way around.

At the same time, too much stimulation, activity, or pressure to learn may upset the confused person, may upset you and may accomplish nothing. The key to this is balance:

1 Accept that lost skills are gone for good (the woman who has lost the ability to cook will not learn to prepare a meal), *but* know that repeatedly and gently giving information within the person's abilities will help him function more comfortably (the person going into a strange day care setting will benefit from frequent reminders about where he is).
2 Realise that even small amounts of excitement – visitors, laughter, changes – can upset the confused person, *but* plan interesting, stimulating things within his capabilities – a walk, visiting one old friend.
3 Look for ways to simplify activities so that a person can continue to be involved within the limits of his abilities (the woman who can no longer prepare a whole meal may still be able to peel the potatoes).
4 Look for things the person is still able to do and focus on them. A person's intellectual abilities are not all lost at once. Both of you will

benefit from carefully assessing what he can still do and making the best use of those abilities. For example:

Mrs Baldwin often cannot remember the words for things she wants to say but she can make her meaning clear with gestures. Her daughter helps her by saying 'Point to what you want.'

5 Consider having a trained person visit the confused person at home, or trying a group programme such as day care for people with dementia. Day care offers the right level of stimulation for some confused people and gives you time off as well.

Memory problems

People with dementing illnesses forget things quickly. For the person with a memory impairment, life may be like constantly coming into the middle of a film performance: one has no idea what happened just before what is happening now. People with dementing illnesses may say they will call a friend and forget to do so, may start to prepare a meal and forget to turn off the cooker, may forget what time it is or where they are. Forgetfulness of recent events can seem puzzling when the person seems to be able to remember clearly events long past. It has to do with the way the brain stores and receives information; *it is not something the person does deliberately.*

Some specific suggestions for memory aids are given throughout this book. You may think of others that will help you.

The success of memory aids depends on the severity of the dementia. A mildly demented person may devise reminders for himself, while a severely impaired person will only become more frustrated by his inability to use aids. People who are able to read can do simple tasks if you write out instructions. Writing down names and often used phone numbers also helps. If you are going out, write down where you are going. If you will be out at a mealtime, leave a written reminder to eat.

Have clocks and calendars in view to help the confused person remember what time and day it is. Mark off the days as they pass. It is often helpful to put a simple list of the day's activities where the patient can easily see it. A regular daily routine is much less confusing than frequent changes.

Leave familiar objects (photographs, magazines, TV, radio) in their usual places where the person can see them easily. A tidy, uncluttered house will be less confusing to an impaired person, and misplaced items will be easier to find. Some families have found that putting labels on things is useful. Labelling drawers 'Mary's stockings', 'Mary's night-gowns' may help.

Remember, however, that with a progressive dementing illness the patient will eventually be unable to read, or will not be able to make sense of what he reads. He may be able to read the words but be unable to act on them. Some families use pictures instead of written messages at that stage. For example, it may help to put a picture of a toilet on the bathroom door if the person is in an unfamiliar place, or has trouble remembering where the bathroom is.

People are often more confused at night and may get lost going to the bathroom. Strips of reflector tape on the wall from the bedroom to the bathroom are useful. Night lights can also be used to show the way.

Pictures of family members and close friends may assist the more confused person to remind himself of who these people are. If you are visiting someone in hospital or in a nursing home, you might try taking along a family photograph album. Looking at the photographs may stir pleasant memories in the confused mind.

Over-reacting or catastrophic reactions

Even though Miss Ramirez had told her sister over and over again that today was the day to visit the doctor, her sister would not get in the car until she was dragged in, screaming, by two neighbours. All the way to the doctor's surgery she shouted for help and when she got there she tried to run away.

Mr Lewis suddenly burst into tears as he tried to tie his shoelaces. He threw the shoes in the wastepaper basket and locked himself, sobbing, in the bathroom.

Mrs Coleman described several incidents similar to this one, where her husband had mislaid his glasses:

'You threw out my glasses,' he told her.

'I didn't touch your glasses,' she answered.

'That's what you always say,' he responded. 'How do you explain that they are gone?'

'You do this to me every time you lose your glasses.'

'I did not lose them. You threw them out.'

Looking back, Mrs Coleman knew that her husband had changed. In the past he would have merely asked her if she knew where his glasses were instead of accusing her and starting an argument.

People with brain diseases often become excessively upset and may experience rapidly changing moods. Strange situations, confusion, groups of people, noises, being asked several questions at once, or being asked to do a task that is difficult for them can precipitate these reactions. The person may weep, blush, or become agitated, angry or stubborn. He may strike out at those trying to help him. He may cover his distress by denying what he is doing or by accusing other people of making things difficult for him.

When a situation overwhelms the limited thinking capacity of a brain injured person, he may over-react. Normal people sometimes do this when they are bombarded with more things at one time than they can manage. Impaired people have the same reaction to simpler, everyday experiences. For example:

Every evening, Mrs Hamilton gets upset and refuses to have a bath. When her daughter insists, she argues and shouts. This makes the rest of the family tense. The whole routine is dreaded by everyone.

Having a bath actually means that Mrs Hamilton must think about several things at once: undressing, unbuttoning, finding the bathroom, turning on taps and climbing into the bath. At the same time she feels insecure without clothes on, and she feels she has lost her privacy and independence. This is overwhelming for a person who cannot remember carrying out the tasks before, who can't remember how to do them, and whose mind cannot process all these activities at once. One way to react to this situation is to refuse to have a bath.

We use the term *catastrophic reaction* to describe this particular behaviour. (The word *catastrophic* is used in a special sense; it does not mean that these situations are necessarily very dramatic or violent.) *Often, a catastrophic reaction does not resemble behaviour caused by a brain illness. The behaviour may appear as if the person is merely being obstinate, critical, or over-emotional.* It may seem inappropriate to become so upset over such a trivial matter.

Catastrophic reactions are upsetting and exhausting for you and for the confused person. They are especially upsetting when it seems as if the person you are trying to help is being stubborn or critical. The person may get so upset that he refuses necessary care. Learning how to avoid or lessen catastrophic reactions is a major key to easier management of them.

Sometimes catastrophic reactions and forgetfulness are the first examples of abnormal behaviour witnessed by family members which make them realise that something is wrong. The mildly impaired person may benefit by being reassured that his panic is not unusual and that you understand his fear.

The methods used to prevent or reduce catastrophic reactions depend on the individual, on you, and on the extent of his limitations. You will gradually learn how to avoid or limit these reactions. *First, you must fully accept that this behaviour is not just stubbornness or nastiness but a response the person with a dementing illness cannot help.*

The person is not just denying reality or trying to manipulate you. You may have to keep reminding yourself of this. Though it seems strange, you may have more control over the person's reactions than he does.

The best way to manage catastrophic reactions is to stop them before they happen. The things that trigger these outbursts vary from one person to another and from one time to another, but as you learn what upsets your family member, you will be able to reduce the number and frequency of outbursts. Some of the common causes of catastrophic reactions are:

- needing to think about several things at once (for example, all the tasks involved in taking a bath);
- trying to do something that the person can no longer manage;
- being cared for by someone who is rushed or upset;
- not wanting to appear inadequate or unable to do things (for example, if the doctor asks a lot of questions that the person cannot answer);
- being hurried (when the person now thinks and moves more slowly);
- not understanding what he is being asked to do;
- not understanding what he can see or hear;
- being tired (none of us are at our best when we are tired);
- not feeling well;
- not being able to make himself understood (see also the next section of this chapter);
- feeling frustrated;
- being treated like a child.

Anything that helps remind the confused person about what is going on, such as following familiar routines, leaving things in familiar places, and written instructions (for people who can manage them), help to reduce catastrophic reactions. Because catastrophic reactions are precipitated by having to think of several things at once, simplify what the confused person has to think about. Take things one step at a time, and give instructions or information one step at a time. For example, when you help a person have a bath, tell the person one thing at a time. Say, 'I'm going to unbutton your shirt,' and then reassure him, 'It's all right.' Say, 'Now I'm going to slip your shirt off. That's fine. You're a big help. Now step into the bath. I will hold your arm.'

Give the confused person time to respond. He may react slowly and become upset if you rush him. Wait for him. If a person is having frequent catastrophic reactions, try to reduce the confusion around him. This might mean having fewer people in the room, having less noise, turning off the TV, or reducing the clutter in the room. The key is to simplify, to reduce the number of signals the impaired, disoriented brain must sort out.

Plan things the impaired person can realistically do. If strange places upset him, you may not want to take him on a trip. If he gets tired or upset quickly, plan shorter visits with friends.

Plan demanding tasks for the person's best time of day. Avoid asking him to do things when he is tired. Know what his limits are and try not to push him beyond them.

You can avert some catastrophic reactions by simplifying the task facing the impaired person. Mr Quinn's family recognised that tying shoelaces had become too difficult for him but that he needed to remain as independent as possible. Buying him slip-on shoes solved the problem. Mrs Coleman's husband often lost things because he forgot where he put them. She found it helpful to ignore his accusations and help him find his glasses. Knowing that accusing her was his way of reacting to his forgetfulness made it easier for her to accept the insult.

Simplify tasks for him. Do the parts he finds difficult yourself. Families often worry they are doing too much for a person and as a result might make him more dependent. A good rule of thumb is to let a person do things for himself until he shows the *first signs* of frustration, then assist him *before* he becomes more upset. Urging him on will usually only upset him more.

If a person seems more irritable than usual, check carefully for signs of illness or pain. *Even minor illness or discomfort can make the person's thinking worse.* Has the person's medication been changed in the past three weeks? Reactions to medicines sometimes cause these outbursts.

Reconsider your approach. Are you unintentionally rushing him? Did you misunderstand him? Did you ignore his protests? Are your behaviour and voice communicating your own frustration to him? Although it is easy to treat a person who is so dependent like a child this may make him angry and precipitate an outburst.

When the person does become upset or resistant, remain calm and remove him from the situation in a quiet, unhurried way. Often the emotional storm will be over as quickly as it began and the confused person usually will be relieved that the upset is over. His short memory may work to your advantage: he may quickly forget the trouble.

As a person with cognitive impairment becomes upset, his ability to think and reason temporarily declines even more. It is useless to argue with him, explain things to him, or even get him to complete a task when he is in the grip of a catastrophic reaction. Arguing, explaining, or restraining him may make things worse. Help him calm down and relax so that he can think as well as possible. Take him away from what upset him, if possible.

You may lose your temper with a person who is having catastrophic reactions or who is unable to undertake what seems like a simple task. This usually will make the person's behaviour worse. Occasionally losing your temper is not a calamity; take a deep breath and try to approach the problem calmly. The person will probably forget your anger much more quickly than you will.

Try not to express your frustration or anger to the confused person. Your frustration will further upset him when he cannot understand your reaction. Speak calmly. Take things one step at a time. Move slowly and quietly. Remember that the person is not being obstinate or doing this intentionally. Avoid trying to reason or argue with an upset individual; this only adds to his confusion and increases his over-reaction.

Gently holding a person's hand or patting him may help calm him. Some people respond to being slowly rocked. Try putting your arms around him and rocking back and forth. Some people will be soothed by this, but others may feel that your arms are restraining them and will become more upset. Physically restraining a person often adds to his panic. Restrain a person only if it is absolutely essential and if nothing else works.

If catastrophic reactions are happening often, keeping a log may help you identify their cause. After the outburst is over, write down what happened, when it happened, who was around and what happened just before the outburst. Look for a pattern: are there events, times, or people that might be triggering upsets? If so, can you avoid them?

These over-reactions are distressing to the confused person as well as to you. After he has calmed down, reassure him. Tell him that you recognise his distress and that you will still care for him.

If you find that catastrophic reactions are occurring frequently and that you are responding with anger and frustration, this is a warning that you are overtired. You are caught in a vicious circle that is bad both for you and the impaired person. It is essential that you have time away from the person. Read Chapter 10, 'Obtaining outside help', and make the effort to arrange some time off for yourself, even if you feel too tired and overwhelmed to do so.

In general, some things can usually be found that will reduce catastrophic reactions in most people with dementia. If you consider that none of the suggestions mentioned above will work; that you are caught in an endless battle this may be an indication of your own depression. See p. 219.

Combativeness

Mrs Frank was having her hair done. The hairdresser was working on the back of her head and Mrs Frank kept trying to turn around. When this happened the hairdresser would turn Mrs Frank's head back. Then Mrs Frank began poking at the hairdresser's hand. She looked as if she were about to cry. Finally, Mrs Frank turned around in the chair and hit the hairdresser.

Mr Williams stood close to a group of nurses who were talking. He bounced up and down on his toes. The nurses ignored him even though he bounced faster and faster. When he began to shout, one of the nurses took his arm to lead him away. He pulled away from her but she held on. When she did not let go he struck her.

When a person with dementia hits (or bites, pinches, or kicks) another, it is upsetting for everyone. In some cases this happens frequently and the care-giver or nursing home may feel they cannot continue to provide care.

Combativeness is almost always an extreme catastrophic reaction. It can be prevented by being alert to the person's signals that his stress level is rising. Perhaps if the hairdresser had talked to Mrs Frank about what he was doing and showed her in a mirror how her hair was progressing, Mrs Frank would have understood what was going on and been less upset. Turning and poking at the hairdresser were signs that she was becoming upset.

Perhaps Mr Williams wanted to join the conversation. If the nurses had kept a log of his outbursts, they might have observed that bouncing on his toes was a sign of his rising agitation. If the nurses had included him in their conversation or suggested something else he might enjoy doing, he might not have become upset. Physically holding or pulling someone is often perceived as an attack and leads to an angry response.

When a person becomes agitated, immediately stop whatever is upsetting him and let him relax. Do not continue to push him. Reread the material on catastrophic reactions in this chapter and in other books (see Appendix I). Look for ideas for preventing outbursts or stopping them when they first begin. Sometimes small doses of medication can help people who are upset for much of the time. However, medication is not a substitute for changing events going on around the person or for altering the ways in which care-givers respond to him.

Problems with speech and communication

You may have problems understanding or communicating verbally with the impaired person. There are two kinds of problems of communication: the problems a person with a dementing illness has in expressing himself to others, and the problems he has in understanding what people say to him.

Problems the impaired person has in making himself understood

The nature of communication problems and whether or not they will become worse depends on the specific disease. Do not assume that the situation will deteriorate.

Some impaired people have only occasional difficulty finding words. They may have trouble remembering the names of familiar objects or people. They may substitute a word that sounds similar, such as saying 'tee' for 'tie' or 'wrong' for 'ring'. They may substitute a word with a similar meaning, such as saying 'wedding' for 'ring' or 'music thing' for 'piano'. They may describe the object they cannot name, such as 'it's a thing that goes around' for 'ring' or 'it's to dress up' for 'bow tie'. Such problems usually do not interfere with your ability to understand what the person means.

Some people have difficulty communicating their thoughts.

> *Mr Jones was trying to say that he had never had a neurological examination before. He said, 'I really have not, not really, ever have been done, I have never . . .'*

In some cases people cannot communicate the whole thought but can express a few of the words in the thought.

> *Mr Mason wanted to say that he was worried about missing his transport home. He could only say, 'Bus, home.'*

Sometimes people are able to ramble on quite fluently, and it seems as if they are talking a lot. They will often string together commonly used phrases, so what they say at first seems to make sense, but upon reflection the listener may not be sure he or she understood the thought being expressed.

> *Mrs Simmons said, 'If I tell you something, I might stop in the middle and . . . I'll be sure about what I've done, . . . said, . . . sometimes I stop right in the middle and I can't get on with . . . from . . . that. In past records . . . I can be so much more sure of the . . . After I get my bearings again I can just go on as if nothing happened. We thought it was high time to start remembering. I just love to . . . have to . . . talk.'*

In these examples, it is possible to understand what the person is saying if we know the context.

When the limitations in ability to communicate frustrate the confused person and frustrate you, they can lead to a series of catastrophic reactions. For example, the impaired person may burst into tears or stamp out of the room when no one understands him.

Sometimes a person is able to conceal language problems. When a doctor asks a person if he knows the word for a wristwatch (a common question used to evaluate language problems), the patient may say, 'Of course I do. Why do you ask?' or 'I don't want to talk about it. Why are you bothering me?' when he cannot think of the word.

Some people begin to use swear words, even if they have never used such language before. This disturbing behaviour appears to be a strange quirk of diseases that take away important language skills. It is commonly seen after a stroke to the language area of the brain. It must be like opening a 'mental dictionary' to say something and have only swear words come out. One person who was asked why he cursed the day care staff said, 'These are the only words I have.' This behaviour is rarely deliberate and sometimes upsets the person as much as it does you.

In a severe case, the person may remember only a few key words, such as 'No', which he may use whether or not he means it. Eventually a person may be unable to speak. He may repeat a phrase, cry out intermittently, or mumble unintelligible phrases. In some cases there seems to be no meaning in the jumbled words produced. Family members and care-givers often grieve when this happens and they can no longer communicate verbally with a loved one. We sense that language is the most human of mental skills. In some families the person continues to be a friend and companion – although a forgetful one – for a long time, but when he is unable to communicate any more, the family feels they have lost that companionship. You may worry that the person will be ill or in pain and be unable to tell you.

How you help the impaired person communicate depends on the kind of difficulty he is having. If he has been diagnosed as having suffered a stroke that interferes with language function, he should be seen by a speech therapist as soon as he has recovered from the acute phase of his illness. Much can be done to rehabilitate stroke victims.

If the person is having difficulty finding the right word, it is usually less frustrating for him to have you supply the word for him than it is to let him search and struggle for the word. When he uses the wrong word and you know what he means, it may be helpful to supply the correct word. However, if doing so upsets him, it may be best to ignore it. When you don't know what he means, ask him to describe it or point to it. For example, the nurse did not know what Mrs Kealey meant when she said, 'I like your wrong.' If the nurse had said, 'What?' Mrs Kealey might have become frustrated in trying to express herself. Instead, the nurse said, 'Describe a wrong.' Mrs Kealey said, 'It's a thing that goes around.' 'Point to it,' said the nurse. Mrs Kealey did and the nurse responded, 'Oh, yes, my ring.'

If the person gets lost in the middle of what he is saying, repeat his last few words – this may help him to continue.

When a person is having trouble expressing an idea, you may be able to guess what he wants to say. Ask him if you are guessing correctly. You might guess wrongly and if you act on an erroneous guess you will add to the confused person's frustration. Say, for example, 'Are you worried about catching the bus home?' or 'Are you saying you have never had an examination like this before?'

People with dementia communicate better when they are relaxed. Try to appear relaxed yourself (even if you have to pretend) and create a calm environment. Never rush the person who is trying to make himself understood.

When you cannot communicate in other ways, you can often guess what a person is trying to tell you. Remember that his feeling is usually accurate, although it may be exaggerated or not appropriate to the actual situation, but that his explanation of why he feels a certain way may be confused. If Mr Mason says, 'Bus, home' and you say, 'You aren't going on the bus' you will not have responded to his feelings. If you correctly guess that he is worried about going home, you can reassure him by saying, 'Your daughter is coming for you at 3 o'clock.'

If a person can still say a few words, or shake or nod his head, you will need to ask him simplified questions about his needs. Say, 'Are you in pain?' or 'Does this hurt?' Point to a body part rather than name it.

When a person cannot communicate, you must establish a regular routine of checking his comfort. Make sure that clothing is comfortable, that the room is warm, that there are no rashes or sores on his skin, that he is taken to the toilet at regular intervals, and that he is not hungry or sleepy.

When a person repeats the same thing over and over, try distracting him. Change the subject, ask him to sing a familiar song, or talk about the feelings behind the statement. For example, if the person is searching for his mother, try saying, 'You must miss your mother' or 'Tell me what your mother was like.'

Problems the impaired person has in understanding others

Often people with brain impairments have difficulty comprehending or understanding what you and others tell them. This is a problem that families sometimes misinterpret as unco-operative behaviour. For example, you may say, 'Mother, I am going to the shops. I will be back in half an hour. Do you understand?' Your mother may say, 'Oh, yes,

I understand,' when in fact she does not understand at all and will get upset as soon as you are out of sight.

People with dementing illnesses also quickly forget what they have already understood. When you give them a careful explanation, they may forget the first part of the explanation before you get to the rest of it.

People with dementing illnesses may have trouble understanding written information, even when they can still read the letters or words. For example, to determine exactly what a person can still do, we may hand him a newspaper and ask him to read the headline, which he may be able to do correctly. Then, when we hand him the written instructions, 'close your eyes', he will not close his eyes, although he may correctly read the words aloud. This indicates that he cannot understand what he is repeating.

Jan told her mother that lunch was in the refrigerator. She left a note on the refrigerator door to remind her mother. Her mother could read the note but could not understand what it said, so she didn't eat her lunch. Instead she complained that she was hungry.

This can be infuriating until you consider that reading and understanding are two different skills, one of which may be lost without the loss of the other. It is not safe to assume that a person can understand and act upon messages he can hear or read. You will need to observe him to know whether he *does* act upon them. If he does not act on instructions, assume he has a problem in understanding language.

The person who can understand what he is told in person may not be able to comprehend what he is told over the telephone. When a person with a dementing illness does not understand what you tell him, the problem is not inattentiveness or wilfulness, but an inability of the malfunctioning brain to make sense out of the words it hears.

There are several ways to improve your verbal communication with a person who has a dementing illness:

1 Make sure he does hear you. Hearing acuity declines in later life and many older people have a hearing deficiency.
2 Lower the tone (pitch) of your voice. A raised pitch is a non-verbal signal that one is upset. Also, a lower pitch is easier for the hearing impaired to hear.
3 Eliminate distracting noises or activities. Both because of the possible hearing deficiency and because of the impaired person's inability to sort things out, he may be unable to understand you when there are other noises or distractions around him.
4 Use short words and short, simple sentences. Avoid complex sen-

tences. Instead of saying, 'I think I'll take the car to the garage now instead of in the morning because in the morning I will get caught in the traffic,' just say, 'I'm going to take the car to the garage now.'

5   Ask only one simple question at a time. If you repeat the question, repeat it exactly. Avoid questions like this: 'Do you want an apple or tart for dessert, or do you want to have dessert later?' Complex choices may overload the person's decision-making ability.

6   Ask the person to do one task at a time, not several. He may not be able to remember several tasks or may be unable to make sense of your message. Most of the things we ask a person to do – have a bath, get ready for bed, put on a coat so we can go to the shops – involve several tasks. We help him by breaking down each project into individual steps and asking the person to do one step at a time.

7   Speak slowly and wait for the person to respond. The impaired person's response may be much slower than what seems natural to us. Wait.

You can improve communication with the person and your understanding of his needs without the usual forms of conversation. People communicate both through what they say and through movements of their face, eyes, hands and body. Everyone uses this non-verbal system of communication without thinking about it. For example, we say, 'He looks angry', 'You can tell by the way they look at each other that they are in love', 'You can tell by the way he walks that he's the boss', 'I know you aren't listening to me', etc. These are all thoughts and emotions we communicate without words. Brain-impaired people can remain sensitive to these non-verbal messages when they cannot understand language well, and they often remain able to express themselves non-verbally.

For example, if you are tired, you may send non-verbal messages that upset the impaired person. Then he may become agitated, which will upset you. Your hands, face and eyes will reveal your distress, which further agitates the confused person. If you are unaware of the significance of body language, you may wonder what happened to upset him. In fact, we all do this all the time. For example, you tell your spouse, 'No, I am not upset.' 'But I know you are,' he or she replies. He or she can detect this fact by the set of your shoulders.

If you are living with a person suffering from dementia, you have already learned to identify many of the non-verbal clues that he sends to make his needs known. Here are some additional ways in which to communicate non-verbally:

1   Remain pleasant, calm, and supportive. (Even if you feel upset, your body language will help to keep the confused person calm.)

2   Smile, take the person's hand, put an arm around his waist, or express affection in some other physical way.

3   *Look directly at him.* Look to see if the person is paying attention to

you. If he uses body language to signal that he is not paying attention, try again in a few minutes.

4 Use other signals besides words: point, touch, hand the person things. Demonstrate an action or describe it with your hands (for example, brushing teeth). Sometimes, if you get him started, he will be able to continue the task.

5 Avoid assuming complex reasons for the person's behaviour. Because the person's brain can no longer process information properly, he experiences the world around and within differently from the way you see things. Since non-verbal communication depends on a completely different set of skills from verbal communication, you may be better able to understand him by considering what it *feels* like he is saying rather than what you *think* he is saying, either through actions or words.

Even when a person is severely confused and unable to communicate, he or she still needs and enjoys affection. Holding hands, hugging or just sitting companionably together is an important way to continue to communicate. The physical care that you give a severely impaired person communicates to him your concern and the fact that he is protected.

Loss of co-ordination

Because dementing illnesses affect many parts of the brain, the person with dementia may lose the ability to make his hands and fingers carry out certain familiar tasks. He may understand what he wants to do, but although his hands and fingers are not stiff or weak, the message just does not get through from the mind to the fingers. Doctors use the word *apraxia* to describe this condition. An early sign of apraxia is a change in the way a person walks. Apraxias may progress gradually or change abruptly, depending on the disease. For example, at first a person may seem only slightly unsteady when walking, but he may gradually change to a slow, shuffling gait.

It can be difficult for the person not trained to assess dementing illnesses to separate problems of memory (can the person remember what he is supposed to do?) from the problems of apraxia (can the person not make his muscles do what they are supposed to do?). Both problems occur when the brain is damaged by the disease. It is not always necessary to distinguish between them in order to help the person manage as independently as possible.

When apraxia begins to affect walking, the person may be slightly unsteady. You must watch for this and provide either a handrail or someone to hold on to when the person is using stairs and stepping on or off a curb.

Loss of co-ordination and manual skills may lead to problems in daily living such as bathing, managing buttons or zips, dressing, pouring a glass of water and eating. Dialling a telephone requires good co-ordination, and a person who does not appear to have any motor impairment may in fact be unable to dial a telephone to call for help. A push-button telephone may help, but it may also be difficult for the confused person to learn the new skills involved in using a push-button phone.

Some of the tasks a person has difficulty with may have to be given up. Others can be modified so that the impaired person can remain partially independent. When you modify a task, the key is to simplify, rather than change it. Because of his intellectual impairment, the person with a dementing illness may be unable to learn a new, simpler task. Consider the nature of each task. Ask yourself if it can be done in a simpler way. For example, shoes that slip on are easier than shoes with laces. Soup is easier to drink out of a mug than to spoon from a bowl. Finger foods are more easily managed than those which must be cut with a knife and fork. Can the person do part of the task if you do the difficult part? You may already have discovered that the person can dress himself if you help with buttons or fasteners.

A person may feel tense, embarrassed or worried about his clumsiness. He may try to conceal his increasing disability by refusing to participate in activities. For example:

Mrs Fisher has always enjoyed knitting. When she abruptly gave up this hobby, her daughter could not understand what had happened. Mrs Fisher said only that she no longer liked to knit. In fact, her increasing apraxia was making knitting impossible, and she was ashamed of her awkwardness.

A relaxed atmosphere often helps make the person's clumsiness less apparent. It is not unusual for a person to have more difficulty with a task when he is feeling tense.

Sometimes a person can carry out certain tasks at some times but not at others. This may be a characteristic of the brain impairment and not laziness. Being hurried, being watched, being upset, or being tired can affect a person's ability to do things – just as it does anyone. Having a brain disease makes these natural fluctuations more dramatic. Sometimes a person can undertake one task with no problem, such as zipping up trousers, and may be unable to undertake another similar task, such as zipping up a jacket. It can appear that the person is being difficult, but the reason may actually be that one task is impossible because it is different in some way.

Sometimes a person can carry out a task if you break it down into a series of smaller tasks and tell him to do each step. For example, brushing your teeth involves picking up the toothbrush, putting the toothpaste on it, putting the toothbrush in your mouth, brushing, rinsing, etc. Gently remind the person of each step. It may help to demonstrate. You may have to repeat each step several times. Sometimes it helps to put a familiar tool, such as a spoon or comb, into the person's hand and gently start his arm moving in the right direction. Beginning the motion seems to help the brain remember the task.

An occupational therapist is trained to assess the motor skills the person has retained and how he may make the best use of them. The information gained from the assessment done by the occupational therapist can help you give the confused person the assistance he needs without taking away his independence.

In the later stages of some of the dementing diseases, extensive loss of muscle control occurs and the person may bump into things and fall down. This is discussed in Chapter 5.

People with dementing illnesses may have other diseases as well that interfere with their ability to carry out daily tasks. Part of the problem may be in the muscles or joints and another part of the problem in the impaired brain. Such complicating conditions include tremors (shaking), muscle weakness, joint or bone diseases such as arthritis, or stiffness caused by medication.

There are many techniques and devices to help people with physical limitations remain independent. When you consider such techniques or devices, remember that most of them require the ability to learn to do something in a new way or to learn to use a new gadget. People with dementing illnesses may not be able to learn the new skills needed.

Some people have tremors. These are shaking movements of the hands or body and can make many activities difficult, but an occupational therapist or physiotherapist may be able to show you how to minimise the effects of tremors.

Some people with neurological conditions, especially Parkinson's disease, have difficulty starting a movement or may get 'stuck' in the middle of a movement. This can be frustrating for both of you. If this is a problem, here are some helpful hints:

1   If the person becomes 'glued' to the floor while walking, tell him to walk towards a particular object or to look at a spot on the floor a few feet in front of him. This may help him to move on.
2   It may be easier to get out of a chair that has armrests. Raise the sitting person's centre of gravity by raising the chair seat to suit him. A firm seat is needed. Use a firm cushion or a higher chair, such as a dining-room chair. Avoid low chairs with soft cushions. Instruct the person to move forward to the edge of the chair and spread his feet about one foot apart to give a wider base to stand on. Ask the

person to put his hands on the armrests and then to rock back and
forth to gain momentum. On the count of three, tell him to get up
quickly. Ensure he takes time to get his balance before he begins to
walk.
3   Sitting down in a chair may be easier to do when the person puts his
hands on the armrests, bends forward as far as possible and then sits
down slowly.

Muscle weakness or stiffness may occur when a person does not move
around much. Exercise is important for memory-impaired people.

Occasionally a person who is taking one of the major tranquillisers or
neuroleptic drugs will get stiff and rigid, or may become restless. These
may be side effects of the medication and can be very uncomfortable.
Notify your doctor. He can change the dosage or prescribe some other
medication to overcome this effect.

Loss of sense of time

The uncanny ability individuals have for judging the passage of time is
one of the first losses experienced by a person with a dementia. He may
repeatedly ask you what time it is, feel that you have left him for hours
when you are out of sight for a few minutes, or want to leave a place as
soon as he has arrived. It is not hard to understand this behaviour when
you consider that in order to know how much time has passed, one must
be able to remember what one has done in the immediate past. The
person who forgets quickly has no way of measuring the passage of time.

In addition to this defect of memory, it appears that dementing diseases can affect the internal clock that keeps the rest of us on a reasonably
regular schedule of sleeping, waking and eating. It will be helpful to you
to recognise that this behaviour is not deliberate (although it can be
irritating). It is the result of the loss of brain function.

The ability to read a clock may be lost early in the course of the
disease. Even when a person can look at the clock and say, 'It is 3.15',
he may be unable to make sense out of this information.

Not being able to keep track of the time can worry the forgetful person.
Many of us, throughout our lives, are dependent upon a regular time
schedule. Not knowing the time can make a person worry that he will
be late, be forgotten, miss the bus, overstay his welcome, miss lunch, or
miss his transport home. The confused person may not know just what
he is worried about, but a general feeling of anxiety may make him ask
you what time it is. And, of course, as soon as you answer him, he will
forget the whole conversation, and ask again.

Sometimes a person feels that you have deserted him when you have been gone only briefly. This is because he cannot remember. Sometimes setting a timer or an old-fashioned hour-glass, or writing a note – 'I am in the back garden and will be in at 3 pm' – might help the person wait more patiently for your return. Be sure to select a cue (timer, note) that he can still comprehend. Perhaps you can think of other ways to reduce this behaviour. For example:

> *When Mr and Mrs Jenkins went to lunch at their son's house, Mr Jenkins would almost immediately insist that it was time to go home. When he could be persuaded to stay for the meal, he insisted on leaving immediately afterwards. His son thought he was just being rude.*
>
> *Things went more smoothly when the family understood that this was because the unfamiliar house, the added confusion and Mr Jenkins's lost sense of time upset him. The family thought back over Mr Jenkins's life and hit upon an old social habit that helped them. In earlier years he had enjoyed watching the football match after Sunday lunch. Now his son turned on the TV as soon as Mr Jenkins finished eating. Since this was an old habit, Mr Jenkins would stay for about an hour, giving his wife time to chat, before he got restless for home.*

Symptoms that are better at some times than at others

Families often observe that the person can carry out certain tasks at some times but not at others:

> *'In the morning my mother does not need as much help as she does in the evening.'*

> *'My wife can use the bathroom alone at home; but she insists she needs help at our daughter's house.'*

> *'My husband does not get as angry and upset at day care as he does at home. Is this because he is angry with me?'*

> *'Bill said a whole sentence yesterday, but today I can't understand a thing he says. Was he trying harder yesterday?'*

Fluctuations in ability are common in people who suffer from dementia. Well people also have fluctuations in ability, but they are less noticeable.

People with dementia have good days and bad days; some are better in the morning, when they are rested; some have more problems in less familiar settings; some do better when they feel more relaxed. Some fluctuations have no explanation. Whatever the likely reason, such fluctuations are normal and do not signal a change in the course of the disease.

People with dementia are more vulnerable than others to minor changes in health (see Chapter 6). An abrupt change in the ability to do something or in the overall level of function may indicate a medication reaction or a new illness. If you suspect this kind of change, it is important to contact the person's doctor.

The brain damage itself will account for some changes in ability. It is possible that damaged nerve cells that fail most of the time do work occasionally. It is also possible that less damaged or undamaged areas can intermittently take over and temporarily 'fix' a defective system.

All of these causes for variation in ability are beyond the person's deliberate control. People with dementia are usually trying as hard as they can. You can help them most by learning which aspects of their environment bring out the best in them and which things cause greater disability.

4 Problems in independent living

As a person begins to develop a dementing illness, she may begin to have difficulty managing independently. You may suspect that she is mismanaging her money, worry that she should not be driving, or wonder if she should be living alone. People with dementing illnesses often appear to be managing well, and they may insist that they are fine and that you are interfering. It can be difficult to know when you should take over and how much you should take over. It can also be painful to take away these outward symbols of a person's independence or the confused person may adamantly refuse to move, to stop driving, or to relinquish her financial responsibilities.

Part of the reason why making any change, however small, can be difficult is because it may symbolise giving up independence and responsibility to the confused person. You and other family members will also have strong feelings about making decisions for her. (We will discuss these role changes in Chapter 11.) Making necessary changes will be easier when you understand the feelings involved.

The first step in deciding whether the time has come to make changes in a person's independence is to obtain a proper medical assessment. This will tell you what the person is still able to do and what she is no longer able to do, and it will give you the authority to insist upon necessary changes. For a medical assessment, first contact your GP and ask if your dependant may see a specialist who may be a neurologist, a geriatrician, a psychiatrist or a psychogeriatrician. When a professional assessment is not immediately available, you and your family must analyse each task as thoroughly and objectively as possible, and decide whether the person can still carry out specific tasks *completely*, *safely* and *without* becoming upset.

A dementing illness can bring about many kinds of loss. It means losing control over one's daily activities, losing independence, losing skills, and losing the ability to do those things that make one feel useful or important. A dementing illness limits the possibilities the future can hold. While others can look forward to things improving, the ill person must gradually realise that her future is limited. Perhaps the most terrible loss of all is the loss of memory. Losing one's memories means losing one's day-to-day connections with others and with one's past. The far past may seem like the present. Without a memory of today or an understanding that the past is past, the future ceases to have meaning.

As losses accumulate in anyone's life, it is natural for him or her to cling even more tightly to the things that remain. Understandably, a confused person might respond to such changes with resistance, denial or anger. The confused person's need for familiar surroundings and the determination of most people not to be a burden on anyone, make it understandable that the disabled person will not want to give up these things. To accept that, she would have to face the extent and finality of her illness, which she may not be able to do.

In addition, the person may be unable to make complete sense of what is going on. Even early in the disease, the person may completely forget recent events. If she has no recollection of leaving the stove on or of having a car accident, she may reasonably insist she can take care of herself or that she is still a good driver. She is not 'denying' the reality of her situations; she cannot remember the mistakes that are evidence of her impairment. If she is not able to assess her own limitations, it may seem to her as if things are being unfairly taken away from her and that her family is 'taking over'. By recognising how she may feel, you may be able to find ways to help her make the necessary changes and still consider that she is in control of her life.

When a person must give up a job

The time when the person must give up a job depends on the kind of job she has and whether she must drive as part of her job. Sometimes an employer will tell you or the impaired person that she must retire. Some employers will be willing to maintain a person in a job that is not too demanding. Sometimes the family must make this decision. You may realise that this time has come.

If the person must give up her job, there are two areas that you must consider: the emotional and psychological adjustments involved in such a major change, and the financial changes that will be involved. A person's job is a key part of her sense of identity. It helps her to feel that she is a valued member of society. The impaired person may resist giving up her job or may deny that anything is wrong. Her adjustment to retirement may be a painful and distressing time. If these things happen, your GP or a social worker may be able to help.

It is important that you consider the financial future of the impaired person. (This is discussed in Chapter 15.) Retirement can create special problems. Individuals who are forced to retire early because of a dementing illness should be entitled to the same disability benefits as a person with any other disabling disease.

The demented person, although she may have good skills remaining, may be unable to learn a new job. If she is denied benefits for this reason, you may want to seek legal advice.

When a person can no longer manage money

The impaired person may be unable to balance her cheque book, she may be unable to calculate the correct change, or she may become irresponsible with her money. Occasionally, when a person can no longer manage her money, she may become nasty and accuse others of stealing from her.

Said Mr Roberts, 'My wife has kept the books for the family business for years. I knew something was wrong when my accountant came to me and told me the books were in a terrible mess.'

Mr Rogers said, 'My wife was giving money to the neighbours, hiding it in the wastepaper basket, and losing her purse. So I took her purse – and her money – away from her. Then she was always saying I stole her money.'

Since money often represents independence, people can be unwilling to give up control of their finances.

You may be able to take over the household accounts by simply correcting the person's efforts. If you have to take the person's cheque book away against her wishes, it may help to write a memo such as, 'My son, John, now takes care of my cheque book' and put this note where the confused person can refer to it to refresh her memory.

It can be upsetting when a person accuses others of stealing, but this is easier to understand when you consider human nature. We have been taught all our lives to be careful with money and when money disappears most of us wonder if it was stolen. As a person's brain becomes less able to remember what is really happening, it is not surprising that she becomes anxious and suspicious that her money is being stolen. Avoid getting into arguments over this, since they may upset her more.

Some families find that giving the forgetful person a small amount of spending money (perhaps small change or a pound coin) helps. If it is lost or given away, it is only a minimal amount. Sometimes a person needs to know that she has a little bit of cash in hand, and this is a way around conflicts about money. One peculiarity of the dementing diseases is that a person sometimes loses the ability to calculate the correct change before she loses the knowledge that she needs money.

Mrs Hutchinson had always been fiercely independent about her money, so Mr Hutchinson gave her a purse with some change in it. He put her name and address in it, in case she lost her purse. She insisted on paying her hairdresser by cheque long after she could not responsibly manage a cheque book. So Mr Hutchinson gave her some cheques stamped VOID by the bank. Each week she gave one to the hairdresser. Mr Hutchinson privately arranged with the hairdresser that these would be accepted and that he would pay the bills.

This may seem extreme. It may also seem unfair to dupe the confused person this way. In reality this arrangement allows a sick woman to continue to feel independent, and it allows her tired and burdened husband to manage the finances and keep the peace.

The Disablement Income Group and the Disability Alliance can help sort out the finances and benefits a person is entitled to. Money matters can cause serious problems, especially when the person is also suspicious or when other members of the family disagree. (It may be helpful here to read Chapters 8 and 11.) Your ingenuity can be a great help to you in making money matters less distressing.

When a person can no longer drive safely

The time may come when you realise that your parent or spouse can no longer drive safely. While some people will recognise their limits, others may be unwilling to give up driving. As a group, people with dementia who continue to drive are more likely to have accidents.

For most experienced drivers, driving is a skill so well learned that it is partly 'automatic'. A person can go back and forth to work every day with her mind on other things – perhaps dictating or listening to music. It does not take much concentration to drive, but if the traffic pattern should suddenly change, she can rely on the mind to focus on the road immediately and respond swiftly to a crisis. Because driving is a well-learned skill, a confused person can still *appear* to be driving well when she is not really safe. Driving requires a highly complex interaction of eyes, brain and muscle, and the ability to solve complicated problems quickly. A person who is still apparently driving safely may have lost the ability to respond appropriately to an unexpected problem on the road. She may be relying entirely on the habits of driving and may be unable to change quickly from a habitual response to a new response when the situation demands it.

Often people make the decision themselves to stop driving when they feel that they 'aren't as sharp as they used to be'. But if they do not, you have a responsibility to them and to others to assess carefully whether or not the person's driving is dangerous, and to intervene when it is. This may be one of the first situations in which you take a decision out of the hands of the impaired person. You may feel hesitant to do this, but you will probably be relieved once you have stopped a forgetful person from driving. To decide whether the time has come, look at the skills that a person needs to drive safely and evaluate whether the confused person still has these skills – both in the car and in other situations:

1 **Good vision**:   A person must have good vision, or vision corrected with glasses, and be able to see clearly, both in front and out of the corners of her eyes (peripheral vision) so that she sees things approaching from the sides.

2 **Good hearing**:   A person must be able to hear well or have her hearing corrected with a hearing aid, so that she is alert to the sounds of approaching cars, horns and so forth.

3 **Quick reaction time**:   A driver must be able to react quickly – to turn, to brake and to avoid accidents. Older people's reaction time, when it is formally tested, is slightly slower than that of young people, but in unimpaired older people it is usually not slow enough to interfere with driving. However, if you notice that a person reacts slowly or inappropriately to sudden changes around the house, this should alert you to the possibility of the same limitations when she is driving.

4 **Ability to make decisions**:   A driver must be able to make quick, *appropriate* decisions rapidly and *calmly*. The ability to make the correct decision when a child darts in front of the car, a horn blares and a lorry is approaching all at once necessitates being able to solve complicated, unfamiliar problems quickly and without panicking. People with a dementing illness often rely on habitual responses that may not be the correct responses in a driving situation. Some people also become confused and upset when several things happen at once. If they are occurring, you will notice these problems around the house as well as in the car.

5 **Good co-ordination**:   Eyes, hands and feet must all still work together well to handle a car safely. If a person is becoming clumsy, or if her way of walking has changed, it should alert you to the fact that she may also have trouble operating the brake.

6 **Alertness to what is going on around her**:   A driver must be alert to all that is going on without becoming upset or confused. If a person is 'missing things' that happen around her, she may no longer be a safe driver.

Sometimes driving behaviours alert you to problems. Forgetful people may get lost on routes that would not have confused them previously. Being lost can distract the driver and further interfere with her ability to react quickly. Sometimes driving too slowly is a clue that the driver is uncertain of her skills – but this does not mean that every cautious driver is an impaired driver.

Confused people may become angry or aggressive when they drive, or they may inappropriately believe that other drivers are 'out to get them'.

This is dangerous. Occasionally a person with a dementing illness is also drinking too much. Even small amounts of alcohol impair the driving ability of people with a dementing illness. This is a dangerous combination, and you must intervene.

If you are concerned about a person's driving ability, you might first approach the problem by discussing it frankly with her. Even though a person is cognitively impaired, she is still able to participate in decisions that involve her. How you initiate such a discussion may affect her response. People with brain impairments are sometimes less able to tolerate criticism than when they were well, so you will need to use tact in such a discussion. If you say, 'Your driving is terrible, you are getting lost, and you're just not safe', a person can feel she has to defend herself and may argue with you. By gently saying, 'You are getting absent-minded about traffic lights', however, you may be able to give a person an 'easy way out'. Giving up driving can mean admitting one's increasing limitations. As well as reacting to the need for safety, look for ways of helping the person to save face and maintain her self-image. Try offering alternatives: 'I'll drive today and you can look at the scenery.'

Sometimes a person will absolutely refuse to give up driving, despite your tact. It may be that when the person is shown what her reaction times are, or is asked to demonstrate driving skills by a skilled instructor, she will come to accept that she should give up driving without being told. The Mobility Advice and Vehicle Information Service (MAVIS, The Department of Transport, Crow House, Berkshire, RGII 6AV, tel: 0344 770456) will be able to tell you where the nearest driving centre is.

If she will not give up it may help to enlist the support of the doctor or family solicitor. If your doctor needs guidance, he can telephone the medical section of the Driver and Vehicle Licensing Centre (tel: 0792 304000) and receive advice on a doctor-to-doctor confidential basis so that the legal side can be clarified and future action decided upon. Some doctors will write an order on a prescription pad that says, 'Do not drive.' Families report that portraying the doctor as the 'bad guy' takes great pressure off the care-giver. Often a person will co-operate with instructions from a recognised authority, such as a doctor, when she may regard your own advice as nagging. As a last resort, some families have disconnected the battery or starter wire and told the impaired person that the car cannot be repaired. (A car mechanic can show you how to do this.)

One wife who did not drive sold her confused husband's car and put the money in a biscuit tin. Every week she added the amount the family used to spend on petrol, maintenance and car insurance. She said it was easier now to spend money on taxis, knowing they used to spend it on the car.

Drivers are required by law to inform the licensing authorities if they suffer from any disability which affects their fitness to drive unless it is unlikely to last for more than three months. Some insurance companies require older drivers to undergo medical examinations to assess their fitness to drive. If drivers are convicted of a motoring offence and their ability to drive is questioned, a magistrate may require them to pass a driving test before allowing them to drive.

Orange Badge Scheme

The 'Orange Badge Scheme' grants concessionary parking to people with disabilities. The regulations state that badges will be issued as of right to people receiving the mobility component of the Disability Living Allowance and registered blind people. Other people may also qualify if their disability is permanent and substantial and causes inability to walk or very considerable difficulty in walking. The badge is exhibited on the car's windscreen and can be obtained from the local authority Social Services or Borough Surveyor's Departments. There is usually a fee, and proof of eligibility will be sought – either evidence that the person is in receipt of a mobility allowance or a doctor's note.

The badge can be moved from car to car, depending on who is providing the transport at any one time. The stress on the carer can be very much reduced by being able to use improved parking facilities through this scheme.

When a person can no longer live alone

When a person has lived alone but can no longer continue to do so, the move to live with someone else can be difficult for everyone. Some people welcome the sense of security that living with others provides. Others vigorously resist giving up their independence.

Often people go through a series of stages from complete independence to living with someone. When a gradual transition from independence is possible, it may be easier for the person to adjust and it may postpone the time when she must live with someone. For example, to begin with, the help of neighbours, a home care assistant or provision of meals-on-wheels may be adequate; later, a family member or a paid voluntary helper may spend part of the day with the confused person. A person who is still fairly independent may only need someone to come in to give medication or help with a meal, but not constant supervision.

When you suspect that someone living alone is becoming confused

You need to be alert to the possibility that the person's ability to function alone may change suddenly: some minor stress or even a mild cold can make her worse. Or, you may not notice the gradual, insidious decline until a crisis occurs. Families often wait too long before taking action.

When things do go wrong, the person may react by trying to 'cover up'. Some confused people do not realise they have problems; others may blame the family or withdraw. Close family members may also deny that there are problems. Therefore, it can be difficult to know for sure what is going on. Here are some questions to consider when deciding whether a person who lives alone is in need of help:

Telephone calls

- Have her conversations become increasingly vague? (Details require more memory.)
- Do conversations ramble, or does she seem to forget what she was saying? Does she repeat herself?
- Does she become 'edgy' when talking on the telephone, more than she used to? Is she less tolerant of frustration?
- Are you receiving fewer phone calls from her, too many calls, or calls late at night?
- Does she repeat the same story at each conversation as if it were new?

Changes in personality or habits

- Is she uncharacteristically apathetic, negative, pessimistic, suspicious or unusually fearful of crime?
- Does she insist that everything is fine, or refuse to admit to problems of which you are already aware?
- Is the person able to manage her own personal care and grooming? Some forgetful people wear dirty clothes, forget (or refuse) to bathe or brush their teeth, or in other ways neglect themselves.
- Has she become isolated? Does she say she is going out when she does not?

Letters

- Has she stopped writing letters or notes, or are her letters uncharacteristically rambling?
- Has her handwriting changed?

Meals and medication

Is the person eating her meals and taking her medicines? A forgetful person may not eat, or may eat only sweets even when you have provided a hot meal. The person may take too much medicine or forget her medicine. This can make her mental impairment worse and can jeopardise her physical health. If the person is safe in other ways, and if someone else helps daily with food and medicine, she may be able to live alone, but it has been our experience that people who forget to eat properly are experiencing sufficient cognitive impairment to indicate that they probably cannot safely live alone.

Is the person forgetting to turn off the cooker or burning the food? People who appear to be managing well often forget to turn off the cooker. Is the person using candles or matches? It can be hard to believe that a person is a danger to herself when she looks so well, but fire is a real and serious hazard. Cases of severe or even fatal accidental burns are not uncommon. If you suspect that the person is forgetting to turn off the cooker, you must intervene.

Other problems

Is the person wandering away from home? She may get lost or be robbed or assaulted. Is the person wandering around outside at night? Such behaviour is not uncommon and is dangerous. Have her friends or neighbours called you with concerns about her behaviour or safety? Has she failed to keep appointments or not come to family events? Has she given you confusing reports of a mishap, such as a car accident? Did she retire from work early or suddenly?

Is the person keeping the house tidy, reasonably clean and free of hazards? Forgetful people may spill puddles of water in the kitchen or bathroom and forget to clean them up. A person can slip and fall on a wet floor. Sometimes people forget to wash the dishes, or forget to flush the toilet, or in other ways create unsanitary conditions. If the house is badly cluttered, they can trip and fall. A confused person may pile up newspapers and rags which become a fire hazard. Does the house smell of urine? This is a signal that the person is unable to manage alone or is ill.

Is the person keeping warm? A forgetful person may keep her house too cold or dress inappropriately. Her body temperature can drop dangerously if she does not keep herself warm. In hot weather the confused person may dress too warmly or may be afraid to open the house for adequate ventilation. This can lead to heatstroke.

Is the person acting in response to 'paranoid' ideas or unrealistic suspiciousness? Such behaviour can lead her into trouble in the community. Sometimes people call the police because of their fears and make their neighbours angry. Also, confused elderly people may become the target of malicious teenagers. These problems can occur in suburban neighbourhoods as well as in inner cities.

Is the person showing good judgement? Some confused people show poor judgement about whom they allow in the house and can be robbed as a result, or they may give away money inappropriately.

Who is paying the bills? Often the first indication family members have that something is wrong is when the electricity or gas is cut off because the bill has not been paid or because the person will not let the meter reader in. The person may stop balancing her cheque book or her spending habits may change.

Such clues indicate that *something* may be wrong – but not necessarily that the person has a dementing illness. Once you are aware that there may be a problem, it is essential to obtain a complete assessment for the person. The changes mentioned above can indicate many other treatable conditions.

What you can do

Visit in person to assess the situation and to see whether it is possible to arrange a diagnosis. The GP may already know of the problem – if not, it is important to make sure that he is made aware of what has been happening. Other family members or neighbours might help you to assess the position.

If your relative does have a dementing illness, it will be useful to contact the Alzheimer's Disease Society group or branch in your community. Most groups have had experience helping families who live at a distance and can give you valuable information. Talk first to your relative and discuss what might be done and how you might keep in touch. Talk to a close friend of the person, a neighbour, or the milkman. The postman, bank manager or clergyman may also be aware of the situation. Give these people your telephone number and ask them to alert you if there are problems. The Alzheimer's Disease Society, or Age Concern or the Citizens Advice Bureau in your relative's town, will be able to tell you about local services which are available.

You will gradually build up a picture of her needs and what help may be available. Sometimes a person can continue to live independently for a while if you can arrange for supervision. Perhaps her physician can give you an idea of how capable the person is of continuing to function alone. Through the Social Services Department, it may be possible to arrange for the person to receive help from the Home Care Service. A social worker may be able to help sort financial matters out.

However, you may have to consider other options such as moving to a care home, or perhaps moving to live with your relative or bringing her to live with you. There is much more detail about what help may be available at home or about choosing a care home in Chapters 10 and 16.

Moving to a new home

If the help available in the community cannot support her degree of confusion, you may decide that she can no longer live alone and that other arrangements must be made for her. You might consider full-time help or you may arrange for the person to move into a residential care home, a nursing home or a psychiatric hospital. (These facilities will be described in detail in Chapter 16.)

Mr Sawyer reports, 'Mother simply cannot live alone any more. We hired a housekeeper and Mother fired her – and when I called the employment agency they said they could not send anyone else. So we talked with Mother, told her we wanted her to come and live with us. But she absolutely refused. She says nothing is wrong with her, that I am trying to steal her money. She won't admit she isn't eating. She says she's changed her clothes and we know she hasn't. I don't know what to do.'

If a confused person refuses to give up her independence and move into a safer setting, understanding something of what she may be thinking and feeling may help to make the move easier. A move from living alone to living with someone else may mean giving up one's independence and admitting one's impairment. Moving means more losses. It means giving up a familiar place and often many familiar possessions. That place and those possessions are the tangible symbols of one's past, and reminders when one's memories fade.

The confused person is dependent upon a familiar setting to provide her with cues that enable her to function independently. Learning one's way around a new place is difficult or even impossible. She feels dependent upon familiar surroundings to survive. The person with a dementing illness may forget the plans that have been discussed, or may be unable to understand them. You may reassure your mother that she is coming to live in your house – which is very familiar to her – but all her damaged mind may perceive is that she is going to lose a lot of her possessions.

As you make plans for this person to live with someone else, there are several things to consider:

1   Take into careful consideration the changes that this move will mean in your life, and plan, before the move, for financial resources and emotional outlets and support for yourself.

If the impaired person is to move in with you, what effect will this have on her income or your own? State pensions and benefits will often stay the same but it is advisable to check this at a local advice agency like the Citizens Advice Bureau. For example, if you are receiving Housing Benefit, this may be reduced if she comes to live with you.

If the person is coming to live with you, how does the rest of the family feel about this? If there are children or teenagers in the family, will their activities upset the confused person, or will the 'odd' behaviour of the confused person upset them? How does your spouse feel about this? Is your marriage already under stress? A demented person in the home creates burdens and stresses under the best of circumstances. If the demented person and her spouse are both moving in, you must also consider how the spouse will interact in the household. All the people affected need to be involved in the decision and need the opportunity to express their concerns.

Assuming the care of a forgetful person may mean changes in other aspects of your life: leisure time (you may not be able to go out because there is no one to sit with Mother); peace (you may not be able to read the newspaper or talk to your wife because Mother is pacing the floor); money (you may face higher heating bills or bills for adapting the home); rest (the confused person may wake at night); visitors (people may stop visiting if the person's behaviour is embarrassing). These are the things that make life tolerable and help to reduce your stress. It is important to plan ways for you and your family to relax and get away from the problems of caring for a sick person. Remember also that other problems are not going to go away. You may still worry about your children, come home exhausted from your job, experience problems with the car etc.

Is the person you are bringing into your home someone you can live with? If you never could get along with your mother and if her illness has made her behaviour worse instead of better, having her move in with you may be disastrous. If you have hitherto had a poor relationship with the person who is now sick, that poor relationship can make things more difficult for you.

2   *Involve the person as much as possible in plans for the move, even if she refuses to move.*

The patient is still a person, and her participation in plans and decisions that involve her is important, unless she is too severely impaired to comprehend what is happening. Confused people who have been hoodwinked into a move may become even more angry and suspicious, and it may be extremely difficult for them to adjust to the new setting. Certainly, the extent and nature of the impaired person's participation depend on the extent of her illness and her attitude towards the move.

Keep in mind that there is a major difference between making the decision – which you may have to do – and participating in the planning – which the confused person can be encouraged to do. Perhaps Mr Sawyer's story will continue like this:

'*After we talked it over with Mother she still absolutely refused to consider a move. So I went ahead with arrangements. I told Mother gently that she had to move because she was getting forgetful.*

'*I knew too many decisions at once would upset her, so we would just ask her a few things at a time. "Mother, would you like to take all your pictures with you?" "Mother, let's take your own bed and your lovely bedspread for your new bedroom." Of course, we made a lot of decisions without her – about the cooker and the washing machine, and the junk in the attic. And, of course, she kept saying she wasn't going and that I was robbing her. Still, I think some of it sank in, that she was helping us get ready to move. Sometimes she would pick up a vase and say, "I want Carol to have this." We tried to comply with her wishes. Then, after the move, we could honestly tell her that the vase was not stolen: she had given it to Carol.*'

When a person is too impaired to understand what is happening around her, it may be better to make the move without the added stress of trying to involve her in it.

3   *Be prepared for a period of adjustment.*   Changes are frequently upsetting to people with dementing illnesses. No matter how carefully and lovingly you plan the move, this is a major change, and the person may be upset for a while. It is easy to understand that it takes time to get over the

losses a move involves. A forgetful person also needs extra time to learn her way around a new place.

Reassure yourself that after an adjustment period the person usually will settle into her new surroundings. Signs on doors may help her find her way around an unfamiliar home. An additional sedative may help her sleep at night. Try to postpone other activities or changes until after the period of adjustment.

Moving with a confused person

Sometimes a care-giver will move to a residence where she can manage the confused person more easily: a flat or a retirement home, for example. We have discussed ways of helping a confused person accept a move on page 55. If you are contemplating moving you will want to consider:

1   What are the financial costs of moving, such as the purchase price of a new residence, and the cost of moving furniture?
2   Will moving mean less property for you to clean or maintain? Will help, such as meal preparation or house cleaning be provided for you?
3   Will moving bring you closer to doctors, hospitals, shopping centres, recreation areas?
4   What kind of transportation will you need?
5   Will moving put you closer to or further away from friends and family who can help you?
6   Does the area you intend to move into have good support services?
7   Will moving provide a safe environment for the person (no stairs, call bells, a ground floor bathroom, supervision, lower crime rate)?
8   What will you do if your financial or physical circumstances change?
9   Whose name should the new property be under, and if there is surplus capital from the sale of any home, how should this be handled.

Moving into her home

Sometimes it will be possible to move in with the confused person yourself. This would obviously save the upheaval for her and mean that she will continue to live in the same familiar surroundings. Before doing so, consider all the possible difficulties we have outlined about moving, but if you are giving up your own home there is one other very important issue to consider.

If eventually your relative needs to go into a care home and her resources are inadequate to pay for that care, she may need to turn to the state for help (see Chapter 16). In such a case, if she owns the home, or part of the home, she may be required to sell her asset to pay for care, leaving you homeless. Some people are protected under current arrangements, which are described in a fact sheet obtainable from Age Concern England, but we would advise that you consult a solicitor before moving. You might be equally vulnerable if she were the tenant of a property and we would suggest discussing this with the landlord and obtaining written confirmation of your situation.

Consultation is essential because the legal situation may change. If you decide to move in with her, you must also keep yourself regularly informed about this through a solicitor while you are together.

Occasionally an impaired person never really adjusts to moving. Don't blame yourself. You did the best you could and acted in her best interests. You may have to accept her inability to adjust as being the result of her illness.

5   Problems arising in daily care

Hazards to watch for

A person with a dementing illness is less able to take responsibility for his own safety. He is no longer able to assess the consequences of his actions the way the rest of us do, and, because he forgets so quickly, accidents can easily happen. He may attempt to carry out familiar tasks without realising that he can no longer manage them. For example, the disease may affect those portions of the brain which remembers how to do simple things, such as doing up buttons or slicing meat. This inability to carry out manual tasks is often unrecognised and causes accidents. Since the person also cannot learn, you will have to take special precautions to guard against accidents. Because a person seems to be managing well, you may not realise that he has lost the judgement he needs to avoid accidents. Families may need to take responsibility for the safety of even a mildly impaired person.

Accidents are most likely to occur when you are cross or tired, when everyone is hurrying, when there is an argument, or when someone in the household is ill. At these times you are less alert to the possibility of an accident and the impaired person may misunderstand or over-react to even the slightest mishap with a catastrophic reaction.

Do what you can to reduce the confusion when it arises. This is difficult when you are struggling with the care of a person with a dementing illness. If you are rushing with him to keep an appointment or finish a job, *stop*, even if it means being late or not getting something done. Catch your breath, rest a minute and let the confused person calm down.

Be aware that mishaps can be a warning sign of impending accidents: you banged your shin on the end of the bed, or dropped and broke a cup, and the impaired person is getting upset. This is the time to create a change of pace before a serious accident occurs. Alert others in the household to the relationship between increased tension and increased accidents. At such times everyone can keep a closer eye on the impaired person.

Be sure you know the limits of the impaired person's abilities. Do not take his word that he can heat up his supper or get into the bath alone. An occupational therapist can give you an excellent picture of what the person can do safely. If such an assessment has not been carried out, observe the person closely as he undertakes various tasks.

Have an emergency plan ready in case something does happen. Whom will you call if someone is hurt? How will you get the upset person out of the house in case of a fire? Remember that he may misinterpret what is happening and resist your efforts to help him.

Change the environment to make it safer. This is one of the most important ways to avoid accidents. Go thoughtfully through your home, garden, neighbourhood and car, looking for things a person with a dementing illness could possibly misuse or misinterpret, thereby causing an accident. Contact an occupational therapist at your local Social Services Department to help you with this. She will also be able to tell you about the range of equipment which might assist in making your relative's environment less dangerous and his life more comfortable. Sometimes the equipment will be available through her department or through the Community Nursing Service.

In the house

A neat house is safer than a cluttered one. There are fewer things to trip over or knock over, and hazards are more easily seen. Knick-knacks or clutter may distract or confuse an impaired person.

Remove objects that cause problems. If a person tries to use the iron and leaves it on, causing a fire hazard, put it away where he cannot find it. Whenever possible, take the easiest path to safety without conflict. Does the impaired person have access to power tools, lawn mower, knives, hair dryer, sewing machine or car keys when he can no longer safely use them? You must ensure these are locked away.

Is all medication kept out of the reach of a person who may forget that he has already taken it? Buy a medicine cabinet, or any small cupboard or box, and equip it with an effective lock to keep medicines safely away from the forgetful person and visiting grandchildren.

Are things stored on the stairs? Clutter is always dangerous, particularly when a person is confused, clumsy or misinterprets what he sees. Are extension cords stretched across the floor where a person might trip over them?

Lower the temperature on your water heater so that water is not hot enough to scald the person who accidentally turns it on. People with dementing illnesses can lose the ability to realise that water is too hot and can burn themselves badly as a result. If hot water pipes are exposed, cover them with insulation.

If the confused person readjusts the boiler or water heater, you may need to lock the kitchen or airing cupboard door.

If you have stairs, install a gate at the top. The confused person can easily become disorientated and fall down the steps, especially at night.

Install handrails if there are none. As the person becomes unsteady on his feet, he will need them. Check existing handrails; be sure they are sturdy. Handrails should be anchored into the brick wall or wooden support beams. Such rails will not hold a person's weight if they are not securely fastened. Put away rugs that slip. If stairs are carpeted, check to see that the carpet is securely tacked down.

Remove furniture with sharp corners or sharp edges. Put away or block off large areas of breakable glass; a person can fall against a glass china cabinet and be badly cut. Put away rocking chairs that tip over easily. Remove coffee tables and fragile antiques.

Use stable chairs that are easy to get out of (see page 94). Check if fingers or toes could become caught in parts of recliners. Furniture upholstery should be easy to clean; you may have to wipe up spills. Furnishing fabrics, curtains and cushions should be flame resistant.

A confused person can easily lean too far out of a window or over a balcony rail and fall – a particular danger in high-rise buildings. Install security locks on windows and balcony doors. Inexpensive devices are available that allow you to lock a window in an open position, so that a person cannot get out but fresh air can get in, or to open the window a little at the top and bottom and secure it.

Block off hot radiators by putting sturdy chairs in front of them. You will need to put guards around all fires and stoves.

Can the person lock himself in a room so that you cannot get in? If so, remove the lock, take the levers out, and replace the knob, or tape the latch open.

Never keep insecticides, petrol, paint, solvents, cleaning agents, etc. in other than their original, clearly labelled containers. Store them safely out of reach of the confused person. Child-proof (and patient-proof) cabinet locks are available at hardware shops, at large chemists such as Boots and at Mothercare shops. Mildly confused people may try to use such materials inappropriately.

Impaired people forget what can be eaten and what cannot; they may drink solvents by mistake. These people may also eat other inappropriate items. Put small objects such as pins and buttons out of reach. Give away poisonous house plants. Some people will eat chips of loose paint from walls or furniture. This could be dangerous if the paint is old and contains lead. Watch closely for any behaviour that involves putting things in the mouth.

Most accidents happen in the kitchen and the bathroom. Confused people often try to turn on the cooker but forget they have done so, or try to cook but put empty pans on a hot burner. *This is a serious fire hazard*. You must watch for this and intervene immediately. People left alone at home or those who get up at night are especially at risk.

You may be able to take the knobs off the cooker so that the disabled person cannot operate it. If your cooker is electric, you can have a switch installed behind it so that when the switch is off the burners will not operate. You can remove the fuse when you are not using the cooker.

If you have a gas cooker, ask the gas board to assist you in making the cooker safe. Depending on the cooker and your house, there are several steps you can take.

Confused people often spill water on the kitchen or bathroom floor and forget to wipe it up. It is easy to slip and fall on a wet spot, so watch for this and keep the floor dry. Perhaps you will want to give up polishing the floor. Polishing is work for you and makes the floor slippery. You could also put carpet down on these floors to avoid the person slipping.

Handrails and grab rails should be installed in the bathroom (see page 85). They may be supplied by local authority Social Services and following an assessment by a Community Occupational Therapist, are then installed by the local authority technician. Alternatively, they can be purchased at various hardware shops and chemists (the Disabled Living Foundation Information Service can give addresses of vendors). It is important to try to get expert advice on your requirements before purchasing. An occupational therapist or physiotherapist can help and you should ask your GP for a referral. Put a non-slip mat in the bath or shower. It is sometimes helpful to replace the bath mat with carpeting.

Outdoors

Both adults and children can easily put a hand through the sheet glass in a front or outside door. These doors should be covered with a protective grille. Sliding glass patio doors should be well marked with stick-on indicators.

Check to see if a confused person might fall off a verandah or balcony. If there are steps, paint them in bright, contrasting colours, attach outdoor non-slip tape to the edges and install a handrail.

Check for uneven ground, cracked paving, holes in the lawn, fallen branches, thorny bushes or molehills that the person can trip over.

Take down the clothes line so the person will not run into it.

Make sure the charcoals have cooled on an outside barbecue. If you have a gas barbecue, be sure the confused person cannot operate it.

Lock up garden tools.

Check garden furniture to be sure it is stable, will not tip or collapse, and has no splinters or chipped paint.

Fence in or dispose of poisonous plants.

Outdoor swimming pools are very dangerous. If you have one, be sure it is securely fenced and locked so that the person cannot reach it. Even if he has always been a good swimmer, a confused person may lose his judgement or his ability to handle himself in the water.

In the car

Problems with driving are discussed in Chapter 4. Never leave a confused person alone in a car. He may wander away, fiddle with the ignition, release the hand brake, be harassed by strangers or run down the battery by using the lights. Automatic windows are dangerous for confused people and for children, who may close a window on their head or arm.

Occasionally, a confused person will open the car door and attempt to get out while the car is moving. Locking the door may help. If this continues to be a problem, a third person may need to drive while you keep the impaired person calm. In some cases you can unscrew and remove the knobs on the door locks so that the person cannot unlock the door while you are driving. Alternatively, child-proof locks can be fitted.

Smoking

If the person smokes, the time will come when he puts down lighted cigarettes and forgets them. *This is a serious hazard.* If it occurs, you must intervene. Try to discourage smoking. Many families have taken cigarettes away completely from a patient. Things may be difficult for a few days or weeks, but much easier in the long run.

Other families allow the impaired person to smoke only under their supervision. All smoking materials and matches must be kept out of reach of the forgetful person. (The person who has cigarettes but no matches may use the cooker to light his cigarette and leave the cooker on.)

Main roads and car parks

Main roads are dangerous. If you think the confused person may be walking along a main road, notify the police immediately. They do not mind being alerted unnecessarily. This is much better than not alerting them and having to deal with a tragedy later.

People driving in large car parks often assume that pedestrians will get out of their way. People with dementia may not be aware of cars approaching, or may move slowly. Be especially alert to entrances into enclosed garages. These often put pedestrians directly into the paths of cars.

Nutrition and mealtimes

Good nutrition is important both to you and the chronically ill person. If you are not eating well, you will be more tense and more easily upset. It is not known to what extent a proper diet affects the progress of dementing diseases, but we do know that forgetful people often fail to eat properly and they can suffer nutritional deficiencies as a result. Sometimes this can make symptoms worse. It is important that you and your dependant have a balanced diet and for detailed advice you should consult your GP or health visitor. Generally, however, you should try and have as much variety as possible in your diet and not eat too much of any one thing. There are no foods which you *must* have, and it is best to have several small meals rather than one or two large ones over a day. If your doctor has recommended a special diet for managing other diseases like diabetes or heart disease, it is important to find out from him what foods you should eat in order to maintain a balanced diet. He can refer you to a dietician who can help you plan a special diet. Dieticians run outpatient clinics in most large hospitals and may also conduct clinics in some health centres.

There is no known link between nutrition and Alzheimer's disease and there are no special diets that have been proved to help memory problems.

Meal preparation

When you must prepare meals on top of all your other responsibilities, you may find yourself taking short cuts such as making just a cup of coffee and some toast for yourself and the confused person. If preparing meals is a job you had to take on for the first time when your spouse or relative became ill, you may not know how to serve good nutritious meals quickly and easily, and you may not want to learn to cook. There are several alternatives. We suggest you plan a variety of ways to eat good meals with a minimum of effort. Lunch clubs and meals-on-wheels services exist in most areas. Both provide one hot, nutritious meal a day. You can find out what meal services are available by calling your local Social Services Department or voluntary agency, such as Age Concern. Meals-on-wheels services bring a meal to your home whereas lunch clubs provide lunch and sometimes recreation facilities in the company of other retired people at a community centre. Transport may sometimes be provided.

Some restaurants will prepare takeaway meals if requested. This is useful when a person can no longer eat in public.

There are numerous inexpensive cookery books on the market that explain the basic steps involved in easy meal preparation. Some are in large print. An experienced housewife can show you how to prepare quick, easy meals. Your health visitor may make some suggestions on budgeting, shopping, meal planning and nutrition, and she can also help you understand and arrange menus for someone with a special diet.

Use tinned and frozen snack meals only as an emergency back-up. They are not an adequate regular diet. They are low in vitamins, high in salt and lack the roughage older people need to prevent constipation.

Problem eating behaviours

It may help to leave a meal prepared for someone who will be on their own, leaving them a note about what meal it is and when to eat it. Wide necked Thermos flasks can be bought for hot meals. Forgetful people who are still eating some meals alone may forget to eat, even if you leave food where it can be seen clearly. They may hide food, throw it away or eat it after it has spoiled. These are signals that the person can no longer manage alone and that you must make new arrangements. You may cope for a time by telephoning at midday to remind him to eat lunch now, but this is only a short-term solution. Confused people who live alone are frequently malnourished. Even when they appear overweight, they may not be eating the proper foods. A poor diet can worsen their confusion.

Check that dentures are tight fitting if the person uses them to eat. If they are loose, it may be safer to leave them out until they can be adjusted.

Check the temperature of foods – confused people often lack the judgement to avoid burning themselves.

People with dementing illnesses may develop rigid likes and dislikes, and refuse to eat certain foods. Such people may be more willing to eat familiar foods, prepared in familiar ways. If the person never liked a particular food, he will not like it now. New foods may confuse him. If the person insists on eating only one or two things and if all efforts at persuasion or disguising foods fail, you will need to ask the doctor about vitamins and diet supplements.

If the person has a complicating illness, such as diabetes, which requires a special diet, it may be necessary to put foods he should not eat where he cannot get them, and allow him only those foods he should have. Remember, he may lack the judgement to decide responsibly between his craving and his well-being. Since a proper diet is important to his health, you may have to be responsible for preventing him from eating foods he should not have, even if he vigorously objects. A locksmith can put a lock on the refrigerator door if necessary. But before you invest in locks, ask yourself whether the foods you wish to lock away are really necessary.

Mealtimes

Many of the problems that arise at mealtimes involve catastrophic reactions. Make mealtimes as regular as possible, with as little confusion as you can arrange. This will help prevent catastrophic reactions. Fussy or messy eaters do better when things are calm.

Seat the person comfortably, as close to a normal eating position as possible. Be sure that possible distractions (such as a television or needing to use the toilet) are taken care of. Some people do better with someone else at the table. Others are distracted by companions.

The dining area should be well lit so that the person can easily see his food. Use a plate that contrasts with the table mat and with the food. (For example, it is easier to see a white plate if it is on a bright blue table mat.) Avoid glass if the person has difficulty seeing it. Avoid dishes with patterns if the person is confused by this. If the person is confused by condiments (salt, pepper, sugar, etc.) on the table, remove them. If he is confused by several utensils, put out only one. Some people do better in a dining-room or a kitchen where there are many subtle clues like food smells that remind them to eat. Let the person feed himself as much as possible.

Some people are unable to decide between the foods on their plate. If so, limit the number of foods you put in front of the confused person at one time. For example, serve only his salad, then only his meat. Having to make choices is often what leads to playing with food. Don't put salt, ketchup, etc. where he can reach it if he mixes it inappropriately into his food; season his food for him. Be sure that food is cut into pieces that are small and tender enough to be eaten safely; people with dementing illnesses may forget to chew or fail to cut up meat properly, because the hands and brain no longer work together.

Messiness

If the person has problems with co-ordination, he may lose the ability to carry out tasks. When this happens, he may become a messy eater, and may use his fingers instead of cutlery or spill food. It is usually easier to adjust to this than to fight circumstances.

Use a plastic tablecloth or plastic table mats. Try a clear plastic cloth over a pretty fabric tablecloth. Buy the person an attractive smock to wear, rather than a bib, if spills are a problem. Turn the bottom up into a big pocket to catch crumbs.

Serve meals in a room where the floor can be easily cleaned. Don't scold when the person uses his fingers. Eating with his fingers will postpone the time when he needs more help from you. Serve things that are easy to pick up in bite-size pieces.

Put only the fork or spoon that the person will need at his place. Knives, forks and spoons with large, built-up handles are easier for people with poor co-ordination. You can purchase these or build up your own handle with foam rubber. A heavier fork or spoon will help remind the person that he is holding something. Forgetful people may not remember that they are holding plastic forks or they may bite off pieces of them.

In general, it is easier for a person to manage a bowl than a plate. Use sturdy plastic rather than glass or china dishes. Use dishes that are a different colour from the table mat. Glass is hard to see. To keep a plate from sliding, place a non-slip Dycem mat under the plate or attach a suction pad to the bottom of the plate. Plates with suction pads are available from chemists and are also sold for children. If neither is available, a damp washcloth under the plate will prevent it from sliding. To keep food from being pushed off a dish, a 'plate guard' can be temporarily attached to any plate. A heated plate will also be useful if he now takes a long time to eat a meal. Information about these items can be obtained from the Disabled Living Foundation Information Service and they may be bought from large chemist shops.

Some people lose the ability to judge how much liquid will fill a glass and overfill glasses. They will need your help. If a person dribbles or spills when drinking from a cup, use a feeding cup, which has a spout. Similar spill-proof cups are also sold for children. Don't fill glasses or cups to the brim. This will help prevent spilling. All these appliances may also be supplied by an occupational therapist who can be contacted through your Social Services Department.

If you spoonfeed a person, put only a small amount of food on the spoon at a time, and wait until the person swallows before giving him the next spoonful. You may have to remind him verbally to swallow.

Hoarding food

Some people save food and hide it in their room. This is a problem if it attracts insects or mice. Some people will give this up if they are frequently reassured that they can have a snack at any time. Leave a biscuit jar where they can find it and remind them where it is. Some families give the person a container with a tightly fitting lid in which to keep snacks. You may need to remind him to keep the snacks in the container. Others persuade the person to 'trade' their old, spoiled food for fresh food.

Nibbling

Sometimes the person seems to forget that he has eaten and will ask for food immediately after a meal. Sometimes people seem to want to eat all the time. Try setting out a tray of small, nutritious 'nibbles' such as small biscuits or cheese cubes. Sometimes people will take one at a time and be satisfied. If weight gain is a problem, put out carrots and celery.

Eating things that should not be eaten

People with dementing illnesses may be unable to recognise that some things are not good to eat. You may need to put out of sight foods like salt, vinegar, oil or Worcestershire sauce, a large amount of which can make a person sick. Sometimes people will eat non-food items like soap, soil in plant pots, or sponges. This probably results from damage to perception and memory. If this occurs you will need to keep these objects out of sight. Many people do not develop this problem, so we do not recommend removing these objects until a problem does occur.

Fluids

Be sure that the person takes enough fluid each day. Even mildly impaired people may forget to drink, and inadequate fluids can lead to other physical problems (see page 105).

Don't give the person a cup of tea or coffee that is too hot to drink. He will eventually lose the ability to judge temperature and will burn himself.

Puréed diet

If the person is on such a diet, use a liquidiser or food processor in which to purée normally prepared foods. This saves time and money. Home-cooked foods will be more appealing to the person than baby foods.

Drooling or respiratory problems

If the person drools or has respiratory problems, milk or citrus juice may produce more mucus and aggravate the situation. Check with your doctor to determine the cause of the problem. Then offer tea or fruit squash instead of orange juice or milk.

Not swallowing

Sometimes a person will carry food around in his mouth but not swallow it. This is due to forgetting how to chew or swallow and is an apraxia (see page 39) which is best handled by giving the person soft foods that do not require much chewing, such as chopped meats, jelly and thick liquids.

If the person does not swallow pills, crush the pill and mix it with food.

Weight loss

People with dementia lose weight for all the same reasons that other people do. Therefore, if the person loses weight, the first step is to consult his GP. Weight loss often indicates a treatable problem or a disease unrelated to the dementia. Do not assume that it signals a decline. It is important that the physician searches carefully for any contributory illness. Is the person constipated? Has the person had a new small stroke? Is the person depressed? Depression can account for weight loss even in a person who has dementia. Poorly fitting dentures, or sore teeth or gums often contribute to weight loss. Some specialists believe that weight loss is part of the disease process itself. However, others disagree. Certainly, all other possible causes should be considered.

When a person is still eating and yet losing weight, he may be pacing, agitated, or so active that he is burning up more calories than he is taking in. Offer nutritious, substantial snacks between meals and before bedtime. Some clinicians think that several such small meals and snacks help prevent this kind of weight loss.

Sometimes all that is needed to persuade a person to improve his nutritional intake is a calm, supportive environment. You may have to experiment before you find the arrangement that best encourages the person to eat. Be sure the food tastes good. Offer the person his favourite foods. Offer only one thing at a time and do not rush the person. People with dementia often eat slowly. Frequently offer snacks. Gently remind him to eat.

Eating problems often arise when people are living in care homes. Most people eat better in a small group, or at a table with one other person in a quiet room. A care home may set aside such a space in which to serve a few confused people instead of in a large, noisy dining-room. However, sometimes staff members are too rushed to coax a person to eat; a familiar family member may have better success. Homemade goodies may be more appealing than institutional food. We know of one person who responded by having her back gently stroked while she was being fed. Another reacted favourably to a low dose of medication given one hour before meals.

You may give a person who is not eating well a liquid diet supplement like Complan or BuildUp. You can purchase these from most chemists. They contain the vitamins, minerals and proteins the person needs, and come in different flavours; the person may like some better than others. Offer this beverage with a meal or as a milk drink between meals. Consult your doctor at all stages, and especially if all efforts fail and the person continues to refuse to eat.

Choking

Sometimes people with co-ordination problems begin to have trouble swallowing. If the person has difficulty changing his facial expression, he may also have trouble chewing or swallowing. When this occurs, it is important to guard against choking. Do not give the person foods that he may forget to chew thoroughly, such as small hard sweets, nuts or carrots. Soft, thick foods are less likely to cause choking. Easily handled foods include chopped meat, soft-boiled eggs, tinned fruit and yogurt. Foods can be liquidised in a blender. Seasoning will make them more appealing.

If the person has trouble swallowing, be sure that he is sitting up straight with his head slightly forward – his head should never tilt back while

he is eating. He should sit at the table in the same position as a well
person, and should remain sitting for fifteen minutes after eating.

Do not feed a person who is agitated or sleepy.

Foods like milk and cereal may cause choking. The two textures –
liquid and solid – make it hard for the person to know whether to chew
or swallow.

Some fluids are easier to swallow than others. If a person tends to
choke on fluids like water, try a thicker liquid. A community nurse can
help you cope with this problem.

First aid for choking

A nurse, the Red Cross or the St John's Ambulance Brigade can teach
you a very simple technique that can save the life of a choking person.
It takes only a few minutes to learn this simple skill. Everyone should
know how to do it.

If the person can talk, cough or breathe, *do not interfere*. If the person
cannot talk, cough or breathe (and he may point to his throat or turn
bluish), *you must help him*. If he is in a chair or standing, stand behind
him, then reach around him and lock or overlap your two hands in the
middle of his abdomen (belly) below the ribs. Pull hard and quickly
back and up (towards you). If he is lying down, turn him so he is face
up, put your two hands in the middle of his belly and push. This will
force air up through the throat and cause the food to fly out like a cork
out of a bottle. (You can practise where to put your hands, but you
should not push hard on a breathing person.)

When to consider tube feeding

People with dementia stop eating for many reasons. They may have
difficulty swallowing due to poor co-ordination, to ulcers in the oesophagus, oesophageal obstruction (narrowing) or overmedication. They
may dislike the food being offered, not recognise it as food, lose the sense
of feeling hungry or thirsty, or be sitting in an uncomfortable position.
People with dementia may stop eating when they are experiencing a
concurrent illness; they *may* resume eating when they recover. Even
severely impaired people may suffer from a depression that causes them
to stop eating. However, some people reach a point in their illness when
they are no longer able to eat or swallow. Good care, even in the last
stages, requires that a physician carefully review the person's medical

status. Then, if weight loss cannot be halted and the patient is no longer competent to continue treatment, you and the doctors are left with an ethical dilemma. Should you allow the insertion of a nasogastric (NG) tube (a tube that goes through the nose into the stomach) to feed the patient, or should you allow the insertion of a feeding tube directly into the stomach (a gastrostomy)? Or should you allow the patient to die? Legally, treatment can be given without consent in cases of urgent necessity, eg to save life. So, if in the doctors clinical judgement, some treatment is necessary to keep the patient alive and does not go beyond this, it should be acceptable. A decision not to treat, if a patient were non-competent, could take into account some evidence of the patient's wishes previously expressed. Generally, if there is little or no guidance from the patient, the doctor could reasonably argue that the burden to the patient arising from the treatment outweighs any benefits that could be achieved, taking into account the pain, suffering and likely period of survival of the patient.

It is helpful if you can talk about this issue before it arises. We discuss these ethical dilemmas on page 118. Here we shall discuss the options you have for sustaining life.

Many physicians believe that a gastrostomy tube (a tube placed through the abdominal wall directly into the stomach) is more comfortable for the patient than the more familiar nasogastric tube (a tube that goes through the nose, down the oesophagus and into the stomach). Patients are less likely to pull gastrostomy tubes out and these tubes need to be changed less often. New surgical procedures make inserting them safe and easy. However, these tubes do require a surgical opening through the abdomen and this may present a slightly higher risk to the patient. If the person has dementia, someone will be required to sign a consent form for this procedure. Nasogastric tubes are now quite thin and less uncomfortable than they once were. New machines are available which can continuously feed a person through this tube. They, too, carry some risks. They may cause irritation and bleeding in the nose, throat, or oesophagus or become dislodged.

People with dementia often try, and sometimes succeed, in pulling out nasogastric tubes. It is not known whether this is because they find the tube uncomfortable or because they know that it does not belong there. It may happen because they are restless. People who pull out their tubes may have to have their hands restrained, so adding to their discomfort.

It is important to discuss all aspects of the decision to insert a feeding tube with the physician who knows the patient well. A visiting nurse can show you how to manage either kind of tube at home.

Doctors know very little about the experience of a person with dementia who cannot eat and is not tube fed. There is not enough information to balance the discomfort of a tube against the discomfort of not using tube feedings. While some people believe that a person this seriously ill is comfortable without nourishment and water, others disagree. If kidneys or other organs stop functioning, the person may be more uncomfortable when food and water are forced. Also, knowledge gained from people dying from other causes may not apply to people with dementia. In the end, you and your family must take the decision you feel most comfortable with. If the person has previously written down or stated his preference, this may help guide your decision, but ultimately, in reality, it is likely to be the family member, or whoever holds the power of attorney or guardianship, who makes the decision.

Exercise

Remaining physically fit is an important part of good health. We do not know the precise role that exercise plays in good health, but we do know that it is important both for you and the confused person to get enough exercise. Perhaps exercise will refresh you after the daily burdens of caring for a chronically ill person. The precise relationship between tension and exercise is unclear, but many people who lead intense, demanding lives are convinced that physical exercise enables them to handle pressure more effectively.

Dementia is not caused by inadequate circulation. Therefore, improving circulation with exercise does not prevent or reverse memory disorders, but it does have other useful effects.

Some practitioners have observed that people with dementing illnesses who exercise regularly seem to be calmer. Some have observed that motor skills seem to be retained longer if they are used regularly. Exercise is a good way to keep an impaired person involved in activities, since it may be easier for him to use his body than to think and remember. Perhaps of most importance to you is the fact that sufficient exercise seems to help confused people sleep at night, and it helps to keep their bowel movements regular.

You may have to exercise with the impaired person. The kind of exercise you do depends on what you and the impaired person enjoy. There is no point in adding an odious exercise programme to your life. Consider what the person did before he became ill and find ways to modify that activity so that it can continue. Sometimes exercise can also be a time for you and the impaired person to be close and affectionate without having to talk.

How much exercise can an older person safely do? If you or the impaired person has high blood pressure or a heart condition, check with the doctor before you do anything. If both of you can easily walk around the house, climb steps and shop for groceries, you can cope with moderate exercise. Always start a new activity gradually and build up slowly. If exercise causes either of you stiffness, pain, or swelling, do less of it or change to a gentler activity. Check the person's feet for blisters or bruises if you begin walking.

Simple exercise

Walking is excellent exercise. Try to take the person outside for a short walk in all but the worst weather. The movement and the fresh air may help him sleep better. If the weather is too wet or cold, drive to the shops. Make a game of 'window shopping'. Ensure both of you are wearing comfortable, low-heeled shoes and soft, absorbent cotton socks. You can gradually build up the distance you walk, but avoid steep hills. It may be easier for a forgetful person to walk the same route each day. Point out scenery, people, smells, etc. as you walk.

Dancing is good exercise. If the person enjoyed dancing before he became ill, encourage some sort of movement to music.

Confused people often enjoy doing movement to music as part of a group, for example in a day care setting. If you are doing exercises in a group or at home, encourage the person to imitate your actions. If he has trouble with specific movements, try gently helping him move.

If the person is able to keep his balance, standing exercises are better than those done sitting in a chair. However, if balance is a problem, do the same exercises from a chair.

If the person played golf or tennis, he may be able to exercise by hitting the ball around long after he has become unable to play a real game.

Even people who are confined to bed can exercise. However, exercises for seriously chronically ill patients must be planned by a doctor or physiotherapist so that they do not aggravate other conditions and are not dangerous to a person who has poor co-ordination or poor balance. You should check with your GP.

Lessons in recreational graded movement with music by specially trained leaders are given by EXTEND (Exercise Training for the Elderly and Disabled) who can be contacted at 22 Maltings Drive, Wheathampstead, Herts AL4 8QJ (tel: 01582 832760). Exercise should be done at the same time each day, in a quiet, orderly way, so it does not create confusion that would add to the person's agitation. Follow the same sequence of exercises, starting from the head and working your way down toward the feet. Make the exercises fun and encourage the person to remember them. If the person has a catastrophic reaction, stop and try again later.

The impaired person may have other physical problems that interfere with his ability to exercise. You should notify your doctor of any new physical problems and of marked changes in existing ones.

When a person has been unwell or inactive, he may become weak and tire more easily. He may get stiff joints. Regular, gentle exercise can help keep his joints and his muscles in a healthy condition. When stiffness or weakness is caused by other diseases such as arthritis or by injury, a doctor, physiotherapist or occupational therapist can plan an exercise programme that may help prevent further stiffness or weakness. There is usually a physiotherapist attached to a hospital from whom you can seek advice. However, if your relative is not attending such a unit, your GP can arrange for a physiotherapist to call and see you in your home.

Recreation

Recreation, having fun and enjoying life are important for everyone. A dementing illness does not mean an end to enjoying life. It may mean, however, that you will need to make a special effort to find things that give pleasure to the impaired person.

As the person's illness progresses, it may become more difficult to find things he can still enjoy. In reality, you may already be doing as much as you can, and adding an 'activity' programme may further exhaust you and add to the stress in the household. Instead, look for things that both of you will enjoy. Perhaps something as simple as taking a walk or playing with the dog will be relaxing for both of you.

Consider arranging for the person to attend a day care centre specialising in the needs of the elderly mentally frail, or organising a sitting service within the home. The sheltered social setting of a day care centre may provide just the right balance of stimulation and security. If they are able to adjust to the new setting, people with dementia enjoy the camaraderie with other people who are also confused. Some respite care schemes provide trained staff to care for the person in his own home. Some schemes offer occupational and recreational therapists. These professionals can help you plan exercises or activities that the person will enjoy. Both home visiting and day care schemes offer social activities and opportunities for success and fun. If at all possible, involve the person in such a programme.

People with dementia often lose the ability to entertain themselves. For some, idleness leads to pacing or other repetitive behaviours. The person may resist your suggestions of things to do. Frequently, this is because he does not understand what you are suggesting. Try beginning an activity and then inviting him to join you. Select simple, adult activities rather than childish games, and those designed to be fun rather than purely 'therapeutic'. Look out for activities that a person will enjoy and that he will succeed at (like sanding wood, playing with a child).

The amount of activity a person can tolerate varies widely. Plan activity when the person is rested; help whenever the person becomes anxious or irritable, and break the activity down into simple steps.

Previously enjoyed activities may remain important and enjoyable even for seriously impaired people. However, the things the person used to enjoy, such as hobbies, guests, or going out to dinner, can become too complicated to be fun for someone who is easily confused. These must be replaced by simpler joys, although it can be hard for family members to understand that simple things can now give just as much pleasure.

Music is a delightful resource for many confused people. Sometimes a severely impaired person seems to retain a capacity to enjoy old, familiar songs. He may be able to use a simple cassette player or radio with large controls. Severely impaired people are sometimes still able to play the piano or sing if they learned this skill earlier.

Some memory-impaired people enjoy television. Others get upset when they cannot follow the storyline of a programme. The quick shifts from one scene to another precipitate catastrophic reactions in some people.

Most confused people enjoy seeing old friends, although sometimes visitors upset them. If this happens, try inviting only one or two people at a time, instead of a group. It is often the confusion of several people at once that is upsetting. Ask visitors to stay for shorter periods, and explain to them the reason for the person's forgetfulness and other abnormal behaviour.

Some families enjoy going out to dinner, and many people with dementing illnesses retain their social graces. Others, however, cause embarrassment with their messy eating. It is helpful to order for the confused person and select simple foods that can be eaten neatly. Remove unnecessary glasses and cutlery. Some families have found that it helps to explain discreetly to the waiter or waitress that the person is confused and cannot order for himself.

Consider the hobbies and interests the person pursued before he became ill, and look for ways he can still enjoy these. Often, people who liked to read a newspaper will continue to want to do so as part of their daily routine even if they cannot retain the information or make sense of the text. They might also continue to enjoy leafing through magazines or books. Sometimes a person puts away a hobby or interest and refuses to pick it up again. This often happens with something a person had done well and can no longer do as effectively. It can seem degrading to encourage a person to do a simplified version of a once fine skill unless he particularly enjoys it. It may be better to find new kinds of recreation.

Everyone enjoys experiencing things through his senses. You probably enjoy watching a brilliant sunset, smelling a flower, or tasting your favourite food. People with dementia are often more isolated and may not be able to seek out experiences to stimulate their senses. Try pointing out a pretty picture, a bird singing, a familiar smell or taste. Remember the sense of touch. The person may enjoy stroking a furry animal, touching a smooth piece of wood or putting his hand under running water. Like you, the person will enjoy certain sensations more than others.

Many families have found that confused people enjoy a ride in the car.

If the person has always enjoyed animals, he may respond with delight to pets. Some cats and dogs seem to have an instinctive way with mentally confused people.

Some individuals enjoy a stuffed animal or doll. A stuffed toy can be either childish and demeaning or comforting; much depends on the attitude of the people around the confused person.

As the dementing illness continues and the person develops trouble with co-ordination and language, it is easy to forget his need to experience pleasant things and to enjoy himself.

Never overlook the importance of holding hands, touching, hugging and loving. Often when there is no other way we can find to communicate with a person, he will respond to touching. Touch is an important part of human communication. You may enjoy just sitting and holding hands. It's a good way to share some time when talking has become difficult or impossible.

Satisfying activity

Much of what a well person does during the day has a purpose that gives meaning and importance to life. We work to make money, to serve others, to feel important. We may knit a sweater for a grandchild or bake a cake for a friend. We wash our hair and clothes so we will look nice and be clean. Such purposeful activities are important to us – they make us feel useful and needed.

When the person with a dementing illness is unable to continue with his usual activities, you need to help him find things to do that are meaningful and still within his capabilities. Such tasks should be meaningful and satisfying to him – whether or not they seem so to you. For example, folding and refolding towels might have meaning for some people but not for others. Seeing themselves as 'volunteers' rather than 'patients' is important to some people. This provides both a sense of worth and the benefit of participation. A man may be able to dig the garden for you and for the neighbours. A woman may be able to peel the vegetables or set the table when she is no longer able to prepare a complete meal. Confused people can wind a ball of wool, dust or stack magazines while you do the housework. Encourage the person to do as much as he can for himself, although you can simplify the tasks for him.

Personal hygiene

The amount of help a person with a dementing illness needs in personal care varies with the extent of his brain damage. The person with Alzheimer's disease will be able to care for himself in the early stages of the disease, but may gradually begin to neglect himself and will eventually need total help.

Problems often arise when persuading a person to change his clothes or take a bath. 'I've already changed,' the person may tell you, or he may turn the tables and make it sound as if you are wrong to suggest such a thing.

A daughter says, 'I can't get her to change her clothes. She has had the same clothes on for a week. She sleeps in them. When I tell her to change, she says she has already done so or she yells at me, "Who do you think you are, telling me when to change my clothes?"'

A husband relates, 'She screams for help the whole time I am bathing her. She'll open the windows and yell, "Help, I'm being robbed."'

A person with a dementing illness may become depressed or apathetic and lose any desire to keep clean. He may be losing the ability to remember how much time has passed: it doesn't seem like a week since he changed his clothes. To have someone telling him he needs to change his clothes may embarrass him. (If someone came up to you and told you that you should change your clothes, you might well become indignant.)

Dressing and bathing are personal activities. We each have our own individual way of doing things. Some of us take showers, some take baths, some of us bathe in the morning, some bathe at night. Some of us change clothes twice a day, some every other day, but each of us is quite set in our way of doing things. Sometimes when a family member begins to help the demented person, he inadvertently overlooks these established habits. The change in routine can be upsetting to the confused person. A generation ago, people often did not wash and change as often as we do today. A bath once a week may have been the routine during the person's childhood.

We begin to wash and dress ourselves as small children. It is a basic indication of our independence. Moreover, bathing and dressing are private activities. Many people have never completely bathed and dressed in front of anyone else. Having other people's hands and eyes on our naked, ageing, not-so-beautiful body is an acutely uncomfortable experience. When we offer to help with something a person has always done for himself – something people do for themselves in private – it is an admission that this person is no longer able to manage for himself, that he has, in fact, become like a child who must have help and be told when to dress.

Changing clothes and bathing involve making many decisions. A man must choose from several shirts, ties and pairs of socks to put together a co-ordinated outfit. When he begins to realise he can't do this, when looking at a drawer full of blue, green and black socks becomes over-whelmingly confusing, it can be easier not to change at all.

Such factors as these often precipitate catastrophic reactions. You are still faced, however, with the problem of keeping this person clean. Begin by trying to understand the person's feelings and his need for privacy and independence. Realise that his behaviour is a product of his brain impairment, and is not deliberately offensive. Look for ways of simplify-ing the number of decisions involved in bathing and dressing without taking away his independence.

Bathing

When a person refuses to take a bath, part of the problem may be that the business of bathing has become too confusing and complicated. Try to follow as many of the person's old routines as possible while you encourage him to have a bath, and at the same time simplify the job for him. If a man has always shaved first, then washed, then eaten breakfast, he is most likely to co-operate with your request if you keep to this system.

Be calm and gentle when you help with a bath and avoid discussions about whether a bath is needed. Instead, tell the person one step at a time what to do in preparation for the bath.

Avoid: 'Dad, I want you to take a bath right after breakfast.' ('Right after breakfast' means he has to remember something.)

Avoid: 'I don't need a bath.'
    'Oh, yes you do. You haven't had a bath for a week.' (You would not like him saying that to you, especially if you couldn't remember when you last had a bath.)

Try: 'Dad, your bath water is ready.'
    'I don't need a bath.'
    'Here is your towel. Now, unbutton your shirt.' (His mind may focus on the buttons instead of on the argument. You can gently help him if you see him having difficulty.)

'Now stand up. Undo your trousers, Dad.'
'I don't need a bath.'
'Now step into the bath.'

One daughter drew her father's bath, got everything ready, and then, when he wandered down the landing, said, 'Oh, look at this lovely bath water. As long as it is here, why not take a bath? It would be terrible to waste it.' Her father, who had always been rather penny pinching, yielded. In another case, a wife told her husband, 'As soon as your bath is over, you and I will eat those cakes Janie brought.'

Some families have found that the confused person will let an aide in uniform or another family member bathe him. If all else fails, give partial baths or sponge baths. Watch the person's skin for rashes or red areas.

If the bath becomes a regular routine, done the same way at the same time each day, the person is more likely to expect this and may put up less resistance. If bathing continues to be difficult, it is not necessary for the person to have a bath every day.

Always check the temperature of the bath or shower water, even if the person has been successfully doing this for himself. The ability to gauge safe temperatures can be lost quite suddenly. Avoid using bubble bath or bath oils that can make the bath slippery. These can also contribute to vaginal infections in women.

Showers are more dangerous than baths because the unsteady person may fall. If you must use a shower, install grab rails or use a bath seat. There are several inexpensive appliances that you can borrow or purchase (such as a free-standing or wall-hinged seat) that make bathing much safer and easier (see page 174). These appliances can also be supplied by a community occupational therapist who can be contacted through your local Social Services Department. Many districts are developing joint loan services which means that some equipment can also be obtained through the Community Health Services Unit via the district nurse. Many families have told us that a bath seat and a hand-held shower hose greatly reduces the bathtime crisis. You have control of the water (and the mess). The seat is safer and the controlled flow of water is less upsetting to the confused person.

It can be difficult to get a person in and out of a bath, especially if he is clumsy or heavy. An unsteady person can slip and fall while stepping over the side.

Never leave the person alone in the bath. Use only two or three inches of water. This helps the person feel more secure, and is safer in case he slips. Put a slip resistant bathmat on the bottom of the bath. People can often continue to wash themselves if you gently remind them one step at a time of each area to be washed.

Sometimes it is embarrassing for a family member to see that the genital area is thoroughly washed, but rashes can develop, so ensure that this is done. Be sure that you or the confused person has washed in folds of flesh and under breasts.

Provide a non-slip bathmat for the person to step out onto, and be sure there are no puddles on the floor. It may be helpful to replace bathmats with washable and absorbent non-slip bathroom carpeting. If the person still dries himself, check that no areas are forgotten. If you dry the person, be sure he is completely dry. Use talcum powder or baby powder under women's breasts, and in creases and folds of skin. It is essential that excess powder is removed to prevent clogging of the skin pores, as this may lead to increased irritation.

While the person is undressed, check for red areas of skin, rashes, or sores. If any red areas or sores appear, ask your doctor or community nurse to help you manage them. Pressure sores or decubitus ulcers develop quickly on people who sit or lie down much of the time. Use body lotion on dry skin. Unscented lotions are available for men.

Dressing

If all of the person's clothes are co-ordinated, he doesn't have to decide what goes with what.

Hang shirts or dresses together with their matching ties, scarves or accessories. Eliminate any belts, scarves, sweaters, ties, etc. that are likely to be put on incorrectly.

Laying out clothes in the order in which the person puts them on may also help to avoid confusion.

Put away clothes which are inappropriate for the time of year, or items which are rarely worn, so they do not involve the person in making extra decisions. If the person refuses to change his clothes, avoid getting into an argument. Make the suggestion again later.

As the disease progresses, it becomes difficult for a person to put on clothes the right way round and in the right sequence. Buttons, zips, shoe laces and belt buckles become impossible to manage. If the person can no longer manage buttons, replace them with Velcro tape, which you can purchase in a fabric shop. One wife, sensitive to her husband's need to continue to dress himself independently, bought him clothes that were reversible. She bought attractive T-shirts (which don't have buttons and which don't look too strange if they are worn back to front), trousers with elastic waistbands and seamless socks. (Such socks don't have heels, so it takes less skill to put them on.) Slip-on shoes are easier than shoes with laces or ties.

Women can look pretty in reversible, slip-on blouses and reversible, wrap-around or elastic-waistband skirts or trousers. Loose-fitting clothing is easier to manage.

Select clothing that is washable and that doesn't need ironing; there is no reason to add to your workload.

Sometimes bright, 'busy' patterns confuse and distract the impaired person. Try simpler patterns and pastel colours. Select colours with considerable contrast; these are easier for older people to distinguish.

Women's underwear is difficult for a confused person to manage, and a mystery to many husbands. Buy soft, loose-fitting pants. It won't matter if they are on back to front or inside out. Don't bother with a slip; it is not necessary. If you must put a bra on a woman, ask her to lean forward to settle her breasts in the cups. Tights are difficult to put on but stockings may be easier. Unfortunately pop-socks are bad for people with poor circulation. Warm slippers may be best to wear at home.

Grooming

Have the person's hair cut in an attractive, short style that is easy to wash and care for. Avoid a style that requires setting. People who have always gone to the hairdresser's or barber's shop may still enjoy doing so. If this is too upsetting an experience, such help may be available at the day care centre or it may be possible to arrange for a hairdresser or barber to visit your home.

It may be safer (and easier on your back) to wash hair in the kitchen sink rather than the bath, unless you have a shower attachment. Invest in a hose attachment for the sink. Be sure you rinse hair well. It should squeak when rubbed through your fingers.

You will need to trim fingernails and toenails or check that the person can still do this. Toenails can curl back against the toes and be quite painful. If there are difficulties, you should contact the community health service to find out about a chiropody clinic. Sometimes it is possible to obtain a visit to your own home if this becomes necessary. Do not undertake more than simple nail cutting without consulting your doctor.

Encourage the person to get dressed and to look nice. Moping around in a dressing-gown will not help his morale. If a woman has always worn make-up, it may be good for her to continue to do so. It is not difficult for a husband to apply powder and lipstick to his wife. Use pastel colours and a light touch on an older woman. Don't bother with eye make-up.

When bathing and dressing are finished, encourage the person to look in the mirror and see how nice he looks (even if you are exhausted and exasperated). Ask the rest of the family to compliment him also. Praise and encouragement are important in helping him continue to feel good about himself, even when a task he has always been able to do, such as dressing, has become too much for him.

Oral hygiene

With all the other tasks of caring for a chronically ill person it is easy to forget what we can't see, but good oral hygiene is important for the person's comfort and for his health. A person who appears to be able to care for himself in other ways may, in fact, be forgetting to care for his teeth or dentures.

Dentures are particularly troublesome. If they don't fit correctly, they interfere with chewing. The natural response is to stop eating those things one can't chew. This can lead to inadequate nutrition or constipation. Dentures should be in place when a person is eating. If they don't fit properly or are uncomfortable, insist that the dentist alters them. If a person forgets to take out his dentures and clean them, or if he refuses to let you do it, he can develop painful sores on his gums which also interfere with eating a proper diet.

Since you want the person to be as independent as possible, you can assume the responsibility of remembering about oral hygiene, but you should let the person do as much of the actual care as possible. One reason people stop caring for their teeth or dentures is that these are actually complicated tasks, involving many steps, and they become confused about what to do next. You can help by breaking down the job into simple stages and reminding the person one step at a time. If you take over the care of the person's dentures, you must remove them daily, clean them and check the gums for irritation. The dentist can show you how to do this. If the person has his own teeth, you may have to brush them for him and check the mouth for sores.

Some dentists recommend foam applicators instead of brushes for cleaning teeth. You can clean the teeth more gently with these. If the person will not unclench his teeth, try to clean the outside of the teeth.

Make oral care a part of a regular, expected routine and do it calmly; you will experience less resistance. Select a time of day when the person is most co-operative. If the person does get upset, stop and try again later.

Healthy teeth or properly fitting dentures are critically important. People with dementing illnesses tend not to chew well and to choke easily. Poor teeth increase this risk. Even mild nutritional problems caused by sore teeth can increase the person's confusion or cause constipation.

Bathroom supplies

Your local Social Services Department can provide a variety of bathroom aids which are also stocked by larger chemists, and which make the bathroom safer and easier for the impaired person.

A raised seat can help an impaired person get on and off the toilet. The seat should fasten securely to the toilet so it does not slip when the person sits on it. Padded (soft) toilet seats are more comfortable for the person who must sit for some time. This is especially important for the person who develops pressure sores easily.

You can borrow a portable commode from the Community Health Service which is usually supplied by a district nurse or health visitor. You can also borrow portable commodes from your local Social Services Department, or from the Red Cross for short-term use, or buy them from various suppliers. (Information on these is available from the Disabled Living Foundation Information Service.) A commode can be placed near a person's bed or on the ground floor, so that the person does not have to climb stairs. Urinals and bedpans are available to meet a variety of needs. If possible, discuss your specific problem with an occupational therapist so that she can help you select the appliance that is best for you.

Grab rails are important. There are rails that help a person lift himself on and off the toilet, and rails that he can grasp as he gets in and out of the bath. You can buy rails that attach to the wall, that are free standing or that clamp onto the bath. The latter are helpful if you are renting your home and are unable to drill holes in walls. You can also obtain grab rails from Social Services (and the Social Services technician will install those supplied), or, if you are buying the grab rails, a local carpenter or builder can install them.

In many homes, towel rails and the handle on the soap dish are glued to the wall or fastened only onto the plaster board. They may come loose if a person grabs them for balance or to lift himself up. Ask someone knowledgeable about carpentry to ensure that the fixtures in question are designed to withstand pressure and are anchored into a structural feature of the wall. A seat for the shower or bath can be purchased or supplied by Social Services. Bath seats or bath boards may also be supplied through the Community Health Services Unit. An aid of this kind often makes a person feel more secure, because it raises him so that he can get in and out of the bath more easily and so that you can reach him without so much bending and stretching. Shower hose attachments are helpful for rinsing the person thoroughly and they make washing hair much easier.

Grab rails, bath seats and shower hoses may be supplied by your local Social Services or can be purchased from department stores and various manufacturers (consult the Disabled Living Foundation Information

Service Department). They come in a variety of designs to fit different bathrooms and to meet different needs. If you are seeking equipment from your local Social Services Department, there will be an initial assessment by an occupational therapist. However, in some areas, Social Services are tending to target their resources on people who have a high dependency and who need aids on a long-term basis. Moderate and low dependency category patients may be assessed but may have to purchase their own equipment.

Incontinence (wetting or soiling)

People with dementing illnesses may begin to wet themselves or have their bowel movements in their clothing. This is called, respectively, urinary incontinence and bowel or faecal incontinence. The two are really separate problems, and one often occurs without the other. There are many causes of incontinence, so it is important to begin by assessing the problem.

Urinating and moving one's bowels are natural human functions. However, as children we are taught that these are private activities. Many of us are also taught that they are nasty, dirty, or socially unacceptable. In addition, we associate caring for our own bodily functions in private with independence and personal dignity. When another person has to help us, it is distressing for both the helper and the disabled person. Often, too, people find urine or bowel movements disgusting and may feel sick when cleaning up. It is important for both family members and professional care-givers to be aware of their own strong feelings in these areas.

Urinary incontinence

Urinary incontinence has many causes, some of which respond well to treatment. Ask yourself the following questions:

● If the person is a woman, does she leak, especially when she laughs, coughs, lifts something, or makes some other sudden exertion?
● Do accidents happen only at certain times of a day, such as at night? (It is helpful to keep a diary for several days of the times accidents occur, the times the person successfully uses the toilet, and the times the person eats or drinks.)
● How often does the person urinate?

- Is the urination painful?
- Did the incontinence begin suddenly?
- Has the person's confusion suddenly become worse?
- Does the incontinence occur occasionally or intermittently?
- Is the person living in a new place?
- Is the person urinating in improper places, such as in cupboards or in flower pots? (This is different from the person who wets himself and his clothing wherever he happens to be.)
- Do accidents happen when the person cannot get to the bathroom on time?
- Are they happening on the way to the bathroom?

Whenever incontinence begins, it is important to consult the doctor. You can help him diagnose the problems by giving him answers to these questions. If the person has a fever, report this to the doctor at once. Do not let a physician dismiss incontinence without carefully exploring all treatable causes.

Incontinence may be brought on by either chronic or acute bladder infections, uncontrolled diabetes, severe constipation, faecal impaction, an enlarged prostate, dehydration, medication, or many other medical problems (see Chapter 6: 'Medical problems'). A leakage can be caused by weakening muscles and other conditions that arc potentially treatable.

'Common sense' might suggest that taking less fluid would reduce incontinence, but this can be dangerous, because it can lead to dehydration. A first step in addressing incontinence is to ensure that the person is taking enough fluid to adequately stimulate the bladder to work. Both too little and too much fluid can be bad. It may be helpful to consider the pattern of fluid intake and to take small regular amounts rather than sudden large volumes. This puts less stress on the bladder. If you are uncertain how much fluid the person should take, ask your doctor or nurse. A doctor or nurse can also determine if the person is dehydrated.

If the problem is that the person who moves slowly, or uses a walking aid, or who is clumsy, cannot get to the bathroom in time, you can bring the toilet closer to the person. For example, if a person must go upstairs to the toilet, buying or borrowing a commode for the ground floor may solve the problem. You can invest in a portable urinal that will help when you travel. You can also simplify clothing so the person can manipulate it faster. Try Velcro tape instead of zips or buttons. Consider extending the fly opening and using an elasticated waistband rather than belts and buttons to hold up trousers. Can the person easily get up out of his chair? If he is sunk into a deep chair, he may not be able to get up in time.

Sometimes people cannot find the bathroom. This often happens in a new setting. A clear sign or a brightly painted door may help. People who urinate in wastepaper baskets, cupboards and flowerpots may be unable to locate the bathroom or unable to remember the appropriate place. Some families find that putting a lid on the wastepaper basket, locking cupboard doors and toileting the person regularly help. Remember that older people may have been taught as children to urinate outdoors or in a chamber pot by the bed. If so, it may be easier to supply them with a pot than to clean up the wastepaper basket.

Purchase washable chair cushion covers. Slide them on over a large rubbish bag in order to waterproof cushions. If you have a favourite chair or rug that you are afraid will be damaged, take the easy way out and put it where the person will not use it.

Sometimes people need help and are either unable to ask for it or embarrassed to ask for it. People may have used children's words such as 'wee wees', 'pooh pooh' or 'widdle piddle', or even obscure euphemisms such as 'go for a walk'. The person with language problems may say 'I want tea'. If the care-giver (particularly someone unfamiliar with the patient) does not understand what the person is asking for, accidents can result. Learn what the person means and be sure that sitters or other care-givers know also.

If the person is incontinent at night, limit the amount of fluid he drinks after supper unless there is some medical reason why he needs extra fluid. (During the rest of the day, ensure he is getting plenty of fluids.) Get him up once at night. It may be helpful to obtain a bedside commode he can use easily, especially if he has trouble moving around. Night lights in the bathroom and bedroom greatly help, too.

Falls often occur on the way to the bathroom at night. Make sure there are adequate lights and non-slip mats, that the person can get out of bed, and that he has slippers that are not slippery or floppy. It is highly dangerous to place polythene sheeting or newspapers on the floor next to the bed as this predisposes a person to falls. If a person has a tendency to urinate immediately they get out of bed, it is better to try to encourage them to wear pads or protective pants rather than to protect the floor.

A diary will provide you with the information you need to prevent many accidents. If you know when the person usually urinates (immediately upon awakening, about 10 am, an hour after he has his coffee), you can take him to the toilet just before an accident is due to occur. This is, in fact, training yourself to the confused person's natural routine. Many families find that they can tell when the patient needs to go to the bathroom. He may become restless or pick at his clothes. Routinely take him to the toilet every two to three hours. A regular schedule will avoid most 'accidents', reduce skin irritations and make life easier for you. If the patient has to take diuretic medication in the morning, it may be necessary to increase the frequency of toileting then until the effect of the tablet has worn off, to maintain continence. While it may be embarrassing to ask the person to go to the bathroom, this routine will save the person the humiliation of wetting himself.

Certain non-verbal signals that tell us it is time or not time to urinate may influence some impaired people. Taking down one's underpants, or opening one's fly, or sitting down on a toilet seat is a clue to 'go'. Dry clothes, and being in bed or in public are signals to 'not go'. (Some people are unable to urinate when there are 'not go' clues, such as in the presence of another person or when using a bedpan.) Taking down pants to undress a woman may cause her to urinate. You may be able to use such non-verbal clues to help a person go at the right time.

One man urinated every morning as soon as he put his feet on the floor. If this is what is happening, you may be able to be prepared and catch the urine in a urinal or bottle. Urinals for women as well as men may be available from Social Services, Community Health Services, or you may purchase these from large chemists. Use a plastic bowl for a standing woman. People may also be inhibited and unable to go when you are in the bathroom with them, or if you ask them to use a commode in a room that is not a bathroom. It is often this involuntary 'no go' response that leads families to say, 'He wouldn't go when I took him and then he wet his pants. I think he is only being difficult'.

Sometimes if a person has trouble urinating, it may help to give him a glass of water with a straw and ask him to blow bubbles. This seems to help the urine start.

Sometimes a person asks to go to the bathroom every few minutes. If this is a problem, it may be necessary to consult a urologist to determine whether there is a medical reason why the person feels he needs to urinate frequently. A urinary tract infection or other local causes can give a person this feeling. If you have ruled out medical reasons and are sure the person is completely emptying his bladder when he urinates, take him to the toilet every two to three hours and try to distract him in the interim period. The Alzheimer's Disease Society produces an advice sheet on managing incontinence.

Some doctors and nurses may still dismiss incontinence as inevitable. It is true that some people with dementia will eventually lose independent control of their functions, but many do not, and many causes of incontinence can be controlled. Even when the person has lost independent function, there is much you can do to make your workload easier and to reduce embarrassment for him. If you are having problems, ask for a referral to a nurse or physician with experience in managing incontinence in a person with dementia. You can also get advice on the telephone by calling the helplines run by either the British Association for Continence Care (tel. 0753 656716), the National Action on Incontinence (tel. 091 2130050) or the Association for Continence Advice (tel. 071-266 3704).

Faecal incontinence

Faecal incontinence, like urinary incontinence, should be discussed with the doctor. Temporary incontinence may be the result of an infection, diarrhoea or constipation (see Chapter 6: 'Medical problems').

Ensure that the bathroom is comfortable and that the person can sit without discomfort or instability long enough to move his bowels. His feet should rest on the floor and he should have something to hold onto. A bar, made from a broom handle and crossing in front of the person between two professionally installed supports, will give him something to hold and will encourage a restless person to stay put. Try giving him something to do or letting him listen to music.

Learn when the person usually moves his bowels and take him to the toilet at that time. Using a stool softener may help (see page 105). Keeping the person as mobile as possible and encouraging him to drink plenty of fluids can reduce the tendency towards developing constipation.

Avoid reprimanding the person who has accidents.

Cleaning up

A person who remains in soiled or wet clothing can quickly develop skin irritation and sores. It is important to watch for these. Keeping the skin clean and dry is really the best protection against skin problems. The skin must be washed after each accident. Unscented powder will keep the skin dry. It is essential that excess powder should be removed to prevent clogging of the pores of the skin and resulting increased irritation. It is important to ensure that powder does not enter the entrance of the penis (the urethra) because this can lead to ulceration if the patient has a catheter or sheath in place. Using a catheter as a continuing way to manage incontinence should be avoided if possible.

The personal care of an incontinent person can seem degrading for him and unpleasant or disgusting to you. Therefore, some families have made a deliberate effort to use the clean-up time as a time to express affection. This can help to make a necessary task less unpleasant.

Special clothing is available for incontinent people. Should you use it? Professionals disagree over the use of incontinence wear. Some think that incontinence pads are demoralising and encourage infantile behaviour, and may exacerbate the problem in patients who have an urgent need to pass urine. Some find that scheduled toileting is easier than managing incontinence wear. The answer lies in your own feelings about this matter and in the confused person's response. Incontinence clothing may make things easier for you and more comfortable for the confused person. However, no care home home should routinely use incontinence pads as a cost-saving exercise without estimating the impact on the individual. We believe a toileting schedule is ideal when it works, but we recognise that some people resist it and others are incontinent even when a schedule is introduced. The doctor or nurse will help you decide what is right for you.

Disposable adult nappies, pads and plastic outer pants are sold in chemists and can be obtained from firms by mail order. Some are more comfortable and effective if special stretch pants are worn over them. Some are designed so that one size fits all with a range of absorbancies; for others, size is by hip or waist measurement. The type of filler used determines how much urine the pad will absorb. Products with a 'gelling property', such as super-absorbent polymers, hold much more than fibre-filled materials. Before you buy any pads, pants or aids, check what is available from the Community Health Service. Some units will supply pads free of charge.

There are both disposable and washable garments. Some washable garments, which are usually lined with soft materials, are more accept-able to the confused person. One type consists of an outer washable part that holds a disposable pad. Many families find that totally disposable pads are better because they minimise the need for laundry. Remember that too liberal a use of barrier creams on the skin can reduce the effective absorption of urine into incontinence pads.

Garments that don't fit or that are too saturated may leak. Don't expect the garment to hold more than one urination. Pads may say how much fluid they will hold. One full bladder may empty eight to ten ounces (one cup) of urine.

If a body worn garment is not suitable (because the person will not tolerate using it or urgency is a problem) then the alternative could be to protect bedding by use of disposable, or washable and reusable, incontinence sheets. Disposable incontinence sheets may be supplied through the district nurse. You can also buy washable absorbent sheets, which will contain the urine, at large chemists or by mail order.

Use a draw sheet in bed. This is a regular sheet folded in half lengthwise and tucked in across the bed. It can be used to hold a plastic incontinence underpad in place between it. Should the patient have an accident, you have only the draw sheet and the pad to change. Absorbent bed pads used in combination with a draw sheet and rubber pad will help keep the bed dry. Follow the manufacturer's washing and drying instructions.

There may be an incontinence laundry service in your area which would save you the burden of washing bed linen and draw sheets. Enquire at your local Social Services Department about this.

It is not a good idea to use plastic pants, plastic bags, or rubber sheets that are not shielded by a layer of cloth next to the skin. They cause moistness to stay in contact with the skin and lead to irritation and rawness.

Problems in walking and balance

As the person's illness progresses, he may become stiff or awkward, and have difficulty getting out of a chair or out of bed. He may develop a stooped or leaning posture, or a shuffling walk. He will need close supervision when he is at risk of falling.

A family member writes, 'His steps are very slow now. As he walks, he often raises his feet high, for he has little sense of space. He clutches door frames or chairs. Sometimes he just grasps at the air. His gaze is unfocused, like that of a blind man. He stops in front of mirrors, and he talks and laughs with the images there.'

A wife says, 'He sometimes falls down. He trips over his own feet or just crumples up. But when I try to lift him – and he is a big man – he yells and struggles against me.'

Any of these symptoms may be caused by medication. Discuss with the doctor the onset of any change in walking, posture, stiffness, repetitive motions, or falling. He needs to be sure that there is not a treatable cause for them, such as medication, a delirium, or a small stroke. These same symptoms will occur when the dementing process has damaged the areas of the brain which control muscle movements. But do not assume this as the cause until the doctor has eliminated other causes.

Watch for the time when the person can no longer safely negotiate stairs, or when he trips or has other difficulties walking. If a person is unsteady on his feet, get him to take your arm, if he will, rather than you grasping his. Hold your arm close to your body. This maximises your ability to keep your balance. Or you may steady him by walking behind him and holding his belt.

Put away mats which may slide when the person steps on them. Install handrails, especially in the bathroom. Pad the steps with rug samples. Staple or tack down rug edges. Round off shelf corners or pad them with foam rubber scraps. Be sure that chairs or other items of furniture that the person tends to lean on are sturdy; put unstable or antique furniture away. Move things out of the way in areas where the person usually walks. Stair rails and banisters in many homes are inadequately anchored, and will come loose if a person leans on them heavily. Ask someone who is knowledgeable about carpentry to check this for you.

Some people fall when they first get out of bed. Encourage the person to sit on the edge of the bed for a few minutes before walking. Many slippers and shoes have smooth soles that can cause falls. Some people will stumble more in crêpe soled shoes. Others benefit from the grip crêpe gives. Some people can learn to use a stick or a Zimmer frame. Others cannot learn this new skill. If people cannot learn to use an appliance properly, it is safer for them not to use it.

A harness can help a person sit up in a chair if he cannot do so unassisted (see page 94). Walking frames and advice should be sought from a physiotherapist or occupational therapist.

It is important that when you help the person, you don't hurt yourself or throw yourself off balance. A physiotherapist, occupational therapist or nurse can show you ways of assisting a person without strain. Avoid leaning forward or bending over when you lift. If you must bend to lift something, bend at the knees, not at the waist. Take your time; accidents happen when you rush yourself or the confused person. If you lift a person, lift from under his arms in the armpit. Avoid pulling him up out of bed by the arms. Avoid trying to put an awkward or heavy person in the back seat of a two-door car.

When a person falls:

1 Remain calm.
2 Check to see if he is visibly injured or in pain.
3 Avoid precipitating a catastrophic reaction.
4 Watch the person for signs of pain, swelling, bruises, agitation, or increased distress, and call the doctor if these symptoms appear, or if you think there is any chance that he has hit his head or hurt himself.

Instead of trying to get her husband up, one wife trained herself to sit down on the floor with him. (Obviously it took an effort to calm her own distress.) She would pat him and chat with him gently until he calmed down. When he was relaxed she was able to encourage him to get himself up one step at a time rather than having to lift him.

Becoming chairbound or bedbound

As the disease progresses, many people gradually lose the ability to walk. This begins with occasional stumbling and falling, progresses to taking smaller and smaller steps, and develops, usually after years, into the person's being unable to stand. Eventually the person may not be able to straighten his legs to the floor when held upright by others. This is sometimes called an apraxia of gait. (See pages 39–42.)

In contrast to this gradual progression, an abrupt loss of ability to stand or walk, or the sudden onset of falling, means that the person has another illness or a medication reaction. This should be investigated promptly by a physician.

The gradual loss of the ability to walk or stand is the result of progressive brain damage; the person has forgotten how to walk. Keeping people as active as possible helps to maintain their muscle strength and general health, but there is no evidence that exercise or activity can postpone or prevent the loss of ability to walk.

Even though a person cannot walk, he may be able to sit up. Sitting in a chair much of the day enables him to continue to be part of the family or institutional life. If the person has a tendency to fall forward or out of the chair, you can prop him with pillows or use a seat belt. You can purchase one or you can make one. It is a padded belt several inches wide, which can be adjusted so that it will not be tight. It should be easy to unfasten from the back in an emergency.

An alternative is a reclining chair. The Disabled Living Foundation Information Service will give you a list of suppliers of suitable chairs if you need to purchase one. If possible, try to get independent advice from the occupational therapist before buying and give your relative an opportunity to try sitting in the chair. Most private suppliers will give a home demonstration without an obligation to buy and the Disabled Living Centre will carry a range of these chairs. When a chair is kept in the reclined position, it protects the person from falling forward. You may prop him with pillows so that he is comfortable. You may want to move the person from chair to chair to bed so that his position changes. Use pieces of 'egg crate' sculptured polyurethane foam to cushion him. The district nurse can supply special cushions such as Spenco, RoHo and Gel cushions to help prevent pressure sores. These can also be purchased through medical equipment catalogues.

Some people eventually become unable to sit. They usually have contractures – stiffened tendons that do not allow their joints to fully open or extend. Contractures may be postponed or reduced by keeping people physically active and with physiotherapy, but they can occur late in Alzheimer's disease or following a stroke, even when the person's joints are moved and exercised by others.

When patients are no longer able to move voluntarily and are confined to bed, they require almost constant physical attention. They are at high risk of developing bedsores or pressure sores (see page 103) and taking food, saliva and other substances into their lungs because they cannot swallow or are lying down.

Bedbound patients should be carefully moved from one side to the other every two hours. Your doctor may recommend more frequent turning. Care must be taken to avoid putting undue pressure or weight on any part of the body, because such patients tend to have brittle bones and fragile skin. Satin or silk sheets and pyjamas can make it easier to move someone who cannot move independently. When the person is lying on his side, he should be propped up with a pillow. A pillow or pad is sometimes necessary between the knees to prevent sores from forming. Skin must be kept clean and dry.

Moving a totally bedbound person requires skill and training. Visiting nurses and physiotherapists can be helpful in teaching you how to move and turn the person.

The district nurse or Social Services Department may also be able to supply you with a special mattress to help prevent pressure sores developing.

Wheelchairs

If the time comes when the person needs a wheelchair, the local Wheelchair Service can give guidance in selecting and using it. You can be referred to the wheelchair service by your GP. If, after assessment, it is felt that an Alzheimer's disease sufferer qualifies for a wheelchair, then this will be supplied free of charge on loan. It will also be maintained free of charge. Cushions of various types are also supplied through the Wheelchair Service. You will be shown a variety of NHS wheelchairs by the Wheelchair Service. To find out about a wider range of wheelchairs, some of which you would have to pay for, you can contact the Disabled Living Foundation Information Service or visit your Local Disability Living Centre.

Wheelchairs can be uncomfortable for people who sit in them for long periods. The seats of many chairs are hard and can cause pressure sores. Chairs that do not support the patient's body correctly can cause muscle and nerve damage as well. Sometimes a patient slumps in the chair or is left sitting with an arm hanging so that the fingers go numb.

There are different kinds of wheelchairs. A qualified person should help you select a chair that is comfortable and supports the patient. A reclining back or special attachment may be required. You will also need a chair that meets your needs in weight (can you lift it?), portability (will you need to take it in the car?) and width (will it go through your doorways?). When selecting a chair at the Wheelchair Service all these questions should be discussed and you should be shown how to help the patient in and out of the chair and how to support the person correctly. If you only require the occasional use of a wheelchair, the Red Cross may be able to loan you a chair for a limited short period.

Changes you can make at home

There are many changes you can make at home which might make life easier for you and for the confused patient. While they may help, gadgets are not the total solution. When you consider changes, ask yourself whether you can live with them comfortably. Also, remember that people who have dementing illnesses may not be able to learn even simple new tasks and sometimes cannot adjust to minor changes. You might purchase a new telephone that is easy for you to operate, only to find that the person cannot learn to use it; or you might rearrange the furniture and then realise this upsets the person more.

Some of the products we mention here are sold for other purposes and it takes a little imagination to apply them to the care of people with dementia. It is important to remember that no single suggestion will work in all situations. However, most of the items are helpful and low in cost.

Products that promote safety

These include non-slip mats (for the bath, under rugs and elsewhere), grab rails (for bath, hall, bedroom), a temperature control on the water heater, fire and smoke alarms, and shower seats. We have discussed these elsewhere in the book. Look for them in hardware and electrical shops, or large chemists. Disabled Living Centres are also able to order these units and can demonstrate them if you are able to visit their Centres.

Long-reach lighters work like cigarette lighters with long nozzles. They make lighting a gas cooker safer and mean that it is unnecessary to have matches lying around. Some people with dementia will be unable to learn how to operate them – which is another advantage.

Timers can be fitted on electric cookers so that they will operate only between certain hours and will shut off automatically.

Sound-activated switches can be used to turn on lights when you or the patient get up at night.

Gadgets that make life easier for older people

These include recliners, special cushions for thin people or those with sensitive skins, all sorts of lights (to make vision easier in, for example, the bathroom or bedroom), heating pads, magnifying glasses, amplifiers, and lights that alert people with hearing problems to sounds such as the telephone or doorbell.

Catalogues advertised in magazines that cater for older people carry many such products; but try to obtain some expert advice on your requirements before purchasing.

Tools that help people with arthritis

Many devices are available which enlarge the size of handles on cutlery, pens and pencils, and any other item that must be grasped. There are also long-reaching devices for picking up things off the floor or for reaching up to high shelves. There are several devices for opening jars.

Gadgets for telephones

Used in conjunction with a tape recorder, a 'record adapter' or 'record control' will turn on the tape recorder when the telephone is picked up and turn it off when the handset is replaced. Such a device will allow you to monitor calls the confused person is receiving or making. There are also telephones that have large numbers for people with co-ordination or vision problems; there are telephones with built-in microphones and loud speakers for people who cannot pick up the receiver. However, people with dementia may not be able to learn to use these. Electrical and specialist telephone shops should be able to advise you on a suitable unit for your needs.

Devices that alert you that the person is up at night or is going out of the door

There are many inexpensive ways to be warned that the person is opening a door or moving about. A handyman can install them. (Expensive 'wandering devices' are seldom needed.) Most of these are sold as burglar alarm devices in electrical shops and from catalogues.

Such devices can be sensitive to motion or sound (when the person approaches or is moving around); to pressure (a pressure pad beside the bed will warn you that the person is up; one by the door will alert you that he may be going out); an open or closed circuit (a pair of small magnetic switches on the door or window will activate a low-voltage buzzer); a switch recessed into the wall will also activate a buzzer when the door is opened; or light (a person passing through a light beam will trigger a buzzer).

Gadgets that turn on lights

These devices can be wired to turn on lights outside (to ward off burglars) or inside (a light going on in the bathroom may help the person find his way without you having to get up).

Gadgets that provide sound for you or him

A headset will allow you to listen to music while the person listens to the television (or vice versa). A clock radio will play soothing music at bedtime and turn itself off. Some gadgets play 'white noise', soothing background sounds that help some people fall asleep. Test them before purchasing.

Gadgets for security

You might consider some of the low-cost devices mentioned above for security purposes. Lighting and electrical shops sell small switches that will turn on your house lights from outside as you approach.

Gadgets that monitor sound

Originally designed for parents of small babies, these systems enable you to hear what is going on while you are in another room or in the garden. You place a small transmitter in the person's pocket and carry a small receiver with you which picks up the sounds of whatever the person is doing.

Home videos

Home video use is limited only by one's imagination. Some people with
dementia enjoy watching films (especially from their own era); nursing
homes use videos for staff training; staff members sometimes videotape
each other interacting with patients, and then study the film for ways of
improving care; home movies can be converted to videotape so that
family members can reminisce together. You can tape yourself giving a
message to the person, which can be used by someone coming in to see
him. For example, 'John, this is Mary, your wife. I have gone to work.
Mrs Lamb will be with you until I come home at six. She will make
your lunch and then you will go for a walk. I want you to stay with her.
I love you. See you at 6.'

Should environments be cluttered or bare?

How cluttered should the environment be? People with dementia often
have difficulty focusing on one thing in a cluttered room. Order, routine,
and simplicity are helpful to the person who has trouble concentrating
or thinking. However, some environments are so barren that they add
to sensory deprivation and disorientation. Some people urge families to
put away many things; others say that patients need stimulation. Some
people argue that pictures on the wall or patterned wallpaper can cause
hallucinations or disorientation. How do you know what is right? The
answer depends on the individual person and the kind of clutter or
interest the room offers.

Observe the person: Does he tend to grab at everything in the bathroom? Does he put his hands into serving dishes or play with the condiments in the centre of the table? Does he seem unable to decide what food
to eat first or what piece of cutlery to pick up? If you observe these things,
try simplifying. Remove unnecessary things from the bathroom; leave
serving dishes in the kitchen or only put one item of food on his plate at a
time. An occasional person will talk to the pictures on the wall or try to
pick the flowers off the wallpaper. However, most people will not do this.
One lady in a nursing home was proud of the wallpaper 'her husband put
up'. If a picture or mirror is distressing a person, remove it; but there is no
reason to move it if he just talks to it and is not distressed by it.

In general, people, animals, noise, lights and action in a room are
more distracting than the decor. If the person is restless, irritable, or
having difficulty attending to you, consider reducing these distractions,
but do be sure that plenty of meaningful, focused, one-to-one interactions
are provided in their place.

Forcing a person to choose between more than one item (like several bottles of shampoo in the shower or several kinds of food on a plate) can cause more problems than things that are 'just there', like several cushions on the sofa. If the person stacks the cushions or carries them around, there is no need to put them away. Remove things only if they are causing a problem.

In contrast to family homes, care homes may not offer enough stimulation, interest, or environmental cues. Whatever the setting, observe the person's response to it. People who pace, fiddle, or repeat the same thing over and over may stop if they are encouraged to carry out an activity on which they can focus.

There are many ways in which we can help a confused person function by changing the physical environment. For example, as we age, we need more light to see; therefore, ensure there is enough light. People with dementia are doubly handicapped because they may not think to turn on a lamp or go over to the window for light. Colours with considerable contrast are easier to see than pastels or colours similar in intensity. To the person with some visual impairment, it may be impossible to see light-coloured food on a white plate. If the bathroom mat is deep blue, the person may have more success targeting the white toilet than if the rug is also white.

Just as colour can be used to help people notice things, it can be used to hide things. Paint a door (frame and all) to match the adjoining walls if you want the person to ignore it. A curtain over a door also helps.

Hearing aids magnify background noise, and people with dementia often cannot learn to compensate for this. Eliminate background noise whenever possible, unless the person is enjoying and focusing on it.

6 Medical problems

People with dementing illnesses can also suffer from other diseases, ranging from relatively minor problems like flu to serious illnesses. They may not be able to tell you they are in pain (even if they are able to speak well) or they may neglect their bodies. Cuts, bruises or even broken bones can go unnoticed. People who sit or lie for long periods of time may develop pressure sores. Their physical health may gradually decline. *Correction of even minor physical problems can greatly help people who suffer from dementing illnesses.*

You may have experienced a feeling of mental 'dullness' when you have been ill. This phenomenon can be worse in the demented person, whose system seems to be especially vulnerable to additional troubles. A delirium can be brought about by other conditions (flu, a minor cold, pneumonia, heart trouble, reactions to medication and many other things), and it may resemble a sudden worsening of the dementia. However, the delirium (and the symptoms) usually goes away when the condition is treated. You should check routinely for signs of illness or injury and call them to the attention of your doctor.

People who cannot express themselves well may not be able to answer yes or no when you ask them specific questions such as, 'Does your head hurt?' Even people who express themselves well may fail to remember, or may be unable to report pain.

All indications of pain or illness must be taken seriously. It is important to find a doctor who is gentle, who understands the patient's condition and who will take care of general medical problems. Do not let a doctor dismiss a patient because she is 'senile' or 'old'. Insist that her infection is treated and her pains diagnosed and relieved. Because of the impaired person's vulnerability to delirium, it is wise to check with the doctor about even minor conditions such as a cold.

Signals of illness include:

- abrupt worsening of behaviour, refusal to do certain things she was previously willing to do (behaviour changes often signal illness);
- moaning or shouting;
- fever (temperature over 37.5°C (100°F)). When taking a temperature, be careful that the person does not bite the thermometer. You can use a paper thermometer that is placed on the forehead, or you can take an approximate temperature by holding the thermometer in the person's armpit for three to five minutes. Alternatively, use the new liquid crystal thermometers that are placed against the skin, or thermometers with plastic-coated 'probes'. These are available from chemists. Older people may not have a significant fever even

when they are seriously ill. Lack of fever does not mean that the person is well;
- flushing or paleness;
- a rapid pulse over 100 (not obviously associated with exercise). Normal for most people is between 60 and 100 beats per minute. Ask your doctor or a nurse to show you how to find a pulse in the wrist. Count for 20 seconds and multiply by 3. It is helpful to know what a normal pulse is for the individual;
- vomiting or diarrhoea;
- changes in the skin (it may lose its elasticity, or look dry or pale);
- dry, pale gums or sores in the mouth;
- thirst or refusal of fluids or foods;
- a change in personality, increased irritability, or increased lassitude or drowsiness;
- headache;
- sudden onset of convulsions, hallucinations or falls; swelling of any part of the body (check especially hands and feet);
- coughing, sneezing, signs of respiratory congestion or difficulty in breathing.

Ask yourself the following questions:

- Has the person had even a minor fall?
- Has she moved her bowels in the last seventy-two hours?
- Has she had a recent change within the past month in medication?
- Do mild pain killers such as aspirin relieve her?
- Is she suddenly not moving an arm or leg?
- Is she wincing in pain?
- Does she have other health problems, such as heart disease, arthritis, or a cold?

If a person begins to lose weight, this may indicate the presence of a serious disease. It is important that your doctor determines the cause of any weight loss. A person who has lost 10 per cent of her weight needs to be seen by a doctor as soon as possible.

Pain

Families ask if people suffer pain as part of a dementing illness. As far as is known, Alzheimer's disease does not cause pain, and multi-infarct dementia causes pain only very rarely. People with dementing illnesses do suffer pain from other causes, such as stomach and abdominal cramps; constipation; hidden sprains or broken bones; sitting too long in one position; flu; arthritis; pressure sores, bruises or cuts; sores or rashes resulting from poor hygiene; sore teeth or gums; and clothes or shoes that rub or are too tight. Indications of pain include a sudden worsening of behaviour, moaning or shouting, refusal to do certain things, and increased restlessness. All signals of pain must be taken seriously. If the person cannot tell you where or whether she is in pain, a doctor may have to search for a cause of the pain.

Falls and Injuries

People with dementing illnesses may become clumsy. They can fall out of bed, bump into things, trip or cut themselves. It is easy to overlook serious injuries for several reasons:

1 Older people are more vulnerable to broken bones from seemingly minor injuries.
2 They may continue to use a fractured limb.
3 Demented people may not tell you they are in pain or may forget they have fallen. A bruise may not be in evidence for several days. Even minor head injuries can cause bleeding within the skull, which must be treated promptly to avoid further brain damage.

Check the person routinely for cuts, bruises and blisters that may be caused by accidents, falls, pacing or uncomfortable clothing. Changes in behaviour may be your only clue to an injury.

Pressure sores

Pressure sores (decubitus ulcers) develop when a person sits or lies down for prolonged periods, as a result of wearing tight clothing, from swelling or from inadequate nutrition. Older people's skin may be quite sensitive to them. Pressure sores begin as red areas and can develop into open sores. They are more common over bony areas: heels, hips, shoulders, shoulder blades, spine, elbows, knees, buttocks and ankles. You must watch for these, even in people who are able to walk, if the person spends a lot of time sitting or lying down. If any reddening appears, make sure the person does not lie on that spot. Continue to turn her so other sores do not form. The doctor can show you how to treat existing sores or the district nurse may be required to dress the sores. You will need to take steps to prevent further problems.

Encourage the person to change position: ask her to change the TV channel, go for a walk, set the table. Ask her to come into the kitchen to see if the cake is baking correctly or to come to the window to see something.

Pressure sores are always a risk in people who are no longer able to move or who are bed- or chairbound. Develop a schedule in which you move the patient from one side to the other or change her position every two hours.

If the person does not change position often enough, you can protect vulnerable areas. Pressure relief cushions can be obtained from statutory authorities. A wide variety of cushions are available and information on the one most suitable for you can be obtained from a community occupational therapist in the Social Services Department or the Disabled Living Foundation Information Service. Cushions can be purchased from private sources but it is important to get professional advice on the type of cushion most suitable. The Wheelchair Service can be a useful source of advice and help. Ask your GP for a referral. It is also possible to obtain from your local community nurse, or via private purchase, heel and elbow pads made of sheepskin or soft synthetic materials that protect those bony areas.

Dehydration

Even people who can walk and appear to be able to care for themselves may become dehydrated. Because we assume that they are caring for themselves, we may not watch for the signs of dehydration. Look for this problem, especially in people who have vomiting, diarrhoea or diabetes, or who are taking diuretics (water pills) or heart medication. Symptoms include: thirst or refusal to drink; fever; flushing; rapid pulse; a dry, pale lining of the mouth or a dried, inelastic skin; dizziness or light-headedness; and confusion or hallucinations.

The amount of fluid a person needs varies with the individual and with the season. People need more fluids during the summer months. If you are uncertain whether the person is taking enough fluid, ask your doctor how much the patient should be drinking.

Pneumonia

Pneumonia is an infection of the lungs caused by bacteria or a virus. It is a frequent complication of dementia, but may be difficult to diagnose because symptoms such as fever or cough may be absent. Delirium may be the earliest symptom, so pneumonia should be suspected when a person with dementia deteriorates suddenly.

Constipation

When a person is forgetful, she may not be able to remember when she last moved her bowels, and she may not realise the cause of the discomfort that comes from constipation. Some people move their bowels less frequently than others; however, they should still have a bowel movement every two or three days.

Constipation can cause discomfort or pain, which can cause a worsening of the person's confusion. Constipation can also lead to a faecal impaction, in which the bowel becomes partially or completely blocked and the body is unable to rid itself of wastes. You should consult a doctor or nurse if you suspect this. (Diarrhoea may accompany a partial impaction.)

Many factors contribute to the development of constipation. One important factor is that most British people eat a diet high in refined, easy-to-prepare foods and low in fibre-containing foods that encourage bowel activity. Often when a person has a dementing illness, or her dentures fit poorly, or her teeth hurt, she makes further changes in her diet that aggravate the problem of constipation. The muscles of the bowel that move wastes are believed to become less active as we age, and when we are less physically active, our bowel is even less active. Some drugs and diet supplements (given to people who are not eating) tend to increase constipation. Ask your pharmacist whether the drugs the person is taking can cause constipation.

If a person has a dementing illness, you cannot assume that she is able to keep track of when she last moved her bowels, even if she seems to be only mildly impaired or if she tells you she is taking care of herself. If a confused person is living alone, she may have stopped eating things that require detailed preparation and may be eating too many cakes, biscuits and other low-fibre, highly refined foods. If you do not live with the person, it may be impossible to find out how regularly her bowels move. If you suspect that she may be constipated, you will need to keep track for her. Do this as quietly and unobtrusively as possible, so that you do not inadvertently make her feel that you are 'taking over'.

Most people are private about their bodily functions and a confused person can react angrily to your seeming invasion of her privacy. Also, keeping track of someone else's bowel movements is distasteful to many of us, and we tend to avoid doing it. These two feelings can conspire to cause a potentially serious problem to be overlooked.

When a demented person cannot talk and appears to be in pain or has a headache, do not overlook constipation as a possible cause. Bloating or 'gas' also signals problems. In the midst of providing care for a seriously impaired person, it is easy to forget to keep track of bowel movements. If you think the person may be constipated, because symptoms such as fever or cough may be absent, you may wish to talk this over with the doctor. He can quickly determine whether the person's bowels are working properly, and, if they are not, he can help manage the problem.

Regular or frequent use of laxatives is not recommended. Instead, increase the amount of fibre and water in the diet, and help the person take more exercise (perhaps a daily walk). The person should drink at least eight cupfuls of some form of beverage every day. Increase the amount of vegetables (try putting them out as nibbles), fruits (including prunes, apples as more nibbles, or on cereal), whole-grain cereals (bran, wholemeal bread, whole-grain breakfast cereal), and salads she eats.

Ask your doctor whether you should add more fibre by giving ispaghula husk preparations (sold under various brand names, such as Regulan, Fybogel or Isogel). Do not use any such product without medical supervision.

Medication

Medication is a two-edged sword. It may play a vital part in helping the patient to sleep, in controlling her agitation, or in the treatment of other conditions. At the same time, people suffering from a dementing illness (and older people in general) are vulnerable to overmedication and to reactions from combinations of drugs. A sudden increase in agitation, a slow stooped walk, falling, drowsiness, incontinence, leaning, stiffness, or strange mouth or hand movements may be a side effect of medication and should be called to the doctor's attention. Doctors cannot always eliminate all the side effects of the medication and at the same time get the required results. You and your doctor must work together to achieve the best possible balance. Many people will need behaviour-controlling medication to help them through some phases of their illness. However, because it can cause serious side effects, including more confusion, it must be used cautiously. Behaviour-controlling drugs are best used when they are aimed at specific symptoms such as sleeplessness, hallucinations, suspicion, and severe irritability. They do not perform well at controlling aimless wandering or restlessness. Whenever the physician raises the dosage of a behaviour-modifying drug, ask yourself if there are any non-drug changes that might also help. (See pages 121–122.) Perhaps if you had more time to yourself, you might be able to tolerate more restlessness on the part of the patient. Is it possible to respond more calmly to her behaviour or divert her before problems develop? Ask whether the drug can be given so that it has greatest effect at the person's worst time of day.

Much of the responsibility for medication will fall on you. Here are some ways you can help. Be sure that all of the doctors involved in the persons's care know about all the drugs she is taking. Sometimes combinations of drugs can make her confusion worse. Your pharmacist will be highly trained in the effects and interactions of drugs. You may want to take all the patient's prescription drugs and over-the-counter medication to your pharmacist, discuss them with him and ask him to make up a card listing all of them. Ask the pharmacist if any of the drugs should be listed on the patient's identification bracelet. (See the Medic Alert information on page 126.) Whenever the physician prescribes a new drug, ask him to review all current medication to see whether any can be discontinued. This will help reduce drug interactions. Ask him to start the new drug in as low a dose as possible, and to increase the dose later if necessary. People with brain injuries like dementia often develop side effects at a low or regular adult dose. Ask how long the drug stays in the body and whether another, similar drug would have fewer side effects.

Ask what side effects to watch for. Side effects can appear even three weeks or a month after the person begins taking the drug. By then, you and the doctor may not attribute new symptoms to the medication. Ask if there are any possible side effects that you should report to your doctor immediately.

Some drugs must be taken before meals, some after. Some have a cumulative effect (that is, they gradually build up their effectiveness), some don't. Older people and people with a dementing illness are especially sensitive to incorrect dosages, so it is imperative that you see that the patient receives the correct amount of medication and at the times specified by the doctor. If a medicine makes the person drowsy, ask if it can be given at bedtime when it will help her sleep and not in the morning when she should be active.

Find out what you should do if you miss a dose or accidentally give a double dose.

Some patients do not understand why you want them to take a particular drug and may have a catastrophic reaction. Avoid arguing about it. Instead, tell the person one step at a time what is happening: 'This is your pill. Dr Brown gave it to you . . . Put it in your mouth . . . Drink some water . . . Good.' If the person becomes upset, try again later. Some people will take pills more easily if you routinely put each dose in a cup or envelope instead of handing the person the whole bottle.

Patients may fail or refuse to swallow pills. They may carry the pill around in their mouth and spit it out later. You may find the pills much later on the floor. Persuading the person to drink something with the medication helps. If this continues to be a problem, ask the doctor if the medication is available in another form. Pills or a liquid may be easier to get down than capsules. Sometimes pills can be crushed and mixed into food or given with a spoonful of jam. If you are not sure whether a person actually took her pill, find out from the doctor what you should do. If pills are going on the floor, be sure that grandchildren or pets don't find and swallow them.

Never assume that a forgetful person is able to manage her own medication. If you must leave a person alone, put out one dose for her and take the bottle away with you. Even people with mild memory impairments (and sometimes well people) forget whether they have taken their pills.

When you are tired or upset, you may forget the person's pills. Some local chemists sell plastic containers with compartments labelled 'Monday', 'Tuesday', 'Wednesday', etc. You can tell at a glance whether today's pills have been taken. (This device is helpful for you: do not trust the patient to be able to use it.) If your local chemist has never heard of such pill dispensers, contact the Disabled Living Foundation Information Service for addresses of suppliers. It is also possible that the hospital the person is attending may have information on pill dispensers and supply you with one. You can also obtain easy-to-open pill bottles if the child-proof ones are difficult for you to manage. However, the child-proof caps may keep the confused person from taking pills she should not have. You must, of course, store medication where the confused person cannot reach it.

Dental problems

It is important that the person receives regular dental check-ups. Sores in her mouth may be hard for you to find and she may not be able to tell you about them. She may refuse to let you look in her mouth. Even mildly forgetful people may neglect their dentures and develop oral infections. The person's teeth must be pain-free and any dentures must fit well. Poor teeth or ill-fitting dentures can lead to poor nutrition, which can significantly add to the person's problems. If the person is in a nursing home, ensure that arrangements are made for continued dental care.

People with dementia tend to lose dentures and partial plates. Ask the dentist to consider alternatives that cannot be removed and lost. Because people with dementia have a shortened life expectancy, a speedy solution allowing for ease of management may be preferable to a long course of treatment (for example, a removable bridge may be better than a fixed crown).

Many people resist going to the dentist. Find a dentist who understands these patients, and who works slowly and gently. Some dentists say they rarely have problems with confused patients. If the dentist recommends a general anaesthetic to care for teeth, carefully balance the need for care against the risks of the anaesthetic. If your local dentist finds difficulty managing your relative, she can be referred to the Community Dental Service provided by the District Health Authority. These dentists are specially trained to care for cognitively impaired people.

Vision problems

Sometimes it appears that the person cannot see well or is going blind. She may bump into things, pick her feet up very high over low curbs, be unable to pick-up her food on her fork, or become confused or lost in dim light. One of several things may be happening. She may have a problem with her eyes, such as long sightedness or cataracts. Arrange for her to be seen by an ophthalmologist. A correctable vision problem should be treated, if possible, so that her impaired brain can receive the best possible information from her eyes. If she is both not seeing well and not thinking well, she will be even less able to make sense of her environment and will function more poorly as a result. Do not let a doctor dismiss her vision problems because she is 'senile'. Even if he cannot help, he should explain to you what the problem is.

Brain-impaired people may be less able to distinguish between similar colour intensities. Thus light blue, light green and light yellow may all look similar. A white handrail on a white wall may be hard to see. It may be hard for some people to tell where a light green wall joins a blue green carpet. This may cause the person to stumble into walls.

Some people have difficulty with depth perception. Prints and patterns may be confusing. A black and white bathroom floor can look as if it is full of holes. It may be difficult to know whether one is close enough to a chair to sit down. It may be hard to tell how high a step or curb is. It can be difficult to see where to step on stairs. Glare from a window tends to obliterate the detail of objects near it. The older eye may adjust more slowly to sudden changes from bright light to darkness or vice versa.

When the brain is not working well, the person will be less able to compensate for these vision problems, but you can help her. She needs to see as well as possible so that she can function at her best level. Paint a handrail dark if the wall is light. Paint skirting boards dark if the walls are light. The dark line will help the person see the change from floor to wall. Cover the bathroom with washable carpeting that is secured so that it does not slip. Delineate the edges and bottom of the bath with colourful strips of waterproof tape. Paint stair risers and treads in contrasting colours. The contrast will help. Outline doors, mantelpieces and other objects the person bumps into with bright tape in a contrasting colour and colour intensity (light on dark or dark on light).

Increase the light in rooms in the daytime and evening, and leave night lights on at night. Install lights in dark cupboards. Cover chairs in bright, contrasting colours without patterns. Put a towel or bedspread over a chair if you don't want to re-cover it. Leave chairs in their familiar places.

People with dementing illnesses can also lose the ability to *know* what they see. In this instance the eyes work correctly but the brain no longer accurately uses what the eyes tell it. For example, the person may bump into furniture, not because she has a vision problem but because her brain is not working properly. What seem like vision problems may be part of the dementia. This condition is called agnosia and is discussed in Chapter 8. When problems are caused by agnosia, the ophthalmologist will not be able to help. In fact, it may be difficult for him to test the vision of a person with thinking or language impairments. Obviously, when this is the problem, it will do no good to tell the person to watch where she is going. She will need increasing care to protect her from injuries she cannot avoid, and you may need to check her frequently for cuts and bruises.

If the person is putting down her glasses and forgetting them, it often helps to persuade her to wear them on a chain. Always make sure she has a spare pair in case she loses her glasses. Carry her prescription and your own with you if you travel away from home. With a prescription, you can replace lost or broken glasses with less trouble and expense.

If the person wears contact lenses, you may need to replace them with glasses before the person reaches a point where she is unable to manage lenses. If she continues to wear them, you must watch for irritations to the eye and be sure she cares for her lenses properly.

Hearing problems

Failing to hear properly deprives the confused brain of information needed to make sense of the environment, and hearing loss can cause or worsen suspiciousness or withdrawal. (See Chapter 8.) It is important to correct any hearing loss if possible. Ask your GP to refer the patient to an Ear, Nose and Throat (ENT) clinic. An audiologist can determine the cause of the hearing loss and help you select an appropriate hearing aid. As with vision problems, it can be difficult for you to separate problems in thinking from problems in hearing. People with Alzheimer's disease develop problems understanding or comprehending what is said to them (see page 36). An audiologist and your physician should be able to distinguish between this and the type of hearing loss that can be corrected.

Since the ill person cannot learn easily, she may not be able to adjust to using her hearing aid. Hearing aids pick up background noises, which can sound loud and be upsetting to the wearer. Most people will get a hearing aid through the ENT department at the local hospital. It may be quicker to obtain an aid privately. If you decide to purchase a hearing aid, then it would be advisable to do so on the understanding that you can return it if the confused person cannot tolerate its use.

If the person uses a hearing aid, you must be responsible for it and must check regularly that the batteries are working.

Here are some other things you can do in addition to correcting the loss with a hearing aid:

1 Reduce background noise, such as noise from appliances, the television, or several people talking at once. It is difficult for the impaired person to distinguish between these and what she wants to hear.
2 Lower the pitch of your voice. High-frequency sounds are harder to hear.
3 Give the person clues as to where sounds are coming from. It can be hard to locate and identify sounds, and this may confuse the person. Remind her, 'That is the sound of the dustman's cart.'
4 Use several kinds of clues at one time: point, speak and gently guide the person, for example.

Visiting the doctor

Visits to the doctor or dentist can turn into an ordeal for you and the patient. Here are some ways to make them easier.

The forgetful person may not be able to understand where she is going or why. This, combined with the bustle of getting ready to go, may precipitate a catastrophic reaction. Look for ways of simplifying the visit for her.

Some people do better if they know in advance that they are going to the doctor. However, with others, it is best if you avoid an argument by not bringing up the subject of the visit until you are almost there. Instead of saying, 'We have to get up early today. Hurry with your breakfast because today you will be going to see Dr Brown, and he has to change your medicine', just get the person up with no comment, serve her breakfast and help her into her coat. When you are almost there, say, 'We are seeing Dr Brown today.'

Rather than get into an argument, ignore or play down objections. If the person says, 'I am not going to the doctor', instead of saying, 'You have to go to the doctor', try changing the subject and saying something like, 'We'll stop and have a cup of tea while we are in town.'

Plan your trip in advance. Know where you are going, where you will park, how long it will take and whether there are stairs or lifts. Allow enough time without rushing, but not so much time that you will be early and have a longer wait. Ask for an appointment at the person's best time of day. Take someone with you to help while you drive.

Talk to the receptionist. She may be able to tell you whether you have a long wait. If the waiting-room is crowded and noisy, she may be able to arrange for you to wait in a quieter place. Take along some snacks or some activity the person enjoys doing. If the receptionist knows that you have a long wait, you may be able to take a short walk if you check in frequently with her. Never leave a forgetful person alone in the waiting-room. The strange place may upset her or she may wander away.

The doctor may prescribe a sedative for the patient if other methods fail. Usually, however, your being calm and matter of fact and giving the person simple information and reassurance are sufficient.

If the ill person must enter hospital

People with dementia often become ill with other conditions and need to go into hospital. This can be a trying time for you and the confused person. The illness that caused the hospitalisation may also cause a temporary decline in the person's cognitive function. The unfamiliar environment, the confusion of a busy hospital and new treatments may precipitate a decline in function as well. It is not unusual for people with dementia to become agitated, scream, or to strike out in such circumstances. Additional behaviour-controlling medication may be necessary, but it can also further impair thinking or worsen behaviour. The person may gradually return to normal when she comes out of hospital.

There are some things you can do to make going into hospital easier, but recognise that you cannot completely prevent problems. *It is important that you do not become exhausted.*

Talk to the doctor in advance about how the dementing illness may complicate the person's admission. Ask if the treatment can be carried out on an outpatient basis. This may be difficult, but it shortens the time the confused person must be in a strange setting. If you do this, arrange for home nursing for the first few days after the treatment. The district nurse can provide this, as can private nursing agencies.

At admission, talk to the nursing staff. Let them know that the person has a dementia. Urge them to tell the person, as frequently as possible, where she is and to be calm and reassuring with her. Write down things the nurses need to know and ask for your notes to be put in the care plan. Mention things that will help staff cope with her, such as nick-names, names of family whom she might ask about, things she will need to have done for her (like filling out the menu and opening milk cartons), and how toileting is managed.

Hospitals can be short-staffed and nurses often work under pressure.

They may not be able to spend as much time with the confused person as they would like. Also, they may not be trained specifically to work with dementia patients.

It is usually comforting for the person to have someone she knows with her as much as possible, and to accompany her to tests and treatments. A family member can help with meals. See that the person takes enough fluid and reassure her about what is going on. Some hospitals will let family members stay overnight with confused patients. *But*, sometimes a family member's own anxiety and nervousness upsets the patient or gets in the way of the staff. Calmness – or nervousness – is contagious. The confused person will be influenced by your feelings. You may want to ask someone else to spend time with the person to give you a break. If you cannot go with the person for tests, explain to the staff how important it is to comfort and reassure her.

You could consider hiring a sitter to stay with the person full-time, if this is affordable, or to be with the person when you or other family members cannot. If possible, arrange a schedule for children, family or understanding close friends to be with the person.

Familiar clothing, a familiar blanket and large photos of family members help reassure the person. Some families write a letter to the person that nurses can use to reassure her when she is anxious. It might read like this:

Dear Mum, You are in the hospital because you broke your hip. You will be coming back home to our house soon. Ted or I will come to see you every night just after you have your supper. The nurses know you have trouble remembering things and they will help you. I love you.
Your daughter, Ann.

If the person must be restrained, ask that the restraint be as mild as possible. For example, mittens can be used to keep her from pulling out tubes. This is usually less frightening than tying her hands.

Do not be alarmed if the person's confusion worsens in the hospital. In most cases the person's level of impairment will return to what it was before the hospitalisation.

Seizures, fits or convulsions

The majority of people with dementing illnesses do not develop seizures. Because they are so uncommon, you are not likely to have to face this problem. However, seizures can be frightening for you if you are not

prepared to deal with them. Various diseases can cause seizures. Therefore, if the person does have a seizure, it may not be related to the
dementia.

There are several types of seizure. In a generalised tonic-clonic seizure
(the kind we usually associate with an epileptic fit), the person becomes
rigid, falls and loses consciousness. Her breathing can become irregular
or even stop briefly. Then her muscles will begin to jerk and she may
clench her teeth tightly. After some seconds the jerking will stop and the
person will slowly regain consciousness. She may be confused, sleepy,
or have a headache. She may have difficulty talking.

Other types of seizure are less dramatic. For example, just a hand or
arm may move in a repetitive manner.

A single epileptic fit is not life-threatening. The most important thing
is to remain calm. Do not try to restrain the person. Try to protect her
from falling or banging her head on something hard. If she is on the
floor, move things out of the way. If she is seated, you may be able to
ease her to the floor, or quickly push a sofa cushion under her to soften
her fall if she should fall out of the chair.

Do not try to move her or stop the seizure. Stay with her and let the
fit run its course. Do not try to hold the tongue and do not try to put a
spoon in the patient's mouth. Never force her mouth open after her teeth
are clenched. You may damage her teeth and gums. Loosen clothing if
you can. For example, unfasten a belt, a tie, or buttons at the neckline.

When the jerking has ceased, ensure that the person is breathing
correctly. If she has more saliva than usual, turn her head gently to the
side and wipe out her mouth. Let her sleep or rest if she wishes.
She may be confused or irritable, or even aggressive after the seizure.
She may know something is wrong, but she will not remember having
the seizure. Be calm, gentle and reassuring. Avoid restraining her,
restricting her, or insisting on what she should do.

Take a few minutes after the seizure to relax and collect yourself.

If the person has a partial fit, nothing need be done. If the person
wanders about, follow her and try to prevent her from hurting herself.
When this type of seizure ends she may be temporarily confused, irritable, or have trouble talking. You may be able to identify the warning
signals that a seizure is starting, such as specific repetitive movements.
If so, you can make sure the person is in a safe place (away from traffic,
away from stairs or cookers, etc.).

Your doctor can be helpful in advising on the management and treatment of epileptic fits. He should be called the first time the person has
any type of seizure, so that he can check her and determine the cause of
the seizure. Stay with the person until the seizure is over and you have
had a chance to collect yourself. Then call the doctor. He can prescribe
medication to minimise the likelihood of further epileptic fits.

If the patient is being treated for seizures, the doctor should be called
if the person has many seizures over a short period of time, if the symp-

toms do not go away after several hours, or if you suspect that the person has hit her head or injured herself in some other way.

Epileptic fits are frightening and unpleasant to watch, but they are usually not life-threatening, nor are they indications of danger to others or of insanity. They can become less frightening for you as you learn how to respond to them. Contact your GP, health visitor, district nurse or an experienced family member with whom you can discuss your distress and who can knowledgeably reassure you.

Jerking movements (myoclonus)

Patients with Alzheimer's disease occasionally develop rapid jerking movements of their arms, legs or body. These are called myoclonic jerks. They are not epileptic fits: in an epileptic fit there are repeated movements of the same muscles, while myoclonic jerks are single thrusts of an arm or of the head.

Myoclonic jerks are not a cause for alarm. They do not progress to epilepsy. The only danger they can cause is possible accidental injury as a result of inadvertently striking an object. At present there is no effective treatment for the myoclonus associated with Alzheimer's disease. Drugs can be tried, but these usually have significant side effects and offer little improvement.

The death of the impaired person

Whenever you have the responsibility for an ill or elderly person, you face the possibility of that person's death. You may have questions you are reluctant to bring up with the doctor. Often thinking about such things in advance will help relieve your mind and can make things easier if you have to face a crisis.

Cause of death

In the final stages of a progressive dementing illness, so much of the nervous system is failing that this profoundly affects the rest of the body. The person may be confined to bed, incontinent and unable to speak. The *immediate* cause of death is often a complicating condition such as

pneumonia, malnutrition (these people sometimes stop eating), dehydration, or infection. Death certificates often list only this immediate
cause of death and do not list the dementing illness as a cause of death.
This has made it difficult for epidemiologists to determine accurately
how prevalent dementing illnesses are. However, reporting practices are
changing as physicians become more knowledgeable about dementia.

Some people will die from stroke, heart attack, cancer, or other causes
even though they also have Alzheimer's disease. These deaths can come
at any time, so some people will be ambulatory and fairly functional up
until their death.

Dying at home

Families sometimes worry that the ill or elderly person will die at home,
perhaps in her sleep, and that they will find her. Because of this, a
care-giver may be afraid to sleep soundly or may get up to check on the
sick person several times a night.

> One daughter said, 'I don't know what I would do. What if one of the children
> found her?'

Perhaps you have heard of someone who found a husband or wife dead,
and you wonder how you would cope with this. Most families find it
reassuring to know what to do. Select a funeral director in advance.
Should a death occur, you have only to call him or your doctor. You
might also call your clergyman. Discuss with these people in advance
whether they can respond to an emergency call late at night. Some
care-givers want a little time to say goodbye; others do not. If you do,
the first thing to do might be to sit or cry a little while with the person,
and then call someone.

Some families value the peacefulness and privacy that death at home
allows, but others worry about what dying looks like and about what to
do. If you want the person to be able to die at home, a district nurse
can show you what care is needed and give you guidance on how to
conserve your own energy. In some areas the MacMillan nurses would
also advise, even though the person is not dying of cancer. You should
contact the Cancer Relief MacMillan Fund, Anchor House, 15/19
Britten Street, LONDON SW3 3TZ, tel: 071-351 7811. Also, books are
available on this topic.

In some areas there are special resources available to people who have
terminal illnesses and who, with their families, wish to die at home. Your

Medical problems   117

GP, district nurse or local hospital will know about the range of home nursing services supplied locally. They will also know about hospices and other terminal care facilities in your area. Hospices will not usually accept severely demented patients, as they care mainly for those dying of cancer, particularly where pain control is a problem. However, each case is judged individually and a demented patient who is dying of cancer with severe pain would, of course, be eligible for admission. The staff in the hospice or terminal care unit may be able to give you information about how to plan for a death, and advice and counselling.

Dying in the hospital or nursing home

Some families are comforted to know that professionals are in charge at this time, and so they choose a nursing home or hospital. Bedside care of a totally dependent person is hard work and is emotionally draining. Do not feel guilty if this is not for you. You may be better able to give loving reassurance if someone else is providing the physical care.

Whatever choice you make, it is the right one for you; but whatever the setting, it is important to do some advance planning. Families have told us that unless you plan in advance, you may have little control over what takes place, and things may be done very differently from the way you and your family member would have wished. Most of these problems revolve around the type and amount of life-sustaining intervention used.

Prolonging suffering?

There is another aspect to consider when a person has a slow, chronic and terminal illness: the question of whether it would be better to allow life to end rather than to prolong suffering. This is a serious question, one with which doctors, judges and ministers struggle as well as the seriously ill and their families. Each person must make that decision for himself, based on his unique background, beliefs and experiences.

There are no 'better' or 'worse' choices, as long as the person receives gentle care and is kept comfortable. Some of the options are described here, to help you select the kind of care that will be right for you and your family member. Some families want to be sure that everything possible has been done; others have felt hassled or upset by medical intervention they did not want.

Occasionally a physician, a social worker, hospital staff or a nursing home will have strong opinions about life support and resuscitation, and will follow these opinions, regardless of your wishes. Some act out of fear of lawsuits and some continue a practice because it is 'the way we have always done it'. Ask your physician and the nursing home what steps they will take. Will they routinely transfer the patient to a hospital? Will they insert tubes or give life-sustaining drugs? What procedures, if any, do they consider 'routine' and carry out without your explicit consent? Will they discourage your presence in the patient's room? If an ambulance is summoned, will the ambulancemen automatically try to resuscitate the person? Will the hospital automatically try resuscitation? Are they open and responsive to your enquiries, or do they avoid your questions and dogmatically state positions?

You might ask a clergyman or a friend to help you make the necessary phone calls to ask these questions. If there is a local hospice organisation, they may be able to acquaint you with the usual practices in your community.

If you are not comfortable with the procedures in your hospital or nursing home, write down details of the care you want the person to receive. Request that these instructions be placed in the person's care plan at the nursing home and hospital. Make one copy for the person's doctor and one copy for the care home to send with the patient to the hospital, and sign each copy. Ask the doctor and the nursing home directly if they will honour these instructions.

Occasionally a family feels so strongly opposed to the care available in a hospital or nursing home that they transfer the person to another nursing home or take her home to die.

What kind of care can be given at the end of life?

When a person has a chronic, terminal illness, the person's family must often make decisions about when to allow treatment and when to accept the declining course of the disease. There are few right or wrong answers, and there are many things that are not understood about the last stages of life. The questions that families often face include whether to use tubes to feed a person who has stopped eating and whether to treat concurrent illnesses with antibiotics or surgery. (You may have faced similar issues earlier in the illness, such as whether to restrain an ambulatory person who might fall. See page 130.)

As you make these decisions, be cautious about accepting dogmatic opinions from 'experts'. Like the rest of us, professionals can easily confuse personal values with fact in this emotion-laden area.

When you consider questions about life-support interventions for terminally ill people, such as the use of feeding tubes or oxygen, the treatment of illnesses such as pneumonia with antibiotics, or surgery for acute problems, recognise that many things are not known about these difficult issues, and we sometimes understand even less about the effects of life-support interventions on patients with dementia. It is difficult to know whether an abrupt decline is part of the dementing illness or whether, if treated, the person might continue comfortably for some time. It is just as difficult to determine when a person with dementia is 'terminally ill' or to predict when a person with late-stage dementia will die. These uncertainties add to the family's burden. Neither you nor the doctors may be able to say whether an intervention will help or will be distressing to a patient close to death.

We often do not know how the ill person experiences treatments – whether the severely impaired person is frightened by feeding tubes, bathing, turning, or restraints; whether lack of food or fluids is painful. We do not know if a patient who tries to pull out tubes does so because they are frightened or uncomfortable. It is risky to generalise about patients with dementia who are dying from other illnesses.

The dementing illnesses are gradually progressive, and you may have to make these painful decisions several times in the course of the illness. Each decision must be made separately. For example, when pneumonia causes an ambulatory and apparently content person to stop eating, you might decide to use tube feeding for a short time while she gets over the infection. Later, when she is severely impaired, you might decide not to use tube feeding if she stops eating.

Pain medication can be given even when a decision has been made not to use antibiotics, forced feeding, or other physical treatments; but pain medication often carries risks. It can impair a person's ability to breathe, for example. Nevertheless, you may decide that the benefit of pain relief outweighs the risk. Discuss this explicitly with the patient's physician and nurses.

Decisions will often be easier if you weigh up the ethical issues *after* you have obtained the best medical information available.

> *Mrs Allen's children argued among themselves over whether or not it was against their religion not to give her food through a tube. She tried to pull out the tube and seemed frightened. When the doctor told them that even with the tube she would live only a few days, it was much easier to decide not to use tube feeding but to give her spoonfuls of ice cream from time to time, to moisten her mouth.*

Ask your physician how likely it is that the person will return to some previous level (that of a week or a month ago, for instance). Is it likely that the person's death will be delayed by hours, days or months by the proposed intervention? What are the available alternatives? Are there any other interventions that might be less distressing?

Who makes the decision? Sometimes the patient has left a written statement about her wishes for life-prolonging care. Other people have told their families how they wish to be cared for, or have made statements such as, 'I never want to be kept alive the way Mabel was.'

If possible, you should arrive at an agreement with the rest of the family on the kind of care to give. Usually, providers must honour the patient's previous statement or wishes, or the request of those close to the patient. Providers are often reluctant to give palliative care to ease the patient's discomfort with strong drugs when the family members are in disagreement.

It can be difficult for family members to discuss these painful issues. Some people may refuse to talk about them; others may get angry. Some feel that it is wrong to 'plan' for death. However, talking things over often relieves feelings of anxiety and dread as death approaches and, as we have said, unless plans are made, the family may have little control over the last days of the person's life.

You might show this section to other family members and ask your physician, social worker or clergyman to help co-ordinate a family discussion. Suggest that family members do not bring up old disagreements but focus on this one issue.

The death of the ill person, even after so long an illness, may be painful, and the practical tasks surrounding death are distasteful to many of us. Still, arranging a gentle and dignified death is one way in which you can give love and care to the ill person, and it will allow you to grieve in the way that is right for you without intrusions from strangers.

The post-mortem

Your doctor may ask you for permission to perform a post-mortem; if you feel you can assent to this request it is helpful for many reasons. A post-mortem is the only way to confirm a diagnosis of Alzheimer's disease and many other causes of dementia. It can be reassuring for you to know the exact illness. In the future, such knowledge may be important when specific treatment is available. Also, individual doctors frequently learn information from the post-mortem that they can use to help others. Finally, post-mortem studies advance our knowledge of the dementing illnesses. Post-mortems do not disfigure the body.

The things people with dementia do – their behaviour – can be the most distressing part of their illness. Chapter 3 discusses some of the common problems, including irritability, anger and agitation. It also discusses why people act as they do: *dementia damages the brain, so the person cannot make sense of what he sees and hears.* This confusion may make the person frightened and anxious. This is why he sometimes insists on 'going home', why he lashes out in anger at you, or resists care. Most of this behaviour is not under his control, and usually he is trying as hard as he can.

Here are some general guidelines for managing difficult behaviour. Ask yourself if such behaviour could result in someone – you or the confused person – being hurt. Or is the behaviour making life intolerable for others (yourself, other residents, or staff) even though it is not dangerous? If the behaviour is potentially harmful, then you probably need to find a way to stop it, even if you must use medication that has serious side effects. If it is not dangerous, you should strongly consider allowing it to continue. This may be easier to tolerate if you can get away from the person once in a while.

The six R's of behaviour management

Some families tell us that the ill person does some things that create serious problems. Do not assume that you will face all or even most of the problems listed in this chapter. But if you do face problems, one of the first places to seek help is the Alzheimer's Disease Society support group in your area. It was from members of such groups that we learned many of the things we suggest in this book. Most Alzheimer's Disease Society branches publish newsletters, as does the national society. You can subscribe to these and they contain excellent ideas.

One husband does not describe problem behaviours as a 'problem'. He calls each difficulty a 'challenge'. This helps him approach it with a positive outlook. Difficult behaviour has different causes in different people and different solutions will work in different households. Some families have found these six Rs helpful in thinking through a problem.

1   **Restrict.**   The first thing we often try is to get the person to stop whatever he is doing. This is especially important when the person

might harm himself or someone else. But trying to make the person stop may upset him more.

2   **Reassess**. Ask yourself: might a physical illness or drug reaction be causing the problem? Might the person be having difficulty seeing or hearing? Is something upsetting him? Could the annoying person or object be removed? Might a different approach upset the person less?

3   **Reconsider**. Ask yourself how things must seem from the patient's point of view. People with dementia are often unaware of the extent of their impairment. When you try to bathe or dress someone who does not understand that he needs help, he may get upset. The person's anxiety is understandable when he can't make sense of what is going on.

4   **Rechannel**. Find a way in which the behaviour can continue in a safe and non-destructive manner. The behaviour may be important to the person in some way that we cannot understand. One man who had been a car mechanic continued to take things apart around the house; but he could not get them back together. His wife had an old carburettor steam cleaned and gave it to him. He was able to enjoy taking it apart for several months and left the household appliances alone.

5   **Reassure**. When a person has been upset, fearful or angry, take time to reassure him that things are all right and that you still care for him. While the person may not remember the reassurance, he may retain the feeling of having been reassured and cared for. Putting your arm around the person or hugging him is a way of reassuring him.
     Take time to reassure yourself as well. You are doing the best you can with a demanding and difficult job. Give yourself a pat on the back for surviving one more challenge. If possible, find some time away from the person to regain your energy; you will solve problems better if you are not exhausted.

6   **Review**. Afterwards, think over what happened and how you managed it. You may face this problem again. What did you learn from this experience that will help you next time? What led up to this behaviour? How did you respond to it? What did you do right? What might you try next time?

Concealed memory loss

People with a deteriorating dementing disease can become skilful at hiding their declining abilities and forgetfulness. This is understandable; no one wants to admit that he is becoming 'senile'.

This tendency to hide limitations can be distressing for families. The person living with someone suffering from a dementing illness may know that the person is impaired, yet receive no support or understanding from others who cannot see the problem. Friends may say, 'He looks and sounds perfectly all right. I don't see anything wrong, and I don't see why he cannot remember to phone me.' Family members may not be able to differentiate between real memory loss and plain contrariness.

When a person has been living alone, family, neighbours and friends may be unaware for a long time that anything is wrong. When the person denies that he has any memory problems, he may manage for years until a crisis occurs. Families are often shocked and distressed by the extent of the problem when they finally learn of it.

You may wonder what the person is still able to do for himself and what needs to be done for him. If he is employed, has responsibility for his own money or is driving, he may not realise or may be unwilling to admit that he can no longer manage these tasks as well as he once could. Some people recognise that their memory is failing. Different people cope with this in different ways. While some people don't want to admit that anything is wrong, others find relief and comfort in talking about what is happening to them. Listen to their thoughts, feelings and fears if this is so. This can be comforting and can give you a chance to correct misconceptions.

Others may successfully conceal their impairment by keeping lists. They may use conversational devices, such as saying, 'Of course I know that' to cover their forgetfulness. Some people get angry and blame others when they forget things. Some people stop participating in activities that they have always enjoyed.

A frequent characteristic of the dementing illnesses is that personality and social skills appear nearly intact while memory and the ability to learn are being lost. This condition enables a person to conceal his illness for a long time. One can talk with such a person about routine matters and fail to recognise that his memory or thinking is impaired. Psychological testing or an occupational therapy assessment can be helpful in such situations because the assessment will give you a realistic measure of how much you can expect from the impaired individual and what things the person can still do. Because dementing illnesses can be so deceiving, even to someone close to the person, the assessment given by professionals is most important in helping you and your family plan realistically.

These professionals may also talk over their findings with the impaired person and show him ways in which he can remain as independent as possible.

Wandering

Wandering is a common and frequently serious problem that deserves thoughtful consideration. Wandering behaviour can make it difficult to manage a person at home. It can make it impossible for day centres, residential homes or certain nursing homes to care for a person. The impaired person is endangered when he wanders into busy streets or into strange neighbourhoods. When a confused person becomes disoriented and lost, he may feel frightened. Because so many people do not understand dementia, strangers who try to help may think the individual is drunk or insane. When wandering occurs at night, it can deprive the family of needed rest. However, often it can be stopped or at least reduced.

Since it appears that there are different kinds of wandering and different reasons why brain-impaired people wander, identifying the cause of the behaviour may help you plan a strategy to manage it.

Reasons why people wander

Wandering may result from getting lost. Sometimes a person sets out on an errand, such as going to the shops, takes a wrong turning, becomes disoriented, and gets completely lost trying to find his way back. Or he may go shopping with you, lose sight of you and get lost trying to find you.

Wandering often increases when a person moves to a new home, starts to go to a day centre or day hospital, or for some other reason is in a new environment.

Some people wander around intermittently for no apparent reason. Some wandering behaviour appears aimless and can go on for hours, and it appears to be different from the wandering associated with being lost or with being in a new place. Some people develop an agitated, determined pacing. When this continues it can be irritating and can also be dangerous when the person is determined to get away. This seemingly incomprehensible pacing may be associated with the damage to the brain. Occasionally continuous pacing and wandering can cause the person's feet to swell.

Some people wander at night. This can be dangerous for the impaired person and exhausting for you. Night wandering can have different causes, from simple disorientation to a seemingly incomprehensible part of the brain injury.

Many of us can sympathise with the confused person's experience of becoming disoriented. We may have lost our car in a car park or become disoriented in a strange place. For a few minutes we feel unnerved until we get hold of ourselves and work out a logical way to find out where we are. The person with a memory impairment is more likely to panic, is less able to 'get hold of himself' and may feel that he must keep his disorientation a secret.

When wandering is made worse by a move to a new home or by some other change in the environment, it may be because it is difficult for a confused, memory-impaired person to learn his way around in a new setting. He may not be able to understand that he has moved and is determined to go 'home'. The stress of such a change may impair his remaining abilities, which makes it harder for him to learn his way around.

Aimless wandering may be the person's way of saying, 'I feel lost. I am searching for the things I feel I have lost.' Sometimes wandering behaviour is the person's way of trying to communicate feelings.

Mr Griffiths was a vigorous man of sixty who kept leaving the day centre. The police would pick him up several miles away, walking along the main road. Mr Griffiths always explained that he was going to Cardiff. Cardiff represented home, friends, security and family to Mr Griffiths.

Wandering may be the person's way of expressing restlessness, boredom or the need for exercise. It may help to fill the need of an active person to be 'doing something'. It may also signal a need to use the toilet.

A constant or agitated pacing or a determination to get away may be difficult to manage. Sometimes this is a catastrophic reaction. Something may be upsetting the person. He may not be able to make sense out of his surroundings or may be misinterpreting what he sees or hears. Sometimes this agitated wandering appears to be a direct result of the brain damage. It is hard to know exactly what is happening to the brain, but we do know that brain function can be seriously and extensively disrupted. Remind yourself that this is not a behaviour that the person can control.

Management of wandering

The management of wandering behaviour depends on the cause of the wandering. If the person is getting lost, and if you are sure he can still read and follow instructions, a card in his pocket may help him. Write *simple* instructions on a card he can carry in his pocket and refer to if he is lost. You might put at the top of the card the written reminder, 'Stay calm and don't walk away.' You might write your telephone number on the card, or put, 'Ask a shop assistant to show you to the men's wear department and stay there. I will come for you.' You may need different cards for different outings. This will make it possible for a mildly confused person to help himself.

It is essential that you buy the person a bracelet with his name and your telephone number on it, together with the statement 'memory impaired'. A bracelet that is securely fastened (so the patient cannot take it off) and too small to slip off is the most practical. This information will help anyone who finds the person if he gets lost. You can have an inexpensive bracelet engraved at a shop that engraves rings, tankards, key rings, etc. Have a 'memory impaired' bracelet made now if there is any possibility that the person will wander or get lost. A lost, confused person will be afraid and upset, and this can cause him to resist help. He may be ignored or be assumed to be crazy by the people around him. Under stress he may function more poorly than usual.

Also available are Medic Alert bracelets and necklaces, and SOS talismans which give information regarding the wearer and a telephone number to contact. These can be obtained from the Medic Alert Foundation, 12 Bridge Wharf, 156 Caledonian Road, London N1 9UU, (tel: 071-833 3034) or Talman Ltd, 21 Grays Corner, Ley Street, Ilford, Essex 1GU 7RQ (tel: 081-554 5579). You could also try recording details in a personal information wallet – bearing a 'disabled' motif and obtained from the Hertfordshire Association for the Disabled (County Office), The Woodside Centre, The Commons, Welwyn-Garden City, Herts. AL7 4DD (tel: 0707 324581).

Some forgetful people are happy to carry a card which gives their name, address and phone number in their pocket or wallet. Others, however, will lose it or throw it away. It is still worth trying.

To reduce increased wandering when the person moves to a new environment, you may want to plan in advance of the move to make it as easy as possible for the impaired person. When a person is still able to understand and participate in what is going on around him, it may help to introduce him gradually to his new situation. If he is moving to a new home, involve him in planning the move (see page 57) and visit the new home as often as possible before he moves. When a person's impairment makes it impossible for him to understand what is happening, it may be easier not to introduce him gradually but simply to make the move as quietly and with as little fuss as possible. Each person is unique. Try to balance his need to participate in decision making with his ability to understand. If you have a choice, make a move early in the illness; it will probably be easier for the person to adjust then and learn his way around.

If you are considering a day care centre, we urge you to do so early in the illness. (See Chapter 10.) Day care centres and care homes have found that people adjust best when

1   they do not stay for a long time on the first few visits;
2   the care-giver stays with them the first few times; and
3   someone from the centre or home visits them at home before the transition.

Leaving a confused person alone to adjust or asking the family not to visit at first may add to the person's panic.

When a confused person finds himself in a new place, he may feel that he is lost, that you cannot find him, or that he is not supposed to be where he is. Reassure the disoriented person often about where he is and why he is there. 'You have come to live with me, Father. Here is your room with your things in it,' or 'You are at the day centre. You will go home at 3.'

Families tell us 'It doesn't work!' when we give this advice. It doesn't work in the sense that the person may continue to insist that he doesn't live here and to keep trying to wander away. This is because he is memory impaired and does not remember what you told him. He still needs to be gently and frequently reassured about his whereabouts. It takes time and patience to get him to accept the move and gradually come to feel secure. He also needs frequent reassurance that you know where he is. A gentle reassurance and your understanding of his confusion will help to reduce his fear and the number of catastrophic reactions he has. Our experience with people who are admitted to hospital for their dementia is that, even with difficult patients, frequent gentle reassurance about where they are sometimes helps them settle down and become easier to manage. However, this may take several (five to seven) days.

A move often upsets a person with a dementing illness, causing him to wander more, or making his behaviour worse for a period of time. It is helpful to know that this is usually a temporary crisis.

Because changes may make the person's behaviour or wandering worse, it is important to consider changes carefully. You may decide that a holiday or an extended visit is not worth the upset to the confused person.

When the wandering seems to be aimless, some professionals suspect that exercise helps to reduce this restlessness. Try taking the person for a long, vigorous walk each day. You may have to continue an activity plan for several weeks before you see whether it is making a difference.

When wandering seems to be the person's way of saying, 'I feel lost' or 'I am searching for the things I feel I have lost', you can help by surrounding the person with familiar things, such as pictures of his family. Make him feel welcome by talking to him or by taking time to have a cup of tea with him.

Agitated pacing or determined efforts to wander away are sometimes caused by frequent or almost constant catastrophic reactions. Ask yourself what may be precipitating such catastrophic reactions. Does this behaviour happen at about the same time each day? Does it happen each time the person is asked to do a certain thing (like take a bath)? Review the way people around the confused person are responding to his wandering. Does their response increase his restlessness and wandering? If you must restrain a person or go after him, try to distract him rather than directly confronting him. Tell him you will walk with him and then lead him around in a big circle. Usually he will accompany you back into the house. Talking calmly can reassure him and prevent a catastrophic reaction that will change aimless wandering into a determination to escape. Wandering can often be reduced by creating an environment that calms the person.

When Mrs Davies came into the hospital, she had been making constant, determined efforts to leave the nursing home. In the hospital, which was also a strange place, the nurses had much less difficulty with her. In both places Mrs Davies felt lost. She knew this was not where she lived and she wanted to go home. Also, she was lonely; she wanted to go back to her job, where her confused mind remembered friends and a sense of belonging. So she wandered towards the door. The overworked nursing staff at the nursing home would yell loudly to her, 'Come back here!' After a few days, one of the other residents in the home began to 'help'. 'Mrs Davies has escaped again!' she would shout. The noise confused Mrs Davies, who doubled her efforts to get out. This brought a nurse on the run; Mrs Davies would panic and run away as fast as she could, straight into a busy street. When an attendant caught her arm and held her, Mrs Davies bit him. This happened several times, exhausting the staff and precipitating almost constant catastrophic reactions. The family was told that Mrs Davies was unmanageable.

Once she was in hospital Mrs Davies headed for the door almost at once. However, rather than attempting to call her back, a nurse approached her quietly and suggested they have a cup of tea together (distraction rather than confrontation). Mrs Davies never stopped wandering to the door, but her vigorous effort to escape and aggressive behaviour did stop.

If you think the person is wandering because he is restless, try giving him some active task like dusting or stacking books. Day centre care may provide things to do as well as companionship and therefore can be beneficial for those who wander.

Medication may reduce the patient's restlessness. However, some drugs can induce restlessness as a side effect so medication must be closely supervised by a doctor. Occasionally, the judicious use of major tranquillisers, under close medical supervision, can lessen wandering significantly. *They should only be used after all non-drug interventions have been tried.*

If incessant wandering causes the person's feet to swell, try sitting down with him and helping him to put his feet up. He may sit still as long as you sit with him. Other measures may be necessary if you still cannot get him off his feet. Ask your GP to examine the patient should he develop swollen or injured feet. The discomfort can make the person's behaviour worse.

Changing the environment to protect the person is an important part of coping with wandering. One family found that the confused person would not go outside if he did not have his shoes on. Taking his shoes away and giving him slippers kept him inside.

It is often helpful to install locks that are difficult to undo or that are unfamiliar to the confused person, so that he cannot go outside unsupervised. Sometimes inexpensive devices such as a spring-operated latch are sufficient because the impaired person cannot learn the new skill of opening them. A confused person is less likely to look for a lock at the bottom of the door. Make sure you can undo the locks quickly in case of a fire. There is an inexpensive plastic gadget available in hardware stores called a child-proof door knob which slips over the existing knob. You can still open the door, but the confused person cannot work out how to operate it.

Check other means of exit as well as doors. Confused people may climb out of upper storey windows. Secure locks protect you as well as ensuring the person's safety. The police can advise you about inexpensive ways of securing your windows and doors.

If the person does go outside, be alert to hazards in the neighbourhood such as busy streets or dogs. The person may no longer possess the judgement to protect himself from these things. You may want to walk through the neighbourhood in which the person lives and look around thoughtfully for things that are dangerous for a person who no longer has the ability to assess his surroundings appropriately. At the same time, you may want to alert people in the neighbourhood to the problem, reassuring them that the person is not crazy or dangerous but just disoriented.

The person himself can be his own worst enemy. When he looks healthy and acts in a reasonable manner, people tend to forget that he may have lost the judgement to keep him from stepping in front of a car.

Other people are also an environmental hazard to the confused person who wanders. In addition to those who don't understand are the cruel and vicious who seek out elderly and frail people in order to harass, torment or rob them. Unfortunately, there seem to be enough such people, even in the 'nicest' neighbourhoods, for you to need to recognise this hazard and protect the confused person from them.

Various physical devices are available to restrain a person in a chair or bed. The decision to use a restraint should be made jointly between you and the health care professional who knows the person best, and it should be used *only after all other possibilities have been tried*. (We are addressing here the use of restraints at home. The use of restraints in a hospital or residential nursing home involves other issues and are discussed in Chapter 16.) Restraining straps used by wheelchair users can be adapted for use with demented people. Contact the Disabled Living Foundation Information Service or your local wheelchair service.

Nurses occasionally find that a restraint, especially at night, provides the person with a firm reassurance that he must stay where he is. However, restraints further agitate some people. Either a restraint or a harness may help to keep a person still and safe long enough for you to take a bath or prepare supper.

Very agitated people can hurt themselves fighting against the bed while in restraints, or may tip over a chair in which they are restrained. People cannot be left unsupervised for long periods in either harnesses or restraints of any kind. Never leave a person alone in the house while he is restrained, because of the possibility of a fire. You should be able to release any restraining device quickly in an emergency.

You may reach a point when the wandering behaviour is more than you can manage or when a person cannot be kept safely in a home setting. If this time comes, you will have done all you can, and will need to plan realistically for institutional care for the person. Many places will not accept a patient who is agitated, aggressive, or a wanderer. See Chapter 6 for a discussion of placement issues.

Sleep disturbances; night wandering

Many people with dementing illnesses are restless at night. They may wake to go to the bathroom and become confused and disoriented in the dark. They may wander around the house, get dressed, try to cook or even go outside. They may 'see things' or 'hear things' that are not there. Few things are more distressing than having your much needed sleep disrupted night after night. Fortunately, there are ways of reducing this behaviour.

Older people seem to need less sleep than younger people. People with dementing illnesses may not be getting enough exercise to make them tired at night, or they may be dozing during the day. Often it seems that the internal 'clock' within the brain is damaged by the dementing illness. Some night-time behaviour problems may result from dreams that the impaired person cannot separate from reality.

If the person is napping during the day, he will be less tired at night. Try to keep him occupied, active and awake in the daytime. If he is taking tranquillising drugs to control his behaviour, these may be making him drowsy during the day. Discuss with the doctor the possibility of giving most of the tranquilliser in the evening instead of spreading the dose throughout the day. This may provide the behaviour control without making the person sleepy during the day. If he must sleep during the day, try to get some rest yourself at the same time.

Often people with dementing illnesses are not very active and don't get much exercise. It may be helpful to plan a regular activity – a long walk, for example – in the late afternoon. This may make the person tired enough to sleep better at night. A car ride makes some people sleepy.

See that the person has been to the toilet before going to sleep.

Older people may not see as well in the dark and this may add to their confusion. As our eyes age, it becomes more difficult to distinguish dim shapes in poor light. The confused person may misinterpret what he sees, so he thinks he sees people or thinks he is in some other place. This can cause catastrophic reactions. Leave a night light on in the bedroom and bathroom. Night lights in other rooms may also help the person orient himself. Reflector tape around the bathroom door may help. Try putting a commode right beside the bed.

Many of us have had the experience of waking from a sound sleep and momentarily not knowing where we are. This sensation may be magnified for the confused person. Your quiet reassurance may be all that is needed.

Ensure that the sleeping arrangements are comfortable, that the room is neither too warm nor too cool, and the bedding is comfortable. Continental quilts are less likely to tangle than blankets and sheets. Cotsides and bedrails help some people remember they are in bed. Other people get upset and try to climb over them, which is dangerous. Cotsides and bedrails can be fitted to most beds and may be loaned or provided by local Social Services or the Community Health Service. Information on the purchase of cotsides and bedrails can be obtained from the Disabled Living Foundation Information Service.

If the confused person gets up in the night, speak softly and quietly to him. When you are awakened suddenly in the night, you may respond irritably and speak crossly. This may precipitate a catastrophic reaction in the impaired person, which will wake everybody in the house. Often all that is needed is gently to remind the person that it is still night-time and that he should go back to bed. A person will often go back to sleep after he has had a cup of warm milk. Encourage him to go back to bed and sit with him quietly while he drinks his milk. A radio playing softly will soothe some people. Quietly remind the disoriented person that it is dark and the curtains are drawn, and therefore it is time to stay in bed.

Sometimes a person who will not sleep in bed will sleep in a lounge chair or on a sofa. If the person gets up in the night and gets dressed, he may sit back down again and fall asleep in his clothes if you don't interfere. It may be better to accept this than to be up part of the night arguing about it.

If the person does wander at night, you must examine your house for safety hazards. Arrange the bedroom so the person can move around safely. Lock the window. Can he turn on the cooker or start a fire while you are sleeping? Can he unlock and walk out through the outside doors? Can he, while trying to go to the bathroom, fall down the stairs? A gate across the stairs may be essential in a house where a disoriented person sleeps.

Finally, if these measures fail, sedative-hypnotics are helpful. However, you cannot simply give the person a sleeping pill and solve the problem. Sedatives affect the chemistry of the brain, which is complex and sensitive. Your doctor faces a series of difficult, interacting problems when he begins to prescribe sedatives. Sedatives can have numerous side effects, some of which are serious.

Older people, including those who have no impairment, are more subject to side effects from drugs than are younger people and elderly brain-injured people are even more sensitive to drugs. Older people are more likely to be taking other drugs that can interact with a sedative or to have other illnesses that can be aggravated by a sedative.

Sedating the person may make him sleep in the daytime instead of at night or it may have a hangover effect that worsens his cognitive functioning during the day. The sedative can make him more confused, more vulnerable to falls, or incontinent. Paradoxically, it may even worsen sleep. Each person is different; what works for one may not work for another.

The effect of the sedative may change – for many reasons – after it has been used for a while. Your doctor may have to try first one drug and then another, carefully adjusting the dosage and the time at which it is given. Drugs may not make the person sleep all night. Therefore, it is important that you do all you can to help the person sleep using other methods. This does not mean that we discourage the use of sedatives; they are a very useful tool, but only one of several tools used to manage a difficult problem. When the person is living at home, the doctor may prescribe sleeping medication for him so that you can get some rest. However, this may not need to be done in a nursing home where adequate, caring staff can use other interventions.

Worsening in the evening

People with dementing illnesses often seem to have more behaviour problems in the evening. We do not know what causes this. It may be that the person cannot see clearly in dim light and misinterprets what he sees, causing catastrophic reactions. Leaving lights on often helps. Telling the person where he is and what is happening may also be useful.

A whole day of trying to cope with confusing perceptions of the environment may be tiring, so a person's tolerance for stress is lower at the end of the day. You are also more tired and may subtly communicate your fatigue to the confused person, so causing catastrophic reactions.

Plan the person's day so that fewer things are expected of him in the evening. A bath (which is often difficult), for example, might be timed for morning or mid-afternoon if this works better.

Sometimes there are more things going on at once in the house in the evening. This may overstimulate the already confused and tired person. For example, do you turn on the TV? Are more people in the house in the evening? Are you busy preparing supper? Are children coming in? Being tired may make it harder for him to understand what is going on and may cause him to have catastrophic reactions.

If possible, try to reduce the number of things going on around the person at his worst times of day, or try to confine the family activity to an area away from the impaired person. It is also important to try to plan your day so that you are reasonably rested and not too pressed for time at the times of day that you observe are worst for the confused person. For example, if he gets most upset while you are getting supper, try to plan meals that are quick and easy, that are left over from lunch, or that you can prepare in advance. Eat the larger meal at midday, if possible.

Sometimes the trouble is that the person wants your constant attention and becomes more demanding when you are busy with other things. Perhaps you can occupy the person with a simple task close to you while you work, or get someone else in the family to spend some time with him.

You may want to talk to the doctor about changing the timing of medication if other methods don't help.

Periods of restlessness or sleeplessness may be an unavoidable part of the brain injury. Reassure yourself that the person is not doing this deliberately, even though it may seem as if he is 'acting up' at the times of day that are hardest for you.

Losing and hiding things

Most people with dementing illnesses put things down and forget where they have put them. Others hide things and forget where they have hidden them. Either way, the result is the same; just when you need them most, the person's dentures or your car keys have vanished and cannot be found.

First, remember that you probably cannot ask the impaired person where he has put the item. He will not remember, and you may precipitate a catastrophic reaction by asking.

There are several things you can do to reduce this problem. A neat house makes it easier to locate misplaced items whereas it is almost impossible to find something hidden in a cluttered cupboard or drawer. Limit the number of hiding places by locking some cupboards or rooms.

Take away valuable items such as rings or silver so they cannot be hidden and lost. Do not keep a significant amount of cash around the house. Make small, easily lost items larger and/or more visible – for example, put your key on a large key ring. Have a spare set of necessary items such as keys, spectacles and hearing aid batteries, if at all possible.

Get into the habit of checking the contents of wastepaper baskets before you empty them. Check under mattresses, under sofa cushions, in wastepaper baskets, in shoes and in desk drawers for lost items. Ask yourself where the confused person used to put things for security. Where did he hide Christmas gifts or money? These are good places to look for lost dentures.

Some people hoard or save food, dirty clothes or other possessions (see page 155). Some people hoard things because they have always collected things. Others seem to need to 'hold on' to something or to 'keep things safe'. If this happens occasionally, it is best to ignore it. If possible, when you tidy up, leave a little of the person's 'hoard'. He may feel less need to add to the collection than he would if he found his supply wiped out.

One daughter said, 'I solved my problem when I decided that it was all right to keep the silver in the laundry basket. Now I look for it there instead of carrying it back to the dining-room several times a day.'

Rummaging in drawers and cupboards

Some people rummage through drawers or take everything out of cupboards. This makes a mess for you to tidy up. It can be particularly upsetting when they rummage through other people's things. You may find it necessary to put hard-to-work latches on some drawers and cupboards. You may need to keep dangerous or valuable things in one lockable drawer, or you may have to move such things to a safer place. If there are young people in the household, they especially will need a private and unmolested place. It may help to fill a top drawer or a box on top of the chest of drawers with interesting things for the person to sort through. Small tools and machine parts will appeal to one person while sewing supplies might interest another.

Inappropriate sexual behaviour

Sometimes confused people take off their clothes and wander naked out into the living-room or down the street. For example:

One teenage boy came home to find his father sitting in the back garden reading the newspaper. He was naked except for his hat.

Occasionally, confused people will expose themselves in public. Sometimes very confused people will fondle their genitals. Or they will fidget in such a way that their fidgeting reminds others of sexual behaviour, which is upsetting.

One man repeatedly undid his belt buckle and unzipped his trousers.

A woman kept fidgeting with the buttons of her blouse.

Sometimes brain damage will cause a person to demand sexual activities frequently or inappropriately. But much more common than actual inappropriate sexual behaviour is the myth that 'senile' people will develop inappropriate sexual behaviour.

One wife who asked for her husband to be referred to the hospital for care confessed that she had no problems managing him but that she had been told that, as he got worse, he would go into his 'second childhood' and start exposing himself to little girls.

There is *no* basis to this myth. Inappropriate sexual behaviour in people with dementing illnesses is uncommon. In a study of patients we found no instances of such behaviour.

Accidental self-exposure and aimless masturbation do sometimes occur. Confused people may wander out in public undressed or partially dressed simply because they have forgotten where they are, how to dress, or the importance of being dressed. They may undo their clothes or lift up a skirt because they need to urinate and have forgotten where the bathroom is. They may undress because they want to go to bed or because a garment is uncomfortable. Urinary tract infections, itching or discomfort may lead to handling the genital area. Check with your doctor.

Don't over-react to this. Just lead the person calmly back to his room or to the bathroom. If you find the person undressed, calmly bring him a dressing-gown and matter-of-factly help him put it on. The man who sat naked in the garden had taken off his clothes because it was hot. He was unable to recognise that he was outside, was in sight of other people, and was not in the privacy of his home. Most confused people will never exhibit this kind of behaviour because their lifelong habits of modesty remain.

Undressing or fidgeting with clothing can often be stopped by changing the kind of clothing the person wears. For example, use trousers that pull on instead of trousers with a fly in them. Find blouses that slip on or zip up the back instead of buttoning in front. If a person's fidgeting is suggestive or embarrassing, try giving him something else to do or something else to fidget with.

In our culture we have strong negative feelings about masturbation and such actions are upsetting to most families. Remember, this behaviour, when it occurs, is a part of the brain damage. The person is only doing what feels good. He has forgotten his social manners. This does not mean that the person will develop other offensive sexual behaviour. If masturbation occurs, try not to appear upset, because it may precipitate a catastrophic reaction. Gently lead the person to a private place. Try distracting him by giving him something else to do.

We know of no case in which a person with a dementing illness has exposed himself to a child and we do not wish to contribute to the myths about 'dirty old men' by focusing on such behaviour. However, should such an incident occur, react matter-of-factly and without creating any more fuss than is absolutely necessary. Your reaction may have much more impact on the child than the actual incident. Remove the person quietly and explain to the child, 'He forgets where he is'.

We have observed that some people with dementing illnesses have a diminished sex drive, and some have more interest in sex than they did previously. If a person develops increased sexuality, remember that, however distressing this is, it is a factor of the brain injury. It is not a factor of personality, or a reflection on you or your marriage (see page 224).

Occasionally a father may make inappropriate advances to his daughter. *This is not incestuous behaviour.* While this can be upsetting for everyone, it usually only means that he is disoriented. Probably he has mistaken his daughter for his wife. Daughters often look much as their mothers did when the mother was young. The confused person may remember that time much more clearly than the present. Such gestures indicate that he does remember his wife and their marriage. Gently redirect him and try not to be too distressed.

Don't hesitate to discuss upsetting sexual behaviour with your doctor, a counsellor, or even other families. They can help you understand and cope with it. The person you choose should be knowledgeable about dementia and comfortable discussing sexual matters. He may make specific suggestions to reduce the behaviour. (Also see Chapters 12 and 16.)

Changing annoying behaviour

Sometimes it is the little things that the impaired person does which really upset you. You may have some success reducing or eliminating this annoying behaviour using the following method.

First, select *one* specific behaviour that occurs often and that you would really like to change. You will have most success with certain kinds of behaviour, such as the annoying habit of repeating questions. Behaviours that arise out of catastrophic reactions are not easily changed by this method but are best managed by eliminating the precipitating cause.

Repeating the question

Many families find that confused people ask the same question over and over and that this is extremely irritating. In part, this may be a symptom of the fear and insecurity of a person who can no longer make sense of his surroundings. The person may not remember things for even brief periods, so he may have no recollection of having asked you before or of your answer.

One husband was particularly upset when his wife asked every night, 'Who are you? What are you doing in my bed?' He stopped trying to explain to her and simply began ignoring the question. He would turn his head away slightly or turn his back on her and pretend she had not said anything. Eventually she stopped asking.

This will work with some people but it will upset others, who will get angry because you did not answer them. Use whatever system works for you.

Sometimes, instead of answering the question again, it is helpful to reassure the person that everything is fine and that you will take care of things. Sometimes the person is really worried about something else, which he is unable to express. If you can correctly guess what this is and reassure him, he may relax. For example:

> *Mr Rockwell's mother kept asking, 'When is my mother coming for me?' When Mr Rockwell told her that her mother had been dead for many years, she would either get upset or ask the question again in a few minutes. Mr Rockwell realised that the question really expressed her feelings that she was lost, and began responding by saying, 'I will take care of you.' This obviously calmed his mother.*

Mr Rockwell might also have tried saying, 'Tell me about your mother' or 'Do you remember when your mother took us to the play?'

Repetitious actions

An occasional and distressing behaviour that may occur in people with a brain disease is the tendency to repeat the same action over and over again.

> *Mrs Weber's mother-in-law folded the laundry over and over again. Mrs Weber was glad the older woman was occupied, but this same activity upset her husband. He would shout, 'Mother, you have already folded that towel five times!'*

> *Mrs Andrews had trouble with baths. She would wash just one side of her face. 'Wash the other side,' her daughter would say, but she kept on washing the same spot.*

> *Mr Barnes paces around and around the kitchen in the same pattern, like a bear in a cage.*

It seems as if the damaged mind has a tendency to 'get stuck' on one activity and has difficulty changing gear to a new activity. When this happens, gently suggest that the person carries out a specific new task, but try not to pressure him or sound upset, because you can easily precipitate a catastrophic reaction.

In the case of Mrs Weber's mother-in-law, ignoring the problem worked well. As Mr Weber came to accept his mother's illness, the behaviour ceased to bother him.

Mrs Andrew's daughter found out that gently patting her mother's cheek, where she wanted her to wash next, would release her from the repetitious pattern. In this example, a stroke had lessened her mother's awareness of one side of her body. Touch is a very good way of transmitting a message to the brain when words fail. Touch the arm you want a person to put into a sleeve; touch the place you want the person to wash next; touch a person's hand with a spoon to get them to pick it up.

Mr Barnes's wife found ways of stopping his pacing by giving him something else to do. 'Here, Joe, hold this,' she would say, and hand him a spoon. She would then say, 'Now hold this' and take the spoon and give him an oven glove. 'Helping' would enable Mr Barnes to stop pacing. It kept him busy and perhaps also made him feel needed.

Distractability

People with dementia may 'get stuck' or be too easily distracted. The person may look elsewhere or grab at other things while you are trying to dress him; he may eat the food on someone else's plate; he may walk off while you are talking to him. Part of our brain filters out things we do not want to pay attention to – this is how you 'tune out' unimportant noises, for example. When the dementing illness damages this ability, the person may be equally attracted to everything that is happening, no matter how unimportant it may be.

If you can identify the things that distract him – people, animals, and sudden noises are common distractions – and reduce them, he may be better able to focus on one activity, such as dressing. Put his plate a little farther from the other plates; have fewer visitors at once; make visits to calm, quiet areas. If he is distracted by the television or radio, turn them off. Plan eating and other activities in an area where other people are not moving about and talking.

Clinging or persistently following you around

Families tell us that forgetful people sometimes follow them from room to room, becoming fretful if the care-giver disappears into the bathroom.

Or they constantly interrupt whenever the care-giver tries to rest or to complete a job. This can be distressing. Few things can irritate more than being followed around all the time.

This behaviour can be understood when we consider how strange the world must seem to a person who constantly forgets. The trusted care-giver becomes the only security in a world of confusion. When one cannot depend on oneself to remember the necessary things in life, a form of security is to stick close to someone who does know.

The memory-impaired person cannot remember that if you go into the bathroom, you will soon be out again. To him, with his confused sense of time, it may seem as if you have vanished. A child-proof door-knob on the bathroom door may give you a few minutes of privacy. Sometimes setting a timer and saying, 'I will be back when the timer goes off' will help. One husband bought a set of headphones so that he could listen to music while his wife continued to talk. (Then he bought her a set because he discovered that she enjoyed the music.)

It is most important that you try not to let annoying behaviours such as these wear you down. You must find other people who will sit with the person so that you can get away and do the things that relax you – go visiting or shopping, take a nap, or enjoy an uninterrupted bath.

Using medication to stop behaviours like this is often unsuccessful and the side effects can be disabling. Unless the behaviour places the person with dementia or someone else in danger, medication should be used only after other solutions have failed.

Find simple tasks that the person can carry out, even if they are things that you could do better or things that are repetitive. Winding a ball of wool, dusting or stacking magazines may make a person feel useful and will keep him occupied while you do your work.

Mrs Hunter's mother-in-law, who has a dementing illness, followed Mrs Hunter around the house never letting her out of her sight and always criticising. Mrs Hunter hit upon the idea of encouraging her mother-in-law to fold up the washing. Since Mrs Hunter has a large family, she has a lot of washing. The older woman folds, unfolds and refolds (not very neatly), and feels that she is a useful part of the household.

Is it being unkind to give a person made-up tasks to keep her occupied? Mrs Hunter doesn't think so. The confused woman needs to feel that she is contributing to the family and she needs to be active.

Complaints and insults

Sometimes people with dementing illnesses repeatedly complain, despite your kindest efforts. The confused person may say things like, 'You are cruel to me', 'I want to go home', 'You stole my things' or 'I don't like you'. When you are doing all that you can to help, you may feel hurt or angry when the confused person says such things. When he looks and sounds well, or when such criticism comes from someone you have looked up to, your first response may be to take the criticism personally. You can quickly become involved in a painful and pointless argument, which may cause him to have a catastrophic reaction and perhaps even scream, cry and throw things at you, leaving you exhausted and upset.

If this happens, step back and think through what is happening. Even though the person looks well, he actually has an injury to his brain. The experiences of having to be cared for, feeling lost, and losing possessions and independence may seem cruel to the confused person. 'You are cruel to me' may really mean 'Life is cruel to me'. Because the person cannot accurately sort out the reality around him, he may misinterpret your efforts to help as stealing from him. He may not be able to accept, understand or remember the facts of his increasing impairment, his financial situation, the past relationship he had with you, and all of the other things you are aware of. For example, he knows only that his things are gone and you are there. Therefore, he feels that you must have stolen his things.

One family member contributed the following interpretations of the things her husband often said. Of course, we cannot know what a brain-impaired person feels or means, but his wife has found loving ways to interpret and accept the painful things her husband says.

He says:	*'I want to go home.'*
He means:	*'I want to go back to the condition of life, the quality of life, when everything seemed to have a purpose and I was useful, when I could see the product of my hands, and when I was without the fear of small things.'*
He says:	*'I don't want to die.'*
He means:	*'I am ill although I feel no pain. Nobody realises just how ill I am. I feel this way all of the time, so I must be going to die. I am afraid of dying.'*
He says:	*'I have no money.'*
He means:	*'I used to carry a wallet with some money in it. It is not in the back pocket of my trousers now. I am angry because I cannot find it. There is something at the shops that I want to buy. I'll have to keep looking.'*
He says:	*'Where is everyone?'*

He means: '*I see people around me, but I don't know who they are. These unfamiliar faces do not belong to my family. Where is my mother? Why has she left me?*'

In coping with remarks such as these, avoid contradicting the person or arguing with him; those responses may lead to a catastrophic reaction. Try not to say, 'I didn't steal your things', 'You are home', 'I gave you some money'. Try not to reason with the person. Saying, 'Your mother died thirty years ago' will only confuse and upset him more.

Some families find it helpful to ignore many of these complaints or to use distractions. Some families respond sympathetically to the feeling they think is being expressed: 'Yes, dear, I know you feel lost', 'Life does seem cruel', 'I know you want to go home'.

Of course, you may become angry sometimes, especially when you have heard the same unfair complaint over and over again. To do so is human. Probably the confused person will quickly forget the incident.

Sometimes the impaired person loses the ability to be tactful. He may say, 'I don't like John' and you may know he never did like this person. This can be upsetting. It helps for those involved to understand that the person is unable to be tactful, that while he may be being honest he is not being purposefully unkind.

Perhaps you can cope with these remarks, but what about other people? Sometimes people with dementing illnesses make inappropriate or insulting remarks to other people. These can range from naive directness, such as telling the minister's wife she has a ladder in her tights, to insults, such as shouting at the neighbour who brings lunch, 'Get out of my house, you're trying to poison us!'

Confused people may tell casual friends or strangers stories such as 'My daughter keeps me locked in my room.' When you take a confused person to visit someone, he may put on his coat and say, 'Let's go home. This place stinks.'

Each brain-impaired person is different. Some will retain their social skills. In others, a tendency toward bluntness may emerge as open rudeness. Some are fearful and suspicious, leading them to make accusations. Catastrophic reactions account for some of this behaviour. The confused person often misjudges who the person is that he is speaking to, or he misjudges the situation.

A secretary was talking with a confused man while the doctor talked to his wife. He was obviously trying to make polite conversation, but he had lost the subtlety he once had. 'How old are you?' he asked, 'You look pretty old.' When she answered another question that no, she was not married, he said, 'I suppose no one would have you.'

People chuckle at this sort of behaviour in a small child because everyone understands that a child has not yet learned good manners. It will be helpful to you if most of the people around you understand that the person has a dementing illness that affects his memory of good manners. Dementing illnesses are common enough now and, as public awareness develops, more people will recognise that this behaviour is the result of specific diseases. Sad as it is, such behaviour is not deliberate.

To those people who see you and the confused person often, such as neighbours, friends, church members and perhaps familiar shop assistants, you may want to give a brief explanation of the person's illness. When you make this explanation, you should reassure people that this illness does not make the person dangerous and that the person is not crazy. Some care-givers have cards printed which say something like: 'Please pardon my family member who has Alzheimer's disease. Although she looks well, this disease has destroyed her memory.' You may want to add a few lines about the disease and how to find out more about it.

Should a confused person create a scene in a public place, perhaps due to a catastrophic reaction, remove him gently. It may be best to say nothing. While this can be embarrassing, you do not necessarily owe strangers any explanation.

Distraction is a good way of extricating a confused person from what might become an embarrassing situation. For example, if he is asking personal questions, change the subject. When a person is telling others that you are keeping him prisoner or not feeding him, try distracting him. Avoid denying statements directly, as this can turn into an argument with the confused person. If these are people you know, you may want to explain to them later. If they are strangers, ask yourself whether it really matters what strangers think.

Sometimes there is a gossip or insensitive person in a community who may build upon the inappropriate remarks of a person with a dementing illness. It is important that you should not be upset by such gossip. Usually other people have an accurate estimate of the truth of this gossip.

Taking things

Confused people may pick up things in shops and not pay for them, or may accuse the shop assistants of stealing their money. One wife reported that her husband was stealing and butchering the neighbour's chickens. He did not realise they were not his own and was proud to be helping with dinner.

If a person is taking things from shops, he may be doing so because he has forgotten to pay for them or because he does not realise that he is in a shop. Several families have found that giving the person things to hold or asking him to push the shopping trolley, so that his hands are occupied, will stop the problem. Before you leave the shop, check to see if he has anything in his pockets. You may want to dress him in something that has no pockets the next time you go shopping.

If the person continues to take items, you might ask your doctor for a brief letter explaining that the person has Alzheimer's disease and sometimes forgets that he has put things in his pockets. If the person does take something and you discover and return it later, or if he is caught by security personnel, you can show them this letter.

The wife of the man who took the chickens arranged for her clergyman to explain things to the neighbours and then arranged to replace any chickens that turned up on her dinner table.

Forgetting telephone calls

Forgetful people who can still talk clearly often continue to answer the telephone or to make calls. However, they may not remember to write down telephone messages. This can upset friends, confuse people, and cause you considerable inconvenience and embarrassment.

Inexpensive telephone call recorders (sold at electrical shops) will record all telephone conversations. (See page 97.) Attaching the device to an extension which the impaired person does not often use may be wise. With this taped record, you can phone people back, explain the situation and respond to their call.

> One husband writes, 'I found out from the tape that she called the dentist five times about her appointment. Since I knew about it, I called them and told them how to manage that.'

You may want to find out from the telephone company under what circumstances it is legal to tape-record calls. Telephone companies can offer a call-forwarding service, which will transfer calls that come to your home to another telephone number. British Telecom Freephone 150 will advise on this and other problems with the use of a telephone.

Demands

> Mr Cooper refused to stop living alone, even though it was clear to his family that he could not manage. Instead, he called his daughter at least once a day

with 'real' emergencies that sent her dashing over to help out. His daughter felt angry and manipulated. She was neglecting her own family and she was exhausted. She felt that her father had always been a self-centred, demanding person, and that his current behaviour was deliberately selfish.

Mrs Dawes lived with her daughter. The two women had never got along well and now Mrs Dawes had Alzheimer's disease. She was wearing her daughter out with demands: 'Get me a cigarette', 'Make me some coffee'. The daughter could not tell her mother to do these things for herself because she started fires.

Sometimes people with dementing illnesses can be demanding and seem to be self-centred. This is especially hard to accept when the person does not appear to be significantly impaired. If you feel that this is happening, try to step back and objectively assess the situation. Is this behaviour deliberate or is it a symptom of the disease? The two can look very much alike, especially when the person had a way of making people feel manipulated before he developed a dementing brain disease. However, what is often happening with an impaired person is *not* something he can control. Manipulative behaviour really requires the ability to plan, which the person with a dementing illness is losing. What you experience are old styles of relating to others which are no longer really deliberate. An assessment can be helpful because it tells you objectively how much of the behaviour is something the person can remember to do or not to do.

Some demanding behaviour reflects the impaired person's feelings of loneliness, fright or loss. For example, when a person has lost his ability to comprehend the passage of time and to remember things, being left alone for a short time can make him feel that he has been abandoned and he may accuse you of deserting him. Realising that this behaviour reflects such feelings can help you feel less angry and it can also help you respond to the real problem (for example, that he feels abandoned) instead of responding to what appears to you to be selfishness or manipulation.

Sometimes you can devise ways in which the confused person can continue to feel a sense of control over his life without being so demanding of you:

Mr Cooper's daughter was able to find a flat for her father in a sheltered housing scheme where meals were provided. This reduced the number of emergencies but enabled Mr Cooper to continue to feel independent.

A medical assessment confirmed for Mrs Dawes's daughter that her mother could not remember her previous requests for a cigarette for even five minutes. With the help of the doctor, she was able to deal with her mother's addiction to cigarettes and coffee.

Families often ask whether they should 'spoil' the person by meeting his demands or whether they should try to 'teach' him to behave differently. The best course may be neither of these. Since he cannot control his behaviour, you are not 'spoiling' him, but it may be impossible for you to meet endless demands. And since the impaired person has limited ability, if any, to learn, you cannot teach him, and scolding may precipitate catastrophic reactions.

If the person demands that you do things you think he can do, check that he really can do these things. He may be overwhelmed by the tasks. Simplifying them may make him willing to do them. Sometimes being very specific and direct with the person helps. Saying, 'I am coming to see you on Wednesday' is more helpful than getting into an argument over why you don't visit more often. Say, 'I will get you a cigarette when the timer goes off. Do not ask me for one until the timer goes off.' Ignore further demands until then.

You may have to set limits on what you can do realistically. But before you set limits, you need to know the extent of the impaired person's disability and you need to find out what other resources you can mobilise to replace what you cannot do. You may need to enlist the help of an outside person – a health visitor or social worker who understands the disease – to help you work out a plan that provides good care for the sick person without leaving you exhausted or trapped. (See Chapter 10.)

When demands make you feel angry and frustrated, try to find an outlet for your anger which does not involve the impaired person. Your anger can precipitate catastrophic reactions, which may make him even more recalcitrant.

Stubbornness and unco-operativeness

'Whatever I want him to do, he won't do it,' said one daughter-in-law. Said another, 'Whenever it's time to dress Dad, he says he has already changed his clothes. He won't go to the doctor, and whatever I serve for dinner he won't eat.'

Families often suspect that a stubborn and unco-operative person with dementia is deliberately trying to frustrate them. It is hard to know whether a person who has always been stubborn is now more so or whether the stubbornness is really a result of the dementia. Some people are more unco-operative than others by nature. However, this kind of behaviour is usually at least partly caused by the illness.

If a person cannot remember when he last took a bath, he may be insulted when he is told to bathe. This is understandable.

The person may not understand what he is being asked to do (go to the doctor, help set the table), and so he refuses. Unco-operativeness may seem a safer course than risking making a fool of one's self. Sometimes a statement such as 'I hate this food' really means 'I am miserable'.

Be sure that requests are understood.'Can you smell our supper cooking? See the roast? It will be delicious. Sit here and I will give you some.'

Focusing on a pleasant experience sometimes helps: 'As soon as we leave Dr Brown's office, we'll celebrate with a big ice cream.'

If strategies like this do not work (and sometimes nothing does), consider that the negative attitudes are often part of the illness rather than a personal attack. The person may be too confused to *intend* to insult your cooking. Take the path of least difficulty. Avoid arguments and accept whatever compromise will work.

When the sick person insults the sitter

When a family is able to arrange for someone to stay with the impaired person, he may fire her. He may become angry or suspicious, insult her, not let her in, or accuse her of stealing. This can make it seem impossible for you to get out of the house, or mean that the impaired person can no longer live in his own home. Often you can find ways to solve the problem.

As with many other problems, this situation may arise out of the impaired person's inability to make sense of his surroundings or to remember explanations. All he may recognise is that a stranger is in the house. Sometimes the presence of a 'baby sitter' means a further loss of his independence, which he may realise and react to.

Make sure that the sitter or housekeeper knows that it is you, not the confused person, who has the authority to hire and fire. If possible, find a sitter the person already knows or introduce the person to the sitter gradually. For the first few times, ask the sitter to come while you remain at home. Eventually the person may become accustomed to the idea that the sitter belongs there. This will also give you an opportunity to teach the sitter how you manage certain situations and to assess how well the sitter relates to the confused person.

Ensure that the sitter understands the nature of a dementing illness and knows how behaviour such as catastrophic reactions are managed. (Finding a sitter is discussed in Chapter 10.) Try to find sitters who are adept at engaging the person's trust and who are clever about managing the person without triggering a catastrophic reaction. Just as there are some people who are naturally good with children and others who are not, there are some people who are intuitively adept with confused people. However, they are often hard to find. If the person will not accept one sitter, try another. Ask yourself if reluctance to use a sitter is part of the problem.

Make sure that the sitter can reach you, another family member, or the doctor in the event of a problem.

Often the confused person will adjust to the presence of a sitter if both you and the sitter can weather the initial, stormy period.

Introduce the sitter as a friend 'who wants to visit you' and not as a sitter. If the person is suspicious of the sitter, his doctor may be able to reduce the suspiciousness with medication or can write a signed note to the impaired person reminding him to stay with the visitor.

In all events, consider your own health. Even if a sitter does upset the person with dementia, it is essential that you get out from time to time if you are to continue to be able to give care. (See Chapter 10.)

Using medication to manage behaviour

This chapter has listed may ways of controlling problem behaviours. You may hear different things about using medication to control problem behaviours. Some people say medication should never be used, while others may see medication as the only solution. Medication is most effective when targeted at specific symptoms. It is usually not helpful when it is given for generalised or annoying symptoms. Since all such medication has potentially harmful side effects, non-drug interventions should be tried first unless the behaviour is potentially dangerous to the patient or others, or unless a condition for which there is a specific treatment, like depression, is causing the problem.

Depression

People with memory problems may also be sad, low or depressed. When a person has memory problems and is depressed, it is very important that a careful diagnosis is made and the depression treated. The memory problems may not be caused by Alzheimer's disease and may disappear when the depression improves. The person may have both Alzheimer's disease and a depression that will respond to treatment.

When a person with an incurable disease is depressed, it can seem logical that she is depressed about the chronic illness. But not all people with Alzheimer's disease or other chronic illnesses are depressed. Some seem not to be aware of their problems. A certain amount of discouragement about one's condition is natural and understandable, but a deep despondency or a continuing depression is neither natural nor necessary. Fortunately, this kind of depression responds well to treatment, so the person can feel better whether or not she also has an irreversible dementing illness.

Researchers are trying to understand why we get depressed, but the complete answer is not yet known. We obviously feel sad or low when something bad happens to us, but this does not entirely explain the phenomenon of depression. For example, researchers are linking some depressions to changes in the brain. It is important that a doctor assesses the nature of each depression and determines whether it is a response to a situation or a deeper despondency, and then treats the depression appropriately. Indications of a deeper despondency include weight loss, a change in sleep patterns, feelings that one has done something bad and deserves to be punished, or a preoccupation with health problems.

It may be impossible for a depressed person to 'snap out of it' by herself. Telling her to do so may only increase her feelings of frustration and discouragement. For some people, trying to cheer them makes them feel that they are misunderstood.

You can encourage a depressed or discouraged person to continue to be with other people. If she has memory problems, be sure that the activities she tries are things she can still do successfully and are of some use, so that she can feel pleased with herself for doing them. Help her avoid tasks that are too complicated. Even small failures can make her feel more discouraged about herself. Ask her to set the table for you. If she doesn't have that much energy, have her set just one place. If that task is too complicated, have her set out just the plates.

If groups of people upset her, encourage her not to withdraw completely but instead to talk with one familiar person at a time. Ask one friend to visit. Urge the friend to talk to the depressed person, to meet her eyes and involve her.

When a person feels discouraged, it may be helpful for her to talk over her concerns with a knowledgeable counsellor, clergyman, physician, psychiatrist or psychologist. This is possible only when she can still communicate well and remember some things. The person chosen must understand dementia.

Complaints about health

If the person often complains about health problems, it is important to take these complaints seriously and have a doctor determine whether there is a physical basis for the complaints. Remember that chronic complainers can become ill. It is easy to overlook real illnesses when a person often focuses on problems with no physical basis. When you and the doctor are sure that no physical illness is present, he can treat the depression that is the underlying cause of the problem. Never let a doctor dismiss a person as 'just a hypochondriac'. People who focus on health problems are, in fact, unhappy and need appropriate care.

Suicide

When a person is depressed, demoralised or discouraged, there is always a possibility that she will harm herself. While it may be difficult for a person with Alzheimer's disease to plan a suicide, you do need to be alert to the possibility that she will injure herself. If the person has access to knives, power tools, solvents, drugs or car keys, she may use them to kill or maim herself.

Alcohol or drug abuse

Depressed people may use alcohol, tranquillisers or other drugs to try to blot out the feelings of sadness. This can compound the problem. In a person with a dementing illness it can also further reduce her ability to function. You need to be especially alert to this possibility in a person who is living alone, or who has used medication or alcohol in the past.

People who are heavy drinkers and who also develop a dementing illness can be difficult for their families to manage. The person may be more sensitive to small amounts of alcohol than a well person, so even one drink can significantly reduce her ability to function. These people often do not eat properly, causing nutritional problems that further impair them. They may also be stubborn or hostile.

It helps to recognise that the brain impairment may make it impossible for the person to control her drinking or her other unpleasant behaviour, and that you may have to provide this control for her. This will include taking steps to end her supply of alcohol. Do so quietly but firmly. Try not to feel that her unpleasant behaviour is aimed at you personally. Avoid saying things that put the blame for the situation on anybody. Do what needs to be done, but try to find ways in which the person can retain her self-esteem and dignity. There should be no alcohol in the house unless it is locked away. One family was able to arrange for the local off-licence to stop serving the patient.

You may need help from a psychiatrist to manage the behaviour of a person with a memory problem who also abuses alcohol or drugs.

Apathy, listlessness

Sometimes people with brain diseases become apathetic and listless. They just sit and don't want to do anything. Such people may be easier to care for than people who are upset, but it is important not to overlook them.

As with depression, we are not sure why some people become apathetic and listless. It is probably due to the effects of the disease on specific areas of the brain. It is important to keep them as active as possible. People need to move around and to use their minds and bodies as much as they can.

Withdrawing may be a person's way of coping when things get too complicated for her, and if you insist on her participation she may have a catastrophic reaction. Try to re-involve her at a level at which she can feel comfortable, can succeed and can feel useful. You could ask her to carry out a simple task, take her for a walk and point out interesting things, play some music, or go for a car ride.

It often seems that getting the body moving helps to cheer a person up. Once a person starts doing something, she may begin to feel less apathetic. Perhaps she can peel only one potato today. Tomorrow she may feel like doing two. Perhaps she can dig the garden. Even if she digs for only a few minutes, it may have helped her to get moving. If she stops a task after a few minutes, instead of urging her to go on, focus your attention on what she has accomplished and compliment her on that.

Occasionally when you try to persuade a person to be more active, she may become upset or agitated. If this happens, you need to weigh up the importance of her being active against her being upset.

Remembering feelings

People with dementia may remember their feelings longer than they remember the situation that caused the feelings. Mrs Bishop stayed angry with her daughter for days, but she forgot that there was a good reason why her daughter had acted as she had.

Similarly, some people constantly restate the same suspicious ideas. Their families understandably wonder why they can't remember other things as well. Our brain probably processes and stores the memory of feelings in a different way than it does memories of facts and, for reasons not as yet understood, emotional memories seem to be less vulnerable to the devastations of the dementing illness. This can have advantages, since people often remember their good feelings longer than the facts surrounding them.

One woman insisted that she had been dancing at the day centre, although she was confined to a wheelchair. She meant that she had had a good time there. One man always remained happy for hours after a visit from his grandchildren even though he forgot the visit itself soon after they had left.

Anger and irritability

Sometimes people with dementing illnesses become angry. They may lash out at you as you try to help them. They may slam things around, hit you, refuse to be cared for, throw food, yell or make accusations. This can be upsetting for you and may cause problems in the household. It can seem as if all this hostility is aimed at you, despite your best efforts to take care of the person, and you may be afraid that the person will hurt herself or someone else when she lashes out in anger. This is certainly a real concern. However, our experience has been that it actually occurs rarely and can usually be controlled.

Angry or violent behaviour is usually a catastrophic reaction and should be handled as you would any other such reaction. (See Chapter 3.) Respond calmly; do not respond with anger. Remove the person from the situation or remove the upsetting stimulus. Look for the event that precipitated the reaction so that you can prevent or minimise a recurrence.

Try not to interpret such anger as you would if it were expressed by a well person. Anger from a confused person is often exaggerated or misdirected. The person may not really be angry with you at all. The anger is probably the result of misunderstanding the situation. For example:

> *Mr Jones adored his small grandson. One day the grandchild tripped and fell, and began to cry. Mr Jones grabbed a knife, began to shout and would allow no one near the child. Mr Jones had misinterpreted the cause of the child's crying and over-reacted. He thought someone was attacking the child. Fortunately, the child's mother understood what was happening. 'I will help you protect the baby,' she said to Mr Jones. She gave Mr Jones a job to do: 'Here, you hold the door for me.' Then she was able to pick up and comfort the child.*

Forgetfulness is an advantage, since the person may quickly forget the episode. Often you can distract a person who is behaving in this way by suggesting an activity you know she enjoys.

> *Mrs Williams's mother-in-law often became angry when Mrs Williams tried to prepare supper. Mr Williams began distracting his mother by spending that time each day talking with her in another part of the house.*

Once in a while a person experiencing a catastrophic reaction will hit someone who is trying to help her. Respond to this as you would to a catastrophic reaction. When at all possible, do not restrain her. If this occurs frequently, you may need to ask the doctor to help you review what is upsetting the person and, if necessary, to consider prescribing medication.

Anxiety, nervousness and restlessness

People with dementing illnesses may become worried, anxious, agitated and upset. They may pace or fidget. Their constant restlessness can become irritating. The person may not be able to tell you why she is upset. Or she may give you an unreasonable explanation for her anxiety. For example:

Mrs Berger was obviously upset over something, but whenever her husband tried to find out what it was, she would say that her mother was coming to get her. Telling her that her mother had been dead for years only caused her to cry.

Some anxiety and nervousness may be caused by the changes within the brain. Other nervousness may come from real feelings of loss or tension. The real feelings that result from not knowing where one is, what one is expected to do and where one's familiar possessions are can lead to almost constant feelings of anxiety. Some people sense that they often do things wrong and they become anxious about 'messing it all up'. Longing for a familiar environment ('I want to go home') or worrying about people from the past ('Where are my children?') can create anxiety. Reassurance, affection and distraction may be all you can offer. Medication occasionally helps relieve these feelings but should be tried only if other options have failed and if the anxiety is severe.

Even severely ill people remain sensitive to the moods of the people around them. If there is tension in the household, the person may respond, no matter how well you try to conceal it. For example, Mrs Powell argued with her son over something minor, and, just when that was solved, her confused mother began to cry because she 'felt that something dreadful was going to happen'. Her feeling was a real response to the mood in the house, but, because she was cognitively impaired, her interpretation of the cause of the feeling was incorrect.

The person may be sad and worried over losing some specific item, such as her watch. Reassuring her that you have the watch may not seem to help. Again, she has an accurate *feeling* (something is lost: her memory is lost, time is lost, many things are lost), but the *explanation* of the feeling is inaccurate. Respond with affection and reassurance to her feeling, which is real, and avoid trying to convince her that what she expresses is unreasonable.

Trying to persuade the person to explain what is troubling her, or arguing with her ('there is no reason to get upset'), may only make her more upset. For example:

Every afternoon at 2 pm, Mrs Novak began to pace and wring her hands at the day centre. She told the staff that she was going to miss the train to London. Telling her she was not going to London only upset her more. The staff realised that she was probably worried about going home, and they reassured her that they would see that she got home safely. This always calmed her down. (They had responded appropriately to her feelings.)

Not all anxiety and nervousness may go away so easily. Sometimes these feelings are inexplicable. Offering the person comfort and reassurance, and trying to simplify her environment may be all that you can do to counteract the effects of her brain disease.

When people with dementing illnesses pace, fiddle with things, resist care, move the furniture around, run away from home or from the day centre, or turn on the cooker and all the taps, they may make others around them nervous. Their restless, irritable behaviour is hard for families to manage without help.

Agitation may be a part of depression, anger or anxiety. It may be restlessness or boredom, a symptom of pain, caused by medication, or an inexplicable part of the dementing illness. Respond calmly and gently; try to simplify what is going on around the person, and avoid 'overloading her mental circuits'. Your calmness and gentleness will communicate to her.

You may find it helpful to give the person who is mildly restless something to fiddle with. Some people will play with worry beads or with coins in their pockets. Giving the person something constructive to do, such as walking to the postbox with you, may help. If the person is drinking caffeinated beverages such as coffee and tea, switching to the de-caffeinated type of these might help, or to drinks that do not contain any caffein. A health food store would advise on these.

> One woman was restless much of the time. She paced, fidgeted and wandered. Her husband stopped telling her to sit down and instead began handing her a pack of cards, saying, 'Here, Helen, play patience.' He took advantage of her lifelong enjoyment of this card game, even though she no longer played it correctly.

Sometimes this behaviour is the result of frequent or almost continuous catastrophic reactions. Try to find ways of reducing the confusion, extra stimulation, noise and change surrounding the confused person. (Read the sections on catastrophic reactions and on wandering on pages 28 and 124.) Medication may help very agitated or restless people.

False ideas, suspiciousness, paranoia and hallucinations

Forgetful people may become unreasonably suspicious. They may suspect or accuse others of stealing their money, their possessions, and even things nobody would take, like an old toothbrush. They may hoard or hide things. They may shout for help or call the police. An impaired person may begin accusing her spouse of infidelity.

People with dementing illness may develop unshakeable ideas that their possessions have been stolen or that people are going to harm them. Carried to an extreme, these ideas can make the person fearful and resistant to all attempts at care and help. Occasionally they develop distressing and strange ideas that they seem to remember and insist upon. They may insist that this is not where they live, that people who are dead are alive and are coming for them, or that someone who lives in the house is a stranger and perhaps dangerous. Occasionally a person will insist that his wife is not his wife – she is someone who looks like his wife, but is an impostor.

A person with a dementing illness may hear, see, feel or smell things that are not there. Such hallucinations may terrify her (if she sees a strange man in the bedroom), or amuse her (if she sees a puppy on the bed).

This behaviour is upsetting for families because it is strange and frightening, and because we associate it with insanity. It may never happen to your family member, but you should be aware of it in case you have to respond to such an experience. When these symptoms occur in the presence of a dementing illness, they are usually the result of the brain injury or a superimposed delirium (see page 302), and are not symptoms of other mental illness.

Misinterpretation

Sometimes these problems are due to the person's misinterpretation of what she sees and hears. If she sees poorly in the dark, she may misinterpret the moving curtains as a strange man. If she hears poorly, she may suspect conversations to be about her. If she loses her shoes, she may misinterpret the loss as a theft.

The cognitively impaired person must be helped to see and hear as well as possible because she may not realise her sensory limitations. Ensure that her glasses and/or hearing aid are working well. If the room is dimly lit, see if improving the lighting helps. If the room is noisy or if sounds are muted, the person may need help identifying sounds (see Chapter 6). Closing the curtains may help if she is 'seeing' someone outside at night.

If you think the person is misinterpreting things, you may be able to help by explaining what she sees or hears. Say, for example, 'That movement is the curtains' or 'That tapping noise is the bush outside your window'. This is different from directly disagreeing with her, which may cause her to have a catastrophic reaction. Avoid saying, 'There is no man in the bedroom' or 'Nobody is trying to break in. Now go to sleep.'

If the person does not hear well, it may help to include her in the conversation by addressing her directly rather than talking about her. Look directly at her. Some people read lips well enough to supplement their hearing. You might say, 'Dad, John says the weather has been terrible lately' or 'Dad, John says the new grandchild is sitting up now.' Never talk about someone in the third person, as if she weren't there, no matter how 'out of it' you think she is. This is dehumanising and can understandably make a person angry. Ask other people not to do it.

Sometimes the impaired person's brain incorrectly interprets what her senses see or hear correctly. This is often what happens when a person becomes unrealistically suspicious. Sometimes you can help by giving the confused person accurate information or writing down reminders. You may have to repeat the same information frequently, since the person will tend to forget quickly what you say.

Failure to recognise people or things (agnosia)

People with dementing illnesses may lose the ability to recognise things or people, not because they have forgotten them or because their eyes are not working but because the brain is not able to put together information properly. This is called agnosia, from the Latin words meaning 'to not know'. It can be a baffling symptom. For example:

Mrs Robinson said to her husband, 'Who are you? What are you doing in my house?'

This is not a problem of memory. Mrs Robinson had not forgotten her husband; in fact, she remembered him quite well, but her brain could not work out who he was from what her eyes saw.

Mr Clark insisted that this was not his house, although he had lived there many years.

He had not forgotten his home, but, because his brain was not working correctly, the place did not look familiar.

You can help by giving the person other information. It may help to say, 'I know it doesn't look familiar, but this is your house.' Hearing your voice may help her remember who you are. Help her focus on one familiar detail. 'Here is your chair. Sit in it. It *feels* familiar.'

'You are not my husband'

Occasionally a person with a dementing illness will insist that her spouse is not her spouse, or that her home is not her real home. She may insist that it looks just like her house, but someone has taken the real one away and replaced it with a fake one. We do not understand exactly what is happening in such situations, but we do know that this distressing symptom is a part of the brain damage.

Reassure the person, 'I am your husband', but avoid arguing. Although this may seem heartbreaking, it is important to tell yourself that it is not a rejection of *you* (the person does remember you), it is just an inexplicable confusion of the damaged brain.

'My mother is coming for me'

Someone with a dementing illness may forget that a person she once knew has died. She may say, 'My mother is coming for me' or she may say that she has been visiting her grandmother. Perhaps her memory of the person is stronger than her memory of the death. Perhaps in her mind the past has become the present.

Instead of either contradicting or playing along with her, try responding to her general feelings of loss, if you feel that that this is what she is expressing.

Telling the confused person outright that her mother has been dead for years may upset her terribly. Her constant focus on these memories probably means that they are important to her. Ask her to tell you about her mother, look through a photo album from those years, or retell some old family stories. This responds to her feelings without hurting her again and again.

Sometimes people feel that this idea is 'spooky' or that the impaired person is 'seeing the dead'. It is much more likely to be just another symptom like forgetfulness, wandering or catastrophic reaction.

You may decide that this issue is not worth an argument.

Suspiciousness

If a person is suspicious or 'paranoid', one must consider the possibility that her suspicions are founded on fact. Sometimes when a person is known to be unusually suspicious, real causes for her suspiciousness are overlooked. In fact, she might be being victimised, robbed or harassed. However, some people with dementing illnesses do develop suspicions that are inappropriate to the real situation.

Paranoia and suspiciousness are not really difficult to understand. We are all suspicious; it is necessary for our survival. The innate naiveté of the child is carefully replaced by a healthy suspicion. We are taught to be suspicious of strangers who offer us sweets, of door-to-door salesmen and of people with 'shifty' eyes. Some of us were also taught as children to be suspicious of people of other races or religions. Some people have always been suspicious, others always trusting. A dementing illness may exaggerate these personality traits.

Ms Henderson returns to her office to find her purse missing. Two other purses have disappeared this week. She suspects that the new filing clerk has stolen it.

As Mr Starr comes out of a restaurant at night, three teenagers approach him and ask for change for the telephone. His heart pounds. He suspects that they plan to rob him.

Mrs Bolton called her friend three times to meet her for lunch and each time the friend refused, giving the excuse that she had extra work. Mrs Bolton worries that her friend is avoiding her.

Situations like these occur frequently. One difference between the response of a well person and that of a brain-impaired person is that the latter's ability to reason may become overwhelmed by the emotions her suspicions raise or by her inability to make sense of her world.

Ms Henderson searched for her purse and actually remembered that she had left it in the cafeteria, where she found it being held for her at the till.

The confused person lacks the ability to remember. Therefore she will never find her purse and will continue to suspect the filing clerk, as would Ms Henderson had she not been able to remember where she had left it.

Knowing that he was in a well-lit, populated area, Mr Starr suppressed his panic and gave a ten pence piece to the three teenagers. They thanked him and ran to the phone.

The confused person lacks the ability to assess his situation realistically and to control his panic. He often over-reacts. In Mr Starr's situation, therefore, he might have called for help, the boys would have run, the police would have been called, etc.

Mrs Bolton discussed her concerns with a mutual friend and learned that her friend had been ill, had got behind in her work and was always eating lunch at her desk.

The confused person lacks the ability to test out her suspicions against the opinions of others and then to evaluate them.

The person with the dementing illness who becomes 'paranoid' has not gone crazy. She lives in a world in which each moment involves beginning again with no memory of the preceding moments, in which things disappear, explanations are forgotten, and in which conversations make no sense. In such a world it is easy to see how healthy suspicion can get out of hand. For example, the person with a dementing illness forgets that you have carefully explained that you have hired a house-keeper. Lacking the information she needs to assess accurately what is going on, she makes exactly the same assumption we would if we found a strange person in the house – that she is a thief.

The first step in coping with excessive suspiciousness is to understand that this is not behaviour the person can control. Secondly, it only makes things worse to confront the person or to argue about the truth of the complaint. Avoid saying 'I've told you twenty times that I put your things in the attic. Nobody stole them.' Perhaps you can make a list of where things are: 'Love seat given to cousin Mary. Cedar chest in Ann's attic.'

When she says, 'You stole my dentures', don't say, 'Nobody has stolen your teeth, you've lost them again.' Instead, say, 'I'll help you find them.' Locating the lost article will often solve the problem. Articles that are mislaid seem stolen to the person who cannot remember where she has put them and who cannot reason that nobody would want her dentures.

One son securely fastened a key to the notice board (so his mother could not remove and hide it). Every time she accused him of stealing her furniture, he replied gently, 'All your things are locked in the attic. Here is your key to the attic.'

Sometimes you can distract a person from her focus on suspicions. Look for the lost articles; try going for a ride or getting her involved in a task. Sometimes you can look for the real cause of her complaints, and respond with sympathy and reassurance to her feelings of loss and confusion.

If most of a person's possessions have to be disposed of when she moves into your home, or into a residential or nursing home, she may insist that they have been stolen. If you have assumed control over a person's finances, she may accuse you of stealing from her. Repeated explanations or lists sometimes help. Often they do not, because the person cannot make sense out of the explanation or will forget it. Such accusations can be discouraging when you are doing the best you can for someone. These accusations are often, at least in part, an expression of the person's overwhelming feelings of loss, confusion and distress, and, although distressing for you, are not really harmful to anyone. When you understand that they occur because of the brain damage, you will be less upset by them.

Few things make us more angry than being falsely accused. Consequently, the impaired person's accusations can alienate sitters, other family members, neighbours and friends, thereby causing you to lose needed sources of friendship and help. Make it clear to people that you do not suspect them of anything and explain that accusatory behaviour results from the confused person's inability to assess reality accurately. Your trust in them must be obvious and strong enough to override the accusations made by the impaired person. Sometimes it is helpful to share with others written material, such as this book, which explains how brain impairment affects behaviour. Part of the problem is that the confused person may look and sound reasonable. It may not appear as if this behaviour were beyond her control, and, because dementing illnesses are often poorly understood, people may not realise what is happening.

Some types of suspicion go beyond this explanation; they cannot be explained by forgetfulness or by the loss of the ability to correctly assess reality. Such suspicion may be caused by the disease process itself. Low doses of medication may help. Treatment not only makes life easier for you but also relieves the ill person of the anxiety and fear that arise from her suspicion.

Hiding things

In a world that is confusing and in which things inexplicably disappear, it is understandable for a person to put precious things in a safe place. The difference between being well and being impaired is that the impaired person forgets where that safe place is more often than the well person. Hiding things often accompanies suspiciousness, but, because it causes so many problems, we have discussed it separately in Chapter 7.

Delusions and hallucinations

Delusions are false ideas unshakeably held by one person. They may be suspicious in nature ('The mafia are after me', or 'You have stolen my money') or self-blaming ('I am a bad person', or 'I am rotting inside and spreading a terrible disease'). The nature of the delusion can help doctors diagnose the person's problem. Self-blaming ideas, for example, are often seen in people who are severely depressed. However, when delusions occur in a person who is known to have a brain impairment resulting from a stroke, from Alzheimer's disease or from another condition, the delusion is believed to arise out of the injury to brain tissue. It can be frustrating to care for a person who seems to be able to remember a false idea and yet is unable to remember real information.

Sometimes delusions appear to come from misinterpreting reality while others are tied to the person's past experiences. (A note of caution: not all strange ideas expressed by older people are delusions.) .

Hallucinations are sensory experiences which are real to the person having them but which others do not share. Hearing voices or seeing things are the most common examples, although occasionally people feel, smell or taste things too.

Mrs Singer sometimes saw a dog asleep in her bed. She would call her daughter to 'Come and get the dog out of my bed.'

Mr Davis saw tiny little men on the floor. They distracted him, and often he sat watching them instead of taking part in activities at the day centre.

Mrs Ellis heard burglars outside her window trying to break in and discussing how they would hurt her. She called the police several times and earned herself the reputation of being a crackpot.

Mr Vaughan tasted poison in all his food. He refused to eat and lost so much weight that he had to be admitted to hospital.

Hallucinations are a symptom, like a fever or sore throat, which can arise from many causes. Certain drugs can induce hallucinations in otherwise well people, and several disease processes can also produce hallucinations. Just as with a fever or sore throat, the first step is to identify the cause of the hallucination. In an elderly person, hallucinations are not necessarily an indication of a dementing illness. They may result from several causes, many of which are treatable. Delirium is one example. If hallucinations or delusions appear in a person who has previously been functioning well, they are probably not associated with dementia. Do not let a doctor dismiss this symptom as 'senility'. The people in the examples given above were not all experiencing hallucinations as a result of dementia.

When hallucinations do develop as an inexplicable part of the dementing illness, your doctor can help. Often these symptoms respond to medication that makes the patient more comfortable and life easier for you.

When delusions or hallucinations occur, react calmly so that you do not further upset the confused person. Although this is not an emergency situation, you will want to seek advice from the doctor as soon as it is convenient. Reassure the person that you are taking care of the situation and that you will see that everything is all right.

Avoid denying the person's experience, or directly confronting her or arguing with her. This will only further upset her. Remember, the experience is real for her. At the same time you should not play along with a delusion or a hallucination. You don't have to agree or disagree; just listen or give a noncommittal answer. You can say, 'I don't hear the voices you hear, but it must be frightening for you.' This is not the same as agreeing with the person. Sometimes you can distract the person so that she forgets her hallucination. Say, 'Let's go into the kitchen and have a cup of warm milk.' When she returns to her bedroom, she may no longer see a dog in her bed and you will have avoided an upsetting confrontation.

It is often comforting to touch the person physically, as long as she does not misinterpret your touch as an effort to restrain her. Say, 'I know you are so upset. Would it help if I held your hand (or gave you a hug)?'

Having nothing to do

As they progress, dementing illnesses greatly limit the things the confused person can do. It becomes impossible to remember the past or to anticipate the future. The confused person cannot plan ahead or organise a simple activity like taking a shower. Many impaired people cannot follow the action on television. While you or the nursing home staff are absorbed with chores, the ill person may have nothing to do but sit with vacant time and empty thoughts.

Restlessness, wandering, trying to go 'home', repetitive motions, asking the same question over and over, scratching, masturbating and many other behaviours begin as an effort to fill this emptiness. But for you the hours are full. We do not believe that a family care-giver, with all the burdens he or she faces, should be expected to take on the additional responsibility of planning recreation. However, we do think activity is important. Enlist the help of other family members, friends, volunteers from groups such as Age Concern or the Alzheimers Disease Society or paid help, if possible.

Whenever you or someone else initiates an activity for a person with dementia, you must walk a fine line between providing meaningful activity and overstressing the person. Move at the confused person's pace. Never let an activity become a test of her abilities; arrange things so that she will succeed. Having fun should be more important than doing something correctly.

Stop when the person becomes restless or irritable.

Anyone can become ill or suffer an accident. If you are tired and under stress from caring for a chronically ill person, your risk of succumbing to illness or having an accident increases. The spouse of a person with a dementing illness, himself no longer young, is at risk of developing other illnesses.

What happens to the confused, forgetful person if you, the care-giver, are injured or become ill? It is important that you have a plan ready. You may never need to put your plan into effect, but because dementia disables a person in such a way that he cannot act in his best interests, you must make advance plans that protect you and the impaired person.

You will, of course, have a GP who is familiar with your health to whom you can turn if you become ill, and who is available quickly in a crisis. In addition, you need to plan in advance for several other kinds of situations: the sudden, severe problems that would arise if you had a heart attack or stroke, or fell and broke a bone; the less sudden problems that would arise if you had a long illness, or required a hospital admission for medical or surgical reasons; and the problems that would arise if you got the flu or were at home, ill, for a few days.

Mrs Brady suddenly began having chest pains and knew she should lie quietly. She told her confused husband to fetch their neighbour, but he kept pulling at her arm and shouting. When, finally, she was able to telephone for help, he refused to let the ambulance men into the house.

Even when an impaired person appears to function satisfactorily as a rule, such a situation may upset him and leave him unable to cope with tasks he can usually do well. Should you suddenly become ill and need assistance, the confused person may not be able to summon help for you. He may misinterpret what is happening and impede efforts to get help.

There are several possible ways you can plan to summon help. If you have a telephone, you can dial emergency services on 999, so try to teach the person to use that number to call for help. Stick the number over the phone. Or give the number of a relative or friend who lives nearby and who will respond to a confused telephone call. Telephones with built-in memories can be pre-programmed so that you can summon assistance by pressing one number. You can paint this digit red with varnish so that it is easily identified.

Telephone alarm systems which you can carry with you and activate

as necessary are also available. Some can be voice activated. The alarm
links via the telephone to a central control. Help the Aged run a national
scheme to provide alarms linked to local authority emergency centres.
They advise on funding and will try to raise money to cover the cost of
an alarm and a year's monitoring, if you need it. For an information
pack contact: Community Alarm Department, Help the Aged, 16–18
St James Walk, London EC1R 0BE, (tel: 071-253 0253).

If you live near someone who is willing to respond in a crisis, you may
be able to use fairly inexpensive walkie-talkies, citizen band radio or
intercoms to summon help. You will need a CB licence which is available
from your local post office.

In some areas there are neighbourhood care schemes which arrange
for someone to telephone you regularly, every day or so, to see if you
are all right. To rely on such a scheme may mean a long delay in
receiving help, but it is better than nothing.

Ensure that the person appointed to respond in a crisis has a key to
your house. The upset, confused person may refuse to let anyone in.

If you must go into the hospital or if you are unwell at home, you will
need to plan carefully in advance for the care of the confused person.
Changes are upsetting for them and it is therefore helpful to minimise
changes as much as possible. The substitute care-giver should be someone the person knows and someone who knows your routines for managing him. (See Chapter 10 for possible sources of temporary help.) Ensure
that the names and telephone numbers of your doctor, the patient's
doctor and social worker, if he has one, your solicitor and close family
members are written down where the person helping out in an emergency
can find them.

Some families have made up a 'cope notebook' in which they have
jotted down the things another person would need to know. For example:
'Dr Brown (tel: 824 8787). John gets a pink pill one hour before lunch.
He will take it best with orange juice. The cooker won't work unless you
turn on the switch that is hidden behind the toaster. John starts to
wander around suppertime. You will need to watch him then.'

In the event of your death

When someone close to you has a dementing illness, you have a special
responsibility to provide for him if you should die. Your plans may never
have to be put into action, but they must, for the sake of the sick person,
be made.

When a family member is unable to take care of himself, it is important
that you draw up a will that provides for his care. Find a solicitor whom
you trust, and have him draw up a will and any other necessary legal

papers. If you do not make a valid will, your estate may be divided against your wishes. To avoid any confusion, you should draw up a succinct summary of your assets for the person who will take over. This should include information on the location of wills, deeds, stocks and share certificates, cemetery plot deeds, and information about the care of the confused person. In addition to the usual matters of disposing of property to one's heirs, the following questions must be addressed, and appropriate arrangements made (see Chapter 15).

What arrangements have been made for your funeral, and who will carry these out? You can select a funeral director in advance and agree with him, in writing, what kind of funeral you will have and how much it will cost. You can also pay for the funeral in advance. Age Concern England has a fact sheet 'Arranging a Funeral' listing the organisations which run such schemes. It is available on receipt of a large stamped addressed envelope. Far from being macabre, this is a considerate and responsible act that ensures that things will be done as you wish. It also saves your family the trouble of making such arrangements in the midst of their grief. Funerals can be expensive and advance plans make it possible for you to ensure that your money is spent as you wish.

What immediate arrangements have been made for the care of the person with a dementing illness, and who will be responsible for seeing that they are carried out? Someone must be available immediately who will be kind and caring. Does the person who will be caring for the person understand his diagnosis and know his doctor? Have you passed on to the new care-giver as much information as possible about how to make the person comfortable?

What financial provisions have been made for the person with a dementing illness, and who will administer them? If he cannot manage his own affairs, someone must be available with the authority to care for him. You will want to select a person whom you trust to do this rather than leave such an important decision to a court or judge. When such decisions are made by a court, they can involve long delays and considerable expense.

Sometimes a husband or wife cares for years for a spouse with a dementing illness and does not want to burden sons or daughters with the knowledge of this illness:

Said a daughter, 'I had no idea anything was wrong with Mum because Dad covered up for her so well. Then he had a heart attack and we found her like this. Now I have the shock of his death and her illness all at once. It would have been so much easier if he had told us about it long ago. And we didn't know anything about dementia. We had to find out all the things he had already learned, and at such a difficult time for us.'

All members of the family need to know what is wrong with the impaired person and what plans have been made. An experience like this is one example of the disservice of 'protecting' other members of the family.

Throughout this book we have emphasised the importance of finding
time for yourself away from the responsibilities of caring for the impaired
person. You may also need other kinds of help: someone to see that a
person who is alone during the day eats her meals; someone to help give
the person a bath; someone to watch the person while you shop, rest or
take a break; someone to help with the housework; or someone with
whom you can talk things over.

You may need someone to stay with the impaired person part of the
day, or to find a place where the person can stay for several days while
you take a holiday or receive medical care. At some point you may need
to find a place where the impaired person can spend time away from
you and where she can make friends of her own. Such help is called
respite, because it gives you a break from care-giving. This chapter will
describe the kinds of services that may be available and some of the
problems you may encounter in looking for them.

Help from friends and neighbours

Usually care-givers who feel that they have the support of others manage
their caring tasks more successfully. It is important that you do not feel
alone in your caring role. Most people first turn to family members,
friends or neighbours for support and help. In many cases people will
offer to help; at other times you may have to ask them.

Family members sometimes disagree, or can't or won't help out. You
may hesitate to ask others for the help you need. In Chapter 11 we
discuss some ways of handling family disagreements and of asking for
help.

Other people are often willing to help in some way. Sometimes a
neighbour will look in on the confused person, the pharmacist will keep
track of prescriptions for you, a clergyman will listen when you are
discouraged, a friend will sit with the person in an emergency, and so
forth. As you plan, you should consider these resources, because they
are important to you.

How much help should you accept or ask for from friends and neighbours? Most people like to help, yet making too many demands on them
may eventually cause them to pull away.

When you turn to friends and neighbours for help, there are several
things you can do to help *them*. Some people are uncomfortable being

with those who are visibly upset. You may not want to express all of
your distress to such people. Close friends may be more willing to share
some of the emotional burden with you than people who do not know
you well.

Although most people have heard of Alzheimer's disease, many need
more information to understand why the person acts as she does. Explain
that the behaviour is the result of the damage to the brain, that it is not
deliberate or dangerous.

People may be reluctant to stay or to visit the person because they do
not know what to do and feel awkward. You can help by suggesting
specific things that the visitor might do with the person. For example,
mention that going for a walk might be more fun than a conversation,
or that reminiscences about old times will be enjoyable for both of them.
Tell the visitor what to do when the impaired person becomes irritable
or restless.

Some groups of the Alzheimer's Disease Society will help family
members or friends to learn more about helping or visiting people with
dementias. Such people can help to bring pleasure to the confused
person, as well as giving you time away from caring.

When you ask people to help you, give them enough advance notice,
if possible, so that they can plan their time. Suggest tasks which helpers
may undertake which they will feel are useful or productive, and which
they can do without upsetting the confused person or bringing about a
catastrophic reaction. Look for things which helpers or visitors will not
find inconvenient. For example, neighbours may not mind 'looking in'
since they live close by, while more distant friends might resent being
asked to make a long journey.

Remember to thank people who help. Try to avoid criticising what
they have done if their efforts appear less than perfect to you.

Finding information and locating other services

At some point, most families or carers look for outside help in obtaining
information, making decisions and planning for the long-term care of
their afflicted family member. Most families also need some time for
themselves away from care-giving. Many families find the help they
need, and manage effectively without extensive professional assistance.
However, the task of caring for a person with dementia is enormous,
and many people have difficulty finding the services that might make
care-giving easier.

The first step in finding out about what may be available is to ask
around. In each area of the country, there are different services, and
different people may have the knowledge which you need. So you may

have to try several possible sources of information before you find the right one for you. This can be particularly difficult if you cannot get out. However, here are some suggestions to point you in the right direction.

People from the *health or social services* may be able to help and advise you. They include:

- your, or your relative's general practitioner;
- the district or community nurse, health visitor, community psychiatric nurse, or practice nurse at the doctor's surgery;
- a social worker, who can be contacted through the Social Services Department, or perhaps through the hospital or general practitioner's surgery;
- the Alzheimer's Disease Society – either a local group or the national organisation;
- MIND – consult the national organisation about local groups which provide day and respite care;
- the Carers' National Association – again, either a local group or the national organisation, for information to support you as a carer;
- Crossroads Care Attendant Schemes – contact either the local or the national organisation for information about its relief schemes for carers;
- other national support groups, such as the Parkinson's Disease Society or Arthritis Care, if your relative has problems additional to dementia;
- Age Concern – local organisations provide many different services and/or advice and support. There is also a national Age Concern in each country of the UK;
- local or national private agencies which offer care or nursing at home.

First steps

You may be lucky and live in an area where there is integrated support already organised for people with Alzheimer's disease. In other areas, however, people have to work quite hard to find out what they need to know, and to obtain the help which they need.

Although there is a range of information sources, it can be difficult to find one place that can give you all the information you need about what services are offered or how to receive them. Even information and referral services often do not have a complete and current list of resources. You will need to be persistent and may need to contact several different people or organisations.

Locating help can be a long and tedious process. If you are providing most of the supervision and care for an impaired person, you may feel too pressed to do this. It may be difficult to make telephone calls in the presence of the confused person. If it is all too much, ask another family member or friend to take on the job of locating outside help. If you are not the person with daily responsibility for care, offer to help the caregiver to find this help.

You may not find what you need; unfortunately, the resources which families of people with dementia need are often not available. Don't blame yourself if you can't find the resources you need. Some agencies have a waiting list or they will take only certain kinds of people, while other agencies may be too expensive. Inadequate resources and services are major problems that can be changed only through public recognition of the dementing diseases and the needs of families, and you may find that obtaining even some help is better than trying to cope alone.

Before you begin, think about what kind of help would be right for you and the confused person. At the end of this chapter is a list of questions to help get you started. Here, however, we will look at changes which are taking place in provision of local services. In years to come, these changes will affect everyone who needs help with care-giving.

The community care changes

In the late 1980s there were some major changes in policy which will gradually take effect during the 1990s. The NHS and Community Care Act has placed a new duty on local authority Social Services Departments (Social Work Departments in Scotland) to arrange assessments for people who appear to them to need community care. This requirement is scheduled to come into force in April 1993. Local authorities will become the 'lead' authority in assessing people for help with care, and arranging community care appropriate to their needs. However, the government has said this must be done within available resources and therefore you may not be able to obtain services even if you need them.

'Community care' means many different things, depending on the group of people in question. For you, it means finding the kind of help and support which you and your relative need for her – and you – to live as independently as possible in your own home. Community care involves many different departments and services. For people with dementia and their carers, it will almost certainly involve 'health' and 'social' support. This means that the general practitioner, the geriatrician or psychogeriatrician, and nurse may all be involved in offering appropriate care, even though the Social Services Department is taking the lead.

If your impaired relative needs a combination of health and social care, and if you need support as well, under the new system you will turn to the Social Services Department, which should arrange an *assessment* of the needs of you *both*. If necessary, carers should be able to have their own needs assessed. This means that you will have a chance to state *your* point of view. This assessment might involve co-operation between all the different people who help you. You should be told the result of the assessment and what services will be arranged. If social services are needed, there may be a fee and your relative will be assessed for her ability to pay.

It will be some time before this new system is well established, but you should gradually notice changes in the way support is offered to you. 'Care management' will gradually be introduced, where people with quite complex needs will have a 'care manager', who will help to arrange a 'package' of appropriate services for the impaired person and her carer. However, you may not be offered help if the person is not considered to be seriously impaired.

Local authority Social Services (or Social Work) Departments also have to publish *community care plans* each year. They must co-operate with health and housing authorities in preparing these plans, which should be publicly available. You and others in similar situations might want to read these plans, to see what is planned in your area for people with dementia and their carers. The plans might refer to different 'client groups' – different groups of people who may have community care needs. The section on 'elderly' people, or 'elderly mentally ill' people might make special reference to people with dementia. It is important for people like you to put forward your views on such plans. You may have some useful information or experience to contribute to the annual planning process. Despite increased awareness of what can be achieved, it is still important to educate communities and policy makers that dementias are diseases – not just 'old age' – and that helping sufferers and their families makes good sense in every way.

Local authority Social Services Departments must have a formal complaints procedure, to allow people to make complaints or comments about services they have received, or about assessment, or about how they have been treated. It is important to make your views known. The local authority should have a designated complaints officer, and should also help you to find someone to help you put your case, if you would like this. People are often afraid to make a complaint, for fear that they or the person they care for will be treated badly as a result. Sometimes people are afraid they will lose a service which has been offered to them. This should not happen. Comments and complaints are a valuable means of allowing authorities and other organisations to evaluate their performance. Complaints should help services to improve, and new complaints procedures should make it easier for you to express your views on the services offered.

Kinds of services

Most of the services described in the rest of this chapter come under the heading of 'health and personal social services'. A checklist of such services is included on pp. 175–6. You shouldn't be limited by this selection. Think about what *you* and the person you care for actually need.

One or two other kinds of services are worth mentioning, however, before we focus in more detail on the major care services. These might help both you and the person you care for. You need to be creative in thinking how they might work in your situation. They include leisure and recreation services – for instance, special hours at the swimming pool for people aged over 50. They also include various concessionary schemes for fares or admission to local places of entertainment, which are vitally important when funds are tight.

Various types of health care can be provided in people's own homes if they cannot go out. These include dental services and sight tests. There may be a fee for these, depending on the person's means.

It may be possible to obtain help with a variety of *housing* needs. Agency services such as 'Care and Repair' or 'Staying Put' give advice and practical assistance to older home owners who need to repair and improve their home, and may be able to advise people who need practical help with gardening or decorating tasks.

There are government grants for home owners, covering all or part of the cost of improvements or repairs. These grants depend on a person's means. There are also disabled facilities grants, covering the cost of, say, installing a downstairs toilet for use by a disabled person. You might be able to get help from the Social Services Department with stair rails, or with locks and safety devices.

These forms of help are not only for people with dementia and their carers, of course. But it is important for you to remember that they may contribute to your overall well-being and ability to manage.

Reflecting on the interests of the forgetful person may give a clue about the kind of help which would be useful:

Mr Gillis had always been active. Now that he had a mild dementia, he was unable to continue his job, and was bored and restless. His daughter arranged for him to work as a volunteer at a nearby nursing home, where he dug the garden and weeded flower-beds. He remained active and useful, and the nursing home staff were able to remind him frequently what to do next.

This example illustrates that help comes not only from *services*, but from thinking creatively about your own needs and those of the person you care for, and looking for opportunities where you live.

A checklist of support which may be available locally

- adaptations to the home – for example ramps, a downstairs toilet;
- adult education classes – lip reading; recreation; active interests;
- aids to daily living – bath aids; modifications to cookers; non-spill cups; non-slip trays;
- alarm systems – to contact a centre or agency in an emergency;
- assessment – arranged by the local authority Social Services Department, in co-operation with other services as necessary;
- bathing service – help with bathing a disabled person;
- care manager – to co-ordinate and arrange a 'care package' after an assessment has been carried out;
- carers' support groups – for mutual help and support;
- chiropody – free from the NHS to anyone over 60;
- clubs – bowls; gardening; photography; sport;
- concessionary schemes – cheap fares, hairdressing, recreation and leisure;
- counselling – for the dementing person and/or carer;
- day care, day centres – sometimes at weekends as well as weekdays; sometimes extended hours so the carer can work;
- day hospitals – arranged through the consultant or specialist;
- dental care – provided at home for people who cannot get out;
- district or community nurse; nursing aide or auxiliary – through GP, clinic or hospital. Includes community psychiatric nursing;
- fostering or family placement schemes – regular breaks or permanent care in a family home;
- general practitioner and 'primary' health care services – includes the offer of an assessment each year for people aged 75 and over;
- health visitors – to advise on a range of health matters;
- holidays – either for the person cared for or for the carer(s) as well;
- home care service – for people who require a lot of personal care and assistance;
- home help – the more traditional cleaning and shopping service;
- home repairs and practical help – decorating, gardening, wiring;
- incontinence services – help with supplies or continence advice;
- key worker – the named person who might have most contact with a dementing person and care-giver;
- laundry service – for people who are incontinent;

- leisure activities and programmes – perhaps through the local health education unit or the local leisure centre;
- library services – including those for housebound people;
- lunch clubs – run by the council, or by voluntary organisations or local groups;
- meals-on-wheels – run by the council, or perhaps by WRVS or Age Concern on behalf of the council;
- nailcutting services;
- night nurses – either from the NHS or a nursing agency;
- occupational therapy – advice on living conditions and other matters – through the Social Services Department for those living at home, or through hospital or day hospital referral;
- physiotherapy – improvement of mobility or recovery from the effects of an operation or illness;
- respite – or short-stay-care – either by arranging for someone to come into your home or by the dementing person going into a home or hospital. Sometimes provided on a regular basis (six weeks out – two weeks in, for instance);
- sitting services – in a person's own home;
- social clubs and activities;
- social work;
- telephones – concessionary rates for low users; special servicing arrangements for people with severe disabilities living on their own;
- twilight service – help with going to bed; also available for getting up in the morning;
- visiting service – someone to drop in from time to time, usually offered by voluntary agencies.

Having someone to come into your home

Many families can continue to care for a person if they are able to arrange for someone to come into their home to help. Such a person may be another family member, a friend, neighbour, church member, paid or volunteer visitor, care attendant, home help, hired housekeeper or nurse. Unfortunately, resources for help at home are limited, and help may not be available in your area or may cost more than you can afford.

Church groups are sometimes involved in neighbourhood care schemes and may organise a team of helpers. Sometimes they will bring in meals for a short period (for example, while you are unwell).

Some voluntary groups are able to find a person who will sit with the impaired person for part of the day and who may prepare meals. Sometimes the helper is paid a small sum or hourly wage. This may make it easier for you to ask for help. New care management arrangements which will gradually be introduced as part of the community care changes may include paying a neighbour or friend for regular specified help.

Another form of support is the meals-on-wheels service, which will bring a hot meal to people who cannot get out. Ask the local Social Services Department who provides this locally. Meals can be brought daily (including weekends), or perhaps just one or two days a week. The person who delivers the meal may also check how well a person living alone is coping, but such care is limited and is no substitute for supervision. Sometimes this service is refused if a person is living with a carer. It is assumed that the carer can cope with the cooking. If this is a problem for you, say so, and explain why the person you care for – and you yourself, if necessary – would benefit from a meal.

Finding a helper

People whom you might employ on an occasional or casual basis are often found through word of mouth. Ask your friends if they know of someone. One person who does this sort of work may be able to recruit some friends. Sometimes a person can be found by advertising in the newspaper. The Social Services Department or Age Concern may know of such people.

Obviously, as with anyone you are taking into your home, you – or the person arranging the care – should check a potential employee's or volunteer's references, and ensure that she understands the confused person's condition and is willing to care for her.

Discuss payment and exact responsibilities before you hire anyone. It may seem too formal to write things down, but that could help to make things clear right from the beginning. For instance, you will want to be clear about what you hope the visitor or helper will do. It may be unreasonable, for instance, to expect someone to clean the house *and* watch an ill person for the same money she would be paid just for cleaning. Realistically, a domestic helper probably cannot look after a confused person and clean the house. It is challenging to do both and often impossible for someone unfamiliar with your home and the impaired person. You may have to settle for a sitter and not a clean house.

It is important for a helper to understand the nature of the person's disability and to know how to avoid or respond to catastrophic reactions. A helper also needs to know how to reach you or another responsible family member in case of an emergency. Explain to the helper what the person can or cannot do, and what special care she needs. Remember that the impaired person might give the helper misleading information. It might help to write down special information: how much assistance will the person need in the toilet or with meals? What does she like for lunch? What cues does she give to show that she is becoming irritable, and how do you respond? What special needs does she have? Invite the helper into your home several times while you are there. This enables the forgetful person to get used to the presence of another person in the house, and gives the helper a chance to learn your routine.

If the sick person has complicating health problems, such as a heart or respiratory condition, a tendency to choke or fall, or epilepsy, you must carefully consider the skills of the helper with whom you leave her. If the person gets upset easily, you may have to discuss with the doctor ways to reduce this behaviour. We discuss the problems which can arise when the confused person rejects the visiting care-giver on pages 182–4.

You may well have to look around to find the help you need. The Social Services Department should be able to offer advice, and may run schemes of their own. They may also be able to set up a package of support for an impaired person living on her own. Such support might include home care several times a day, help with cooking meals and support at weekends. This might be appropriate for a confused person who doesn't wander, for instance.

Sometimes families group together to exchange services, perhaps through a carers' support group. Plans can be simple or elaborate; basically, two or three families agree to take turns sitting. You may sit with the confused people in your home one afternoon, and then the next week someone else will sit while you enjoy an afternoon out. This system works best when the impaired person is not agitated and does not wander. Such a person enjoys the contact with others.

Nursing and other employment agencies may be able to offer private nurses and other staff, such as companions, to help you on a paid basis. Companions – either live-in or non-residential – may provide a variety of services including personal care, meals and shopping. Nursing help may cover certain tasks, such as changing a catheter or bathing an ill person; or may cover longer periods of supervision.

A number of voluntary organisations may be able to help you with support from either paid or volunteer staff. These groups include local Age Concern, the Alzheimer's Disease Society, MIND, the Carers' National Association, the Women's Royal Voluntary Service, Crossroads Care Attendant Schemes, Councils for Voluntary Service, Stroke Association groups and volunteer bureaux. Services offered might include support groups, day care, night sitting, practical jobs and other forms of care.

If you cannot afford to pay for help, it may be possible to obtain some support with the cost from charitable organisations. Age Concern's factsheet on finding help at home, gives information on looking for such help and is available free on receipt of a large s.a.e.

Care outside your home

Another way for you to obtain help with the care of a person with a dementing illness is to arrange for her to have care outside your home for part of the time. Your local Social Services Department, Alzheimer's Disease Society group or Age Concern may be your best sources of information. As with home care services, care providers outside the home may be reluctant to accept people with dementing illnesses. You may have to help them learn how to care for such people.

One quite informal source of support is a *lunch club*, which will provide a hot meal and also serve as a social occasion. Lunch clubs do not, however, provide medical care, give medication, or accept wandering or disruptive people. They can be very helpful for the mildly or moderately confused person.

Lunch clubs may be run by the local authority or voluntary organisations such as Age Concern and the Women's Royal Voluntary Service. Sometimes the voluntary agencies run the service on behalf of the local authority. There is usually a charge, but this varies from area to area.

Day Care Centres

Day care centres offer several hours care a day for frail, older people. Some centres accept only people with mild or moderate dementia and it may be necessary to find a centre which devotes all or part of its time to demented people – if the person you care for is severely demented. Here they will provide a higher staffing ratio and will be able to provide mental stimulation. Services offered will vary from centre to centre, and you should arrange to see the centre organiser. In some areas, day centres care for members of particular ethnic minority groups. Day centres are run by both local authorities and voluntary organisations. There is usually a charge for transport and meals but this may be assessed according to the client's means. Some centres are attached to or are part of a local authority or independent residential homes. Some are part of 'resource centres', which offer a range of services in one building, perhaps including respite care and various social work services. All kinds of day centres can provide good quality care, which depends largely on the skill of the staff and the philosophy of the centre.

It is not unusual for a family to be discouraged by the first visit to a day centre.

Mr Wilson said, 'I went to see the day centre. The social worker told me this was an excellent centre. But I can't put Alice in there. These people are old and sick. One of them was dragging a shopping bag around and mumbling. One was dribbling. Some of them were in these chairs with a tray across them, hanging on the tray or sleeping.'

The sight of other disabled or elderly people can be distressing, and our perception of a person we love is coloured by our memory of how she used to be. You may feel that such a place does not offer the special care that you can give at home. If you find yourself reacting in this way to places you visit, you may find it helpful to talk to other families who are already using the service. They can tell you how they felt, what places they found that they like, and how they have been able to accept things that upset them at first. You may need to weigh up the importance of relaxation for yourself and the benefits of the impaired person's contact with others against this concern. We have observed that getting out of the house and being with other people may be good for the forgetful person. She may feel comfortable in a setting that does not demand much of her and may make friends with other impaired people.

However, it is also important to make your views known to the people providing or arranging the service. It can be easy sometimes for care to fall into a routine which suits the workers rather than the people who use the service. If, after a while, this appears to you to be the case, then it may be helpful to give gentle reminders that the people receiving care may be dependent, but they are still *people*. They should be cared for in a way that helps them to retain as much dignity and independence as possible. It is not acceptable for people to be restrained without good reason or for incontinent people to have to sit in pools of urine. It is important not to ignore these things, but to help constructively to see how they can be improved. It is never easy to complain, or to make comments which could be taken as criticism of a service which is often provided by dedicated, hardworking and very caring staff. But sometimes making a comment or a complaint can be an important way of helping to improve a service.

Day care is one of the most important resources for families. It provides urgently needed respite for the care-giver and it often benefits the person with dementia. For most of us, the pressures of family life can be relieved by getting away to be with friends or to be alone. The person with dementia does not have this opportunity. She must be with her care-giver day after day, but her impairment does not take away her need to have her own friends and time apart. The burden of this enforced togetherness may be difficult for the impaired person as well as for the care-giver.

People with dementia experience failures and reminders of their inadequacies at every turn. But even when they cannot feed or dress themselves, they often retain their ability to enjoy music, laughter, friends and the pleasures involved in pursuing some simple activity. People with dementia may make friends with other people at the centre, even when they are so impaired that they may not be able to tell you about their friend. Day care staff observe that participants regain a sense of humour, appear more relaxed and enjoy the activities. Good day care centres find ways in which people can succeed at little things and thereby feel better about themselves. Day care fills empty time with activities the person can do well. Some centres may not offer much stimulation or socialisation for the impaired person, but they remain a valuable source of time away from you, and you may gradually be able to suggest some changes which will increase the person's enjoyment of the time spent at the centre.

A major aspect of day care is transportation. Transporting people to and from day care is time-consuming and expensive. Some services pick people up, some contract with local transportation or taxi services, and some require you to transport the person. Be sure that you can cope with these arrangements. If you are kept waiting too long, or the service is irregular, see if there is some way in which it can be improved. Be sure that the person will be given enough supervision while on the way to the day centre.

Many families turn to day care or home care only as a last resort. However, the ability of the confused person to adjust to and benefit from such care is usually greater if you seek care early, when the person still has some mental capacity to adjust to and enjoy a new situation. Your continued ability to care also depends on obtaining early relief for yourself.

Day hospitals

Psychogeriatric day hospitals offer medical services, recreational activities and occupational therapy for impaired people who live at home. They are staffed by nurses, social workers, doctors and other professionals. Transport is often provided to the day hospital.

Because a limited number of places is available in most districts, the vacancies in these units are only offered to patients who are moderately to severely demented to give respite to the care-giver and to try to achieve an improvement in behavioural problems. The impaired person will be assessed by a psychiatrist or psychogeriatrician to determine her needs. The mildly confused person can probably manage to attend a day centre, and there are also day care places available in some Part III residential homes (see page 272).

Geriatric day hospitals admit elderly patients with physical problems (for instance, the impaired person may have had a stroke). Usually the patients must have the potential for rehabilitation, so only mild to moderately demented patients are likely to be considered. The time a person may go to this type of day hospital is normally limited to the period of assessment and treatment.

Short-stay respite care

The confused person may need to stay elsewhere for a short period – a weekend, a week or a few weeks – while you take a holiday, receive needed medical care or just rest. Some care-givers are reluctant to use such short-stay respite; they fear that once they give up the burden of care, even temporarily, they will be unable to shoulder it again. You must have a clear understanding with the provider about the length of the stay. As with all respite programmes, short-stay care is more effective if you can begin to use it *before* you reach the breaking point.

Your local Social Services Department should be able to tell you what short-stay respite care is available in your area. This can be in a residential or nursing home, with another family in a family placement scheme or in a hospital. Some local Age Concerns organise respite care schemes, and the local Alzheimer's Disease Society may also be able to offer advice. Health authorities may arrange respite care in a hospital.

New surroundings may cause stress to people with dementia so short-stay respite care should provide enough staff or carers to give skilled attention to the person's needs. It is important to explain the special requirements of your relative to the providers.

Sometimes it is possible for someone to stay in your own home with the impaired person while you have to be away so that her life is not disrupted and she remains in familiar surroundings. Some social services departments will arrange to do this or you may arrange such care through private agencies, although this can prove very expensive.

For many carers, a regular or occasional break is essential for them to be able to carry on. The community care changes mentioned earlier in this chapter are aimed in part at helping carers; ensuring that there is adequate respite care is one way of fulfilling this aim, and local authority community care plans should show how respite care is going to be developed in your area. If you are not happy with what is planned, make your views known along with those of other people in similar situations to yours.

Helping the confused person adjust to care

Families often say, 'I know my husband. He would never go to day care (or accept another carer at home)', but impaired people can surprise their relatives by enjoying day care or the variety of someone else coming into the home. Avoid asking the person if she would like to go to day care. She is likely to answer 'No', because she does not understand what you are suggesting. Some people continue to say they don't want to go, even when they are clearly enjoying themselves. This usually means that they do not understand or do not remember their enjoyment. Continue cheerfully to take the person to day care.

When a family is able to arrange for someone to stay at home with the impaired person, the ill person may fire the sitter or housekeeper, may become angry or suspicious, insult her, not let her in or accuse her of stealing. To the person with dementia, the new person in the house may seem like an intruder.

Be prepared for a period of adjustment. People with dementia adjust to change slowly: it may take a month for a person with dementia to accept a new routine. When you are already exhausted, arguments over respite care may seem overwhelming. Confused people may refuse to go to day care or put up such a fuss getting ready that you are tempted to give up. Do not feel guilty about forcing the person to change their ways so that you can take a break. Make a commitment to yourself to give the programme a good trial. Often the confused person will accept the new plan if you can weather the initial storm.

What you say will make a difference. Refer to the outside care as an interesting activity the person will like. Introduce the home care provider as a friend who has come to visit. Find things the person with dementia enjoys that the two can do together: take a walk, groom the dog, play a game of draughts (even if not by the rules) or have a cookery session. Call day care anything the person will accept, for example, 'the club'. Often mildly impaired people prefer to 'volunteer' at the centre. Most day care programmes will support this. 'Helping' people who are more impaired allows the person to feel successful while reducing the pressure on her to perform.

Write the confused person a note – say why she is there (or why the home care provider is there), when you will return, and that she is to stay there and wait for you. Sign the note and give it to her or to the provider. If this does not work, ask your doctor to write and sign such a note. The provider can read it with the impaired person each time she becomes restless.

Some families make a short videotape about the care of the confused person. This is particularly helpful when the provider will be assisting in personal care such as dressing or eating. You can show the order in which you do things, for example which arm goes in which sleeve first. You might leave written instructions as well.

Day care and home care providers have found that people adjust better when:

1   the first visits to day care are short enough not to tire the confused person. Although many day care programmes ask care-givers to stay

with the person for the first visit or two, a few prefer them not to
remain. For most people, the presence of the care-giver is reassuring,
although a few do better on their own, away from the care-giver's
tension and uncertainty;

2 someone from the day care centre visits the person at home before
   her first visit to day care;

3 the primary care-giver stays with the confused person during a home
   carer's first few visits. This may help the confused person to feel she
   knows the carer. The first few sessions should be quite short.

Remember, for the confused person, each session at day care or with a
home carer is like starting again. However, most people gradually begin
to accept the new routine. Quite frequent visits to day care or from the
home care provider may help the person experience a sense of continuity.

Some care-givers find that the bother of getting the person ready is so
great that day care is pointless. Perhaps you can arrange for a friend or
neighbour to help with this task. Allow plenty of time; feeling rushed
will upset the confused person even more.

Occasionally a person in day care will come home and say to her
husband, 'My husband is at the centre.' Of course, this is distressing for
the care-giving spouse. The person usually does not mean 'husband'.
Perhaps she is trying to say 'friend' but cannot find the word. Perhaps
'husband' is the closest word she can find to mean companion. It does
not imply a romance and has to be accepted as behaviour which is part
of the illness.

Sometimes the confused person will say, 'She hit me' or 'They
wouldn't give me anything to eat' or 'The fat one took my purse'. It is
important to bear in mind that people with dementia can misperceive,
misremember or express themselves inaccurately. Perhaps she cannot
remember having lunch. Ask the staff for the true version of events.

There may be times, however, when you feel there could be a genuine
problem. You may want to talk to other relatives and carers to see how
they feel about care at the centre. It is more difficult to monitor what is
happening at home. If the impaired person remains unhappy or nervous
over a long period of time, it may be that there is a problem which
should be investigated.

You may ask the person, 'What did you do today?' and she may reply,
'Nothing.' 'Well, did you have a good time?' 'No.' Answers like this may
indicate that she can't remember what went on. Don't embarrass her
by continuing to ask. Ask a staff member what she enjoyed today.

If the person says she does not want to go to day care (or have the
home care provider), you do not have to take this literally. She may
mean that she does not understand what you are suggesting. She may
not remember earlier visits at all. Avoid getting into arguments.
Reassure her that this is something she can handle, that you will come
back for her, and that the people there are nice and will help her.

A few people cannot adjust to home care or day care. Try several different providers. Some people have a way with dementia. Ask yourself whether your attitude is affecting her adjustment (see below). If you cannot use a respite programme now, try again in a few weeks or months. Often changes in the person's condition will make it easier for her to accept a new situation.

Your own feelings about obtaining respite for yourself

As we have seen, many families can be discouraged by their first visit to a day centre and some families are reluctant to bring a stranger into their home. You may not like strangers in your home or you may worry about whether they are honest. You may not want anyone to see your house in a mess. And many people feel, 'My family and I are private people. We take care of our own. We just aren't the kind of people who use public help.'

Like you, families provide almost all of the care of frail elderly people. However, a dementing illness can be particularly devastating for family members. Because it is a disease of the mind, you are faced with the grief of losing companionship and communication, as well as with difficult behaviour, and the tasks of dressing, feeding and toileting the person. These diseases last many years, and care-givers cannot leave the ill person for even a few minutes. Many care-givers are doing little more than surviving – just barely hanging on.

If you become ill, as many care-givers do, others will have to assume responsibility for the person you care for. Good care means caring for yourself too. If you are tired or depressed, you may snap at the confused person. She will usually sense your distress and may respond by whining or wandering or arguing even more (she can't help it). Many care-givers find themselves using medication to control these behaviours. This may make the ill person more confused. Ask yourself: am I rushing her? snapping at her? slapping her?

The best prescriptions we know are to talk to other families and to get some time away from the ill person. Arranging time for yourself, and returning rested and in a better humour can allow you to continue caring.

Talking to other families will often reveal that they, too, were reluctant to use respite care but that the time apart helps the confused person as well as themselves. Care-givers have told us that knowing that a professional provider is also having difficulty with the person makes them feel better about their own efforts to manage. And worries about your home are often unfounded – home care workers say they rarely notice whether the house is tidy or not.

Even if the respite situation is not perfect – if the home sitter watches soap operas or the participants in day care seem to just sit for most of the time – you may want to continue with it. It is very common for family carers to worry that others can't care for their relative as well as they can. While this may be true, remember that your continued strength and your ability to keep on providing care may depend on your taking regular breaks from care-giving.

Some home carers urge you to leave the house while they provide care. This is because they think carers need the time away. It can be tempting to stay and talk with the respite worker or to help with the confused person, but you may manage better in the long run if you get away, even if all you do is take a walk or visit a neighbour. If you stay at home, go into another room, away from the patient.

Paying for care

Local authority fees for day and home care vary. What you pay may depend, for instance, on whether your relative receives the Attendance Allowance or care component of the Disabled Living Allowance; or on what other income your relative receives. You should ensure that you and your relative are receiving all the benefits to which you may be entitled. See Chapter 15 for more about financial matters.

Home nursing and home care assistants can be hired from nursing or home care agencies. If you use an agency, find out whether they will replace an employee if she does not arrive, and also ask how much training or experience the staff have had in caring for people with dementia.

Home carers and companions whom you find and employ yourself are usually less expensive than agency staff but you can spend considerable time locating them and some are unpredictable. Remember that it is vitally important to ask for and check on references very carefully before you employ someone to work in your home.

Some charities may be able to assist with part of the cost of home care and adaptations to your home, but these resources are extremely limited, and many families can expect to pay at least part of the cost of care. There is also increasing uncertainty about who pays for nursing home care. There may be a temptation to save money rather than spend it on respite care, in case resources are needed later for residential or nursing home fees. For a full discussion of paying for residential and nursing home care, see Chapter 16.

Should services mix people who have dementia with people who have other problems?

You may have heard that care services which specialise in the care of people with dementia are supposed to be better than those that mix people with different kinds of health problems. Families sometimes worry about what might happen if a frail, elderly person with Alzheimer's disease is at a centre which caters for people with other types of problem.

Services for a group of people whose needs and levels of functioning are similar, can more easily provide specialised programming that meets their needs. However, many programmes in America have successfully mixed people who are confused with people who have head traumas or physical disabilities. In some areas there are not enough people with dementia who have similar needs to make a specialised programme cost effective. Diagnosis does not describe a person's needs and level of function well: the care of an active and younger individual with Alzheimer's disease may be more similar to that of a head trauma patient than the care of a frail, anxious person with Alzheimer's disease. Anger, grief and exhaustion are common to most families, regardless of diagnosis. Staff skill is more important than diagnosis in most cases.

It is best to judge a service on its standards of individual care and how well you think your family member will fit in with the group. A confused person can take great satisfaction from pushing a wheelchair or handing a dish of biscuits to a physically impaired person. On the other hand, a service that offers a lot of discussion groups, reading and film-watching is focusing on activities that will leave out most people with dementia. If you are concerned that your family member will not fit in or is too frail, discuss your concerns with the centre manager. Some programmes are flexible and try to match activities to a person's current abilities. A trial period is often the best idea. People with dementia often surprise us by how well they can fit in.

Determining the quality of services

Since the confused person may not be able to tell you about the care she receives, you must know about the quality of care provided. *Many of the agencies you approach will not have reliable information about the quality of services they recommend.* For instance, hospital social workers are often under pressure from the hospital to place people quickly.

Many people assume that some government agency is responsible for safeguarding the quality of services such as day care and home care. In fact, central government has almost no control over such programmes. There are no national standards for care, nor is there any requirement for such services to be registered and inspected. However, there are moves by home care providers to introduce a voluntary set of standards and code of practice for care in people's own homes. It is possible that inspection units of local authorities may in future inspect day and home care services which they provide or arrange. Day centres must meet certain safety requirements laid down by local fire and environmental health officers. However, existing standards may not take into account the special limitations of people with dementia (for example, that they need more supervision or that they cannot respond to fire alarms).

Never assume that, because you are given the name of a service by an authority, it is a good-quality service, there are standards it must meet, or it has been recently inspected.

In most of the schemes we have seen, providers work because they love the job, and they give good care. However, there is an occasional bad apple. Checking on the quality of a service is up to you.

Workers should be supervised by a professional or very experienced person, and should be trained in the safe care of elderly people and in the special care of people with dementia. Ask the provider what training the helpers are given. Ask questions, check references and monitor the standard of care, particularly in the beginning. In a day centre, ask about meal preparation, supervision of wandering, fire emergency plans and the kinds of activities provided.

People with dementia often misunderstand or misinterpret things. We have already commented on the importance of keeping a balance between believing what might be far-fetched stories and keeping an eye out for problems which might be developing. It can be difficult to know how well another person is caring for your family member. Carers are almost always honest and caring, and it is important that you have some respite time. Do not avoid obtaining help because you worry about the quality of care. At the same time, be alert to potential problems.

In summary

This chapter has been about obtaining outside help. You will probably already know that this isn't always an easy thing to do. It is hoped that the community care changes will increasingly mean that carers of people with dementia should be able to describe what help they *need*, rather than being limited to the services which have traditionally been available. Some of the services described in this chapter may suit your needs, but there may be other ways in which you feel you need help. Find out what is available in your area – even if you don't feel you need the service now – by asking at your local Social Services Department, Citizens Advice Bureau, Alzheimer's Disease Society or local Age Concern. But don't just think along the lines of the 'traditional' services. The person who knows the most about your needs and those of the person you care for is *you*.

Here is a final check-list to help you to start thinking about what kinds of help would be right for you and the confused person:

- Do you need help with financial planning?
- Do you need more information about the disease or about diagnosis?
- Should you try day care or a sitter at home?
- If you use day care, will you need transportation for the confused person?
- Do you need help for specific tasks, such as giving baths?
- Do you want to go out one night a week? Or do you need to get out during the day when you can drive?
- Do you need someone to talk to?
- What kind of help will the confused person need? (If she becomes agitated, wanders, or is incontinent, be sure that the provider can manage this.)
- Does she need help walking or does she need bed care?

Write down your questions before you begin making telephone calls or visits. Keep notes of your conversations. Write down the names of the people you talk to. If you call back later for additional information, this record will be helpful. If the person you speak to does not have the answers to your questions, ask to speak to someone who does. If a person dismisses you abruptly, ask to speak to someone else. In brief, don't give up.

Chapters 2 to 10 have discussed ways of caring and of obtaining help for the sick person. However, you and your family are important too. A chronic dementing illness places a heavy burden on families: it may mean a lot of work or financial sacrifices; it may mean accepting the reality that someone you love will never be the same again; it may mean that responsibilities and relationships within the family will change; it may mean disagreements within the family; it may mean that you feel overwhelmed, discouraged, isolated, angry or depressed.

You and the person with a dementing illness, as well as the other people close to him, all interact as part of a family system. This system can be severely stressed by a dementing illness. It is helpful to consider the changes that may occur in families that are faced with a chronic illness and to identify the feelings you may experience. Sometimes just knowing that what is happening to you has happened to others can make life easier. Often recognising what is happening suggests ways of improving things.

It is important to know that almost all families do care for their elderly and sick relatives as long as possible. It is simply not true that most British people abandon their elderly in hospitals or 'dump' them in nursing homes. Studies have shown that although many older people do not live with their children, they are closely involved with or cared for by them. Families usually do all they can, often at great personal sacrifice, to care for ill elderly members before seeking help. Of course, there are families who do not care for ill family members. There are some who, because of illness or other problems, are unable to care for their elderly; there are a few who do not wish to; there are some elderly people who have no family to help them. But in the majority of cases, families are struggling to do the best they can for their ill and elderly relatives.

Most family members discover a closeness and co-operation as they work together to care for someone with a dementing illness. Sometimes, however, the pressures of caring for an ill person create conflicts in families, or cause old disagreements to flare up. For example:

Mr Higgins said, 'We can't agree on what to do. I want to keep Mother at home. My sister wants her in a nursing home. We don't even agree on what is wrong.'

Mrs Tate said, 'My brother doesn't call and he refuses even to talk about it. I have to take care of Mother alone.'

In addition, the burden of caring for a person with a dementing illness can be exhausting and distressing for you.

> *Mrs Friday said, 'I get so depressed. I cry. Then I lie awake at night and worry. I feel so helpless.'*

Watching someone close to you decline can be a painful experience. This chapter discusses some of the problems that arise in families. Chapter 12 focuses on some of the feelings you may experience.

It is important to remember that not all of your experiences will be unhappy ones. Many people feel a sense of pride in learning to cope with difficult situations. Many family members rediscover one another as they work together to care for an ill person. As you help a forgetful person enjoy the world around him, you may experience a renewed delight in sharing little things – playing with a puppy or enjoying flowers. You may discover a new faith in yourself, in others, or in God. Most dementing illnesses progress slowly, so you and your family member can look forward to many good years.

> *Mrs Morgan said, 'Although it has been hard, it's been good for me in a lot of ways. It's given me confidence to know that I can manage things my husband always took care of, and in some ways my children and I have grown closer as he has become ill.'*

Since this book is designed to help you with problems when they do occur, most of what we discuss are unhappy feelings and problems, although we know that this is a one-sided view that reflects only part of what life is like for you.

The feelings and problems you and your family experience interact and affect one another. However, for simplicity, we have organised them into separate topics: changes in roles within the family, finding ways to cope with changes in roles and the family conflict that can arise, your own feelings, and finding ways to care for yourself.

Changes in roles

Roles, responsibilities and expectations within the family change when one person becomes ill. For example:

A wife said, 'The worst part is writing out cheques. We have been married 35 years and now I have to learn how to write out cheques and balance the bank account.'

A husband said, 'I feel like a fool washing ladies' underwear in the launderette.'

A son said, 'My father has always been the head of the household. How can I tell him he can't drive?'

A daughter said, 'Why can't my brother help out and take his turn looking after Mother?'

Roles are different from responsibilities, and it is helpful to recognise what roles mean to you and to others in the family. Responsibilities are the jobs each person has in the family, whereas roles relate to who you are, how you are seen and what is expected of you. By 'role' we mean a person's place in his family (for example, head of the household, mother or 'the person everyone turns to'). Roles are established over many years and are not always easy to define. Tasks often symbolise our roles. In the examples above, family members describe having to learn new tasks (doing the washing or balancing the bank account) as well as adjusting to changes in roles (money manager, homemaker, head of the household).

Learning a new responsibility, such as balancing the bank account or washing clothes, can be difficult when you are also faced with the many other day-to-day needs of the confused person, yourself and your family. However, changes in roles are often more difficult to accept or adjust to. Realising that each person's responsibilities change, and that roles and expectations of others also change, will help you to understand the other personal feelings and problems that may arise within families. It is helpful to remember that you have coped with changes in roles at other times in your life and that this experience will help you adjust to new responsibilities.

There are many relationships in which role changes occur as the person becomes demented. Here are four examples:

1   *The relationship between a husband and wife changes when one of them becomes ill.* Some of these changes may be sad and painful. Others can be enriching experiences.

John and May Douglas had been married 41 years when John became ill. John has always been the head of the household. He supported the family, paid the bills and made most of the big decisions. May saw herself as a person who always leaned on her husband. When he became ill, she realised that she did not know how much money or insurance they had, or even how to balance their bank account. Bills were going unpaid, yet when she asked John about it, he yelled at her.

For their anniversary, May cooked a small turkey and planned a quiet time together when they could forget what was happening. When she put the electric carving knife in front of John, he threw it down and shouted at her that the knife did not work and she had ruined the turkey. Trying to keep the peace, May took the knife, and then realised that she had no idea how to carve a turkey. May cried and John stormed. Neither of them felt like eating supper that night.

Having to carve a turkey seemed like the last straw for May. She realised that John could no longer do this, nor could he manage their finances, and she suddenly felt overwhelmed and lost. Throughout their marriage, May had looked to John to solve problems. Now she had to learn to do the things he had always done at the same time as facing his illness.

Learning new skills and responsibilities involves energy and effort, and also means extra work for you. You may not want to take on new tasks. Few husbands want to learn to do the washing, and more than one has found himself the owner of shrunken sweaters and pale pink pants before realising that you can't wash red sweaters with white underwear. A wife who has never managed the cheque book may feel that she doesn't have the ability to manage money and may be afraid of making errors.

In addition to having to do the job itself, the realisation that you must take this job away from your spouse may symbolise all of the sad changes that have taken place. For May, carving the turkey symbolised John's loss of status as head of the family.

A spouse may gradually realise that he is alone with his problem – he has lost the partner with whom he shared things. May could no longer see herself as leaning on her husband. She suddenly found herself, at sixty, on her own and forced to be independent with no one to help her. No wonder she felt overwhelmed by the task. But at the same time, learning new skills gradually gave May a sense of accomplishment. She said, 'I was surprised at myself, really, that I could handle things. Even though I felt so upset, it was good for me to learn that I could manage so well.'

Sometimes problems only appear to be insurmountable because they involve changes in roles as well as the need for you to learn new tasks. Having to learn new skills when you are upset and tired can be difficult. As well as recognising the distress that may be caused by changing roles, you may need some practical suggestions about taking on new responsibilities.

If you must take over the housework, often you can do it gradually and learn as you go. But you can save yourself the frustration of burned suppers and ruined laundry by obtaining the advice of experts. Your local Citizens Advice Bureau may be able to direct you to sources of information on shopping, meal preparation, laundry, budgeting and home maintenance, or you can obtain advice from a social worker or a visiting nurse. You may even find useful brochures or recipes in the supermarket.

> *Mrs Stearns says, I know my husband can't manage his money any more, but it seems as though it is taking away the last of his manhood to take away the cheque book. I know I have to, but I just can't seem to do it.'*

Having to take this symbol of independence away from someone you love can be difficult. It can be worse when you are not accustomed to managing money.

If you have never balanced a cheque book or paid the bills, you may find it hard to learn this new responsibility. In fact, managing household finances is not difficult, even for people who dislike maths. Most banks employ staff who will advise you, without charge. They also will show you how to balance a cheque book. There are books in the library on this subject. The fact that you must take over this role, rather than the task itself, is sometimes what makes it hard to do.

The bank or a solicitor can also help you draw up a list of your or the confused person's assets and liabilities. Sometimes a person has been private about financial affairs, has told no one and now can no longer remember the details. Chapter 15 lists some of the financial resources he may have and which you should try to trace.

If you are unable or do not like to drive but would like to take on responsibility for driving, find a driving course designed for adults. Enquire through the police or through ROSPA (Royal Society for the Prevention of Accidents), Cannon House, Queensway, Birmingham B4 6BS (tel: 021 200 2461). ROSPA runs courses and publishes leaflets on defensive driving, which helps people to avoid being involved in accidents. Life will be much easier if you are comfortable behind the wheel.

2   *The relationship between a parent with a dementing illness and his adult children often has to change.* The changes that occur when an adult child has to assume the responsibility and care of a parent are sometimes called 'role reversal'. Perhaps this is better described as a shift in roles and responsibilities, in which the adult son or daughter gradually assumes increasing responsibility for a parent while the roles of the parent change accordingly. These changes can be difficult. You, the adult son or daughter, may feel sadness and grief at the losses you see in someone you love and look up to. You may feel guilty about 'taking over'.

'I can't tell my mother she shouldn't live alone any more,' Mrs Russell says. *'I know I have to, but every time I try to talk to her she manages to make me feel like a small child who has been bad.'*

To varying degrees, many of us as adults still feel that our parents are parents and that we, the children, are less assured, capable and 'grown up'. In some families, the parents seem to maintain this kind of relationship with their adult children long past the time when adult sons and daughters usually come to feel mature in their own right.

Not everyone has had a good relationship with his parents. If a parent has not been able to let his grown children feel grown up, a lot of unhappiness and conflict may develop. Then, as the parent develops a dementing illness, he can seem to be demanding and manipulative. You may find yourself feeling trapped. You may feel used, angry and guilty at the same time.

What seems demanding to you may feel different to the impaired person. He may be feeling that with 'just a little help' he can hold on to his independence, perhaps continue to live alone. As he senses his decline, this may seem the only way he can respond to his losses.

Adult children often feel embarrassed by the tasks of physically caring for a parent – for example, giving their mother a bath or changing their father's underwear. Look for ways of helping your parent retain his dignity at the same time as you give needed care.

3   *The sick person must adjust to his changing roles within the family.* This often means giving up some of his independence, responsibility or leadership, which can be difficult for everyone (see also Chapter 4). He may become discouraged or depressed as he realises his abilities are waning. He may be unable to change or recognise his decline.

The roles a person has held within the family in the past, and the kind of person he is, will influence the new roles he assumes as he becomes ill. You can help him to maintain his position as an important member of the family even when he can no longer carry out familiar tasks. Consult him, talk to him, listen to him (even if what he says seems confused). Let him know by these actions that he is still respected.

4.   *As the roles of the sick person change, the expectations of each member of the family for the others change too.* Your relationships with and expectations of members of the family are based on family roles that have been established over many years. Changes often lead to conflicts, misunderstandings and occasions when people's expectations of each other do not agree. At the same time, adjusting to changes and facing problems can bring families closer together, even when they have not been close for years.

Understanding family conflicts

Mrs Eaton says, 'My brother doesn't have anything to do with Mum now – and he was always her favourite. He won't even come to see her. All the burden is on my sister and me. Because my sister's marriage is shaky, I hate to leave Mum with her for long. So I end up taking care of Mum pretty much alone.'

Mr Cooke says, 'My son wants me to put her in a nursing home. He doesn't understand that, after thirty years of marriage, I can't just put her in a nursing home.' His son says, 'Dad isn't being realistic. He can't manage Mother in that big two-storey house. She's going to fall one of these days. And Dad has a heart condition that he refuses to discuss.'

Mr Vane says, 'My brother says if I kept her more active, she would get better. He says I should answer her back when she gets nasty, but that only makes things worse. He doesn't live with her. He just stays in his own home and criticises.'

Division of responsibility

The responsibility of caring for an impaired person often is not evenly shared by the family. Like Mrs Eaton, you may find that you are carrying most of the burden of care. There are many reasons why it is difficult to divide responsibility evenly. Some members of the family may live far away, may be in poor health, may be financially unable to help or may have problems with their children or marriage.

Sometimes families accept stereotypical ideas about who should help without really considering the best solution. One such idea is that daughters (and daughters-in-law) are 'supposed' to take care of the sick. But the daughter or daughter-in-law may already be heavily burdened and not be able to take on this task. Perhaps she has young children, or a full-time job. Perhaps she is a single parent.

Long-established roles, responsibilities and mutual expectations within the family, even when we are unaware of them, can play an important part in determining who accepts responsibility for the impaired person. For example:

'My mother brought me up. Now I must take care of her.'

'She was a good wife, and she would have done the same for me.'

'I married him late in life. What responsibility is mine and what responsibility is his children's?'

'He was always hard on me, deserted my mother when I was ten, and he's willed all his money to some organisation. How much do I owe him?'

Sometimes expectations are illogical and may not be based on the fairest or most practical way of arranging things.

Sometimes family members fail to help as much as they might because it is difficult for them to accept the reality of the impaired person's illness. Sometimes a person just can't bear to face this illness. It is painful, as you know, to watch a loved one decline. Sometimes family members who do not have the burden of daily care stay away because witnessing the decline makes them feel sad. However, others in the family may view this action as desertion.

Sometimes one family member assumes most of the burden of care. He may not tell other members of the family how bad things are. He may not want to burden them or he may not really want their help.

Mr Newman says, 'I hesitate to call on my sons. They are willing to help, but they have their own careers and families.'

Mrs King says, 'I don't like to call on my daughter. She always tells me what she thinks I am doing wrong.'

Often you and other members of the family have strong and differing ideas of how things should be done. Sometimes this happens because not all family members understand what is wrong with the person who has a dementing illness, or why he acts as he does, or what can be expected in the future.

Family members who do not share the day-to-day experience of living with a person suffering from a dementing illness may not know what it is really like, and may be critical or unsympathetic. It is hard for people on the outside to realise how wearing the daily burden of constant care can be. Often, too, people don't realise how you are feeling unless you tell them.

Occasionally a family member will oppose your efforts to obtain outside help. If this happens, insist that the family member helps to take care of the ill person so that you can get some rest. If the family member lives some distance away, ask him to attend a support group in his community or to volunteer to work in a facility caring for people with dementia so that he will better understand what you are facing. Ultimately, the family must accept that the relative who provides most of the care should make the final decisions about using day care, support in the home or a nursing home, and fewer misunderstandings arise when everyone is kept informed about the cost and availability of resources.

Your marriage

When the ill person is your parent or in-law, it is important to consider the effect of his illness on your marriage. Maintaining a good marriage is often not easy, and caring for a person with a dementing illness can make it much more difficult. It may mean greater financial burdens, and less time to talk, to go out and to make love. It may entail being more involved with your in-laws, having more things to disagree over, often being tired, and not giving the children enough attention. It can mean having to include a difficult, disagreeable, seemingly demanding and sick person in your lives.

A dementing illness can be painful to watch. It is understandable for a person to look at his impaired in-law, and to wonder if his spouse will become like that and if, as a result, he will have to go through this whole process again.

Sons or daughters can easily find themselves torn between the needs of an impaired parent, the expectations of brothers and sisters (or the other parent), and the needs and demands of a spouse and children. It's easy to take out frustrations or fatigue on those we love and trust most – our spouse and our children.

The spouse of an ill parent may also create problems. He may be upset, critical or ill, or he may even desert his ill partner. Such problems can add to the tension in your own marriage, and, if at all possible, should be discussed with everyone involved. It is sometimes easier if sons or daughters discuss the problem with their own relatives first, explaining that it is causing tensions in their own marriage.

A good relationship can survive for a while in the face of stress and trouble, but we believe it is important for the husband and wife to find time and energy for each other – to talk, to get away and to enjoy their relationship as they always have.

Coping with role changes and family conflicts

When family members do not agree, or when most of the burden falls on one relative, it adds to the problems. The burden of caring for a chronically ill person is often too much for one individual. It is important for carers to receive the help of others – to give them 'time out' from constant care, to give encouragement and support, to help with the work, and to share the financial responsibility.

If you are being criticised by your family, or not receiving enough help from them, it is usually not a good idea to let your resentment smoulder. It may be up to you to take the initiative to change things in your family. When families are in disagreement or when long-established conflicts get in the way, this may be difficult to do.

How do you handle the often complex, painful role changes that are set in motion by a chronic, dementing illness? First, recognise these as aspects of family relationships. Just knowing that roles in families are complex, often unrecognised or unacknowledged, and that changes can be painful, will help you to feel calmer and more able to cope. Recognise that certain tasks may be symbolic of important roles in the family and that it is the shift of role, rather than the specific issue, which may be painful.

Find out all you can about the disease. What family members believe to be true about the illness can affect how much help they provide for a person and the frequency with which disagreements arise. Family members who live some distance away can attend Alzheimer's Disease Society meetings in their own community in order to improve their understanding.

Think about the differences between the responsibilities or tasks that an impaired person may have to give up and the roles that he may be able to retain. For example, although a husband's illness means he can no longer make many decisions, his *role* as a loved and respected husband can remain (see p. 191).

Understand what the impaired person is still able to do and what is too difficult for him. Of course, one wants a person to remain as self-reliant as possible, but expectations that exceed his capabilities can upset him. (Sometimes such expectations of how well a person can function come from others; sometimes they come from the impaired person himself.) If he cannot carry out a task independently, try to simplify the job so that he can still do part of it.

Recognise that role changes are not one-off events, but rather continuing processes. As the illness progresses, you may again have to take on new responsibilities. Each time, you will probably re-experience some of the feelings of sadness and of being overwhelmed by your job. This is a part of the grief process involved in caring for someone with a chronic disease.

Talk over your situation with other families. This is one of the advantages of family support groups. You may find it comforting to learn that other families have struggled with similar changes. Laugh at yourself a little. When you have just burned the supper, try to see the humour in the situation. Often, when families of people with dementing illnesses meet they share both tears and laughter over such experiences.

Look for ways of helping each other. When a wife takes on most of the responsibility for daily care of a parent, she may badly need her husband's help with such untraditional jobs as the housework or with sitting with the parent while she goes out. She will certainly need his love and encouragement, and may need his help with the rest of the family.

You may reach a point where the demands of your job are exhausting you. You must be able to recognise this and to make other arrangements when that time comes. Your responsibilities as decision maker may eventually include making the decision to give up your role as primary care-giver.

A family conference

We feel that a family conference is one of the most effective ways of helping families cope. Arrange a family meeting, with help from a social worker or the doctor if needed, to talk over the problems and to make plans. Together you can make definite decisions about how much help or money each person will contribute.

There are ground rules for a family conference which you might suggest at the beginning: everyone attend (including children who will be affected by the decision), each person has his say, uninterrupted, and everyone listens to what the others have to say (even if they don't agree).

If family members disagree about what is wrong with the confused, forgetful person or about how to manage his care, it may be helpful to give other members of the family this book and other written material about the specific disease, or to ask the doctor to talk to them. It is surprising how often this reduces the tensions between family members.

Here are some questions to ask of each other when you meet:

- What are the problems?
- Who is doing what now?
- What needs to be done, and who can do it?
- How can you help each other?
- What will these changes mean for each of you?

Some of the practical questions that need to be discussed might be:

- Who will be responsible for daily care?
- Does this mean giving up privacy? not having friends over? not being able to afford a holiday?
- Does this mean that parents will expect their children to act in a more grown-up way because the parents will be busy with the impaired person?

- Who will make the decision to put a relative in a nursing home or seek hospital care?
- Who will be responsible for the impaired person's money?

If a well spouse of the impaired person is to move into a son or daughter's home with the impaired person, what will this person's roles in the family be? Will she have responsibility for the grandchildren? Will there be two women in the kitchen? An expanded family can be enriching, but it also can create tensions. Anticipating and discussing areas of disagreement in advance can make things easier.

It is also important to talk about several other practical areas which can cause trouble in family relationships. It can seem insensitive even to think about matters of money or inheritance when a loved one is ill but financial concerns are important, and questions about who will receive the inheritance are real – if often hidden – factors in determining responsibility for a family member. They can be the underlying cause of much bitterness, so money matters need to be brought out into the open. Ask yourself the following questions:

1 Does everyone realise the amount of the inheritance likely to be bequeathed? It is surprising how often one son is thinking, 'Dad has those shares he bought twenty years ago, he owns his house, and he has his pension. He ought to be quite comfortable.' The other son, who is taking care of his father, knows 'the house needs a new roof and a new boiler, those old shares are worthless, and he gets barely enough to live on from his pension. I have to dip into my own pocket to pay some bills.'

2 Is there a will? Does someone feel that he may have been short-changed in the will? Do some members of the family feel that others are greedy for inherited money, property or personal possessions? This is not unusual and it can best be handled when it is openly faced. Hidden resentments often smoulder and can emerge as conflicts over the daily care of the person.

3 How much does it cost to care for the impaired person, and who is paying the bills? When a family cares for a person at home, there are many 'hidden' costs to consider: special foods, special door latches, a sitter, transport, another bed, bedroom furniture on the ground floor. You may also have to estimate the loss of a wife's income if she gives up work to care for the confused person.

4 Does everyone know what it costs to care for a person with a dementing illness in a residential or nursing home, and does everyone know who is legally responsible for those costs? (Care home costs are discussed in Chapter 16.) Sometimes when a daughter says, 'Mother

must put Dad in a home', she does not realise that doing so may deprive her mother of most of their joint income and leave her mother nearly destitute.

5   Do some members of the family feel that money has been unequally distributed in the past? For example:

   'Dad put my brother through college and gave him the down payment on his house. Yet now my brother won't take him, so I get the work – and the cost – of taking care of him.'

Families sometimes say, 'It is inconceivable that my family will come together to talk about things like that. My brother won't even discuss it on the phone. And if we did get together it would just be a big fight.' If you feel that your family is like this, you may be discouraged. Although you need your family's aid, you may feel trapped because you feel that your family will not help. It is not unusual for families to need the assistance of an outside person – a counsellor, minister or social worker – to work out their problems and to help them arrive at an equitable arrangement.

   One of the advantages of seeking the assistance of a counsellor is that he can listen objectively. He can also help the family focus on the problems under consideration and not become side tracked by old arguments. Your doctor, a social worker or a counsellor may be able to intervene on your behalf and convince everyone involved of the need for a family meeting to discuss issues of concern to them all. You should be able to trace a local counsellor thorugh the British Association for Counselling, 1 Regent Place, Rugby, Warwickshire, CV21 2RY (tel: 0788 578328/9). Sometimes a family solicitor can help. If you seek the help of a solicitor, ensure that he is genuinely interested in helping resolve conflict rather than in helping you become involved in litigation against other family members. If your family is having problems and you ask a third party to assist you, the first item on the agenda may be to agree that the third party should not take sides.

   You need your family. Now is an excellent time to put aside old conflicts for the sake of the impaired person. If your relatives cannot resolve all their disagreements, you may perhaps, through discussion, discover one or two issues upon which you do agree. This will encourage everyone and the next discussion may be easier.

When you live some distance away

   'My father takes care of my mother. They live about a hundred miles from here and it's hard for me to get back home often. I don't think Dad tells me how bad things really are. It's just terribly hard to be so far away: you feel so guilty and helpless.'

> *'I'm just the daughter-in-law, so I can't say much. They haven't obtained an accurate diagnosis. They keep going to this old family doctor. I worry that there is something else wrong with her. But every time I make a suggestion, they pretend they didn't hear it.'*

Not living in the same community as the confused person and the person who provides daily care creates special problems. Long-distance family members care just as much as those close to home, and they often feel frustrated and helpless. They worry that they do not know what is really happening, that the care-giver has not obtained the best diagnosis or that the care-giver should do things differently. They may feel guilty that they cannot be nearby at a time when their family needs them.

At first, it can be more difficult to accept the severity of a person's limitations if you see the person infrequently. Later, the shock of seeing how a person has declined can be heartbreaking.

The support of the person who provides the daily care is probably the single most important contribution you can make to the ill family member. Dementing illnesses usually last for several years and you need to establish family co-operation for the 'long haul'. If the person who provides daily care rejects your suggestions at first, she may accept them later.

When you are not the primary care-giver, what can you do to help?

British families do not abandon their elderly members, nor do they abandon each other. Despite differences, families usually resolve their disagreements sufficiently enough to pull together.

There are many things family members can do. One care-giver may need a telephone call every day; another may need a sitter so that he can go out one night a week; one may need someone who can come over at short notice when things get difficult; another may just need a shoulder to cry on.

Stay in close touch. Maintain open lines of communication with the care-giver. This will help you sense when the care-giver needs more help. Care-givers manage better and experience less stress when they feel well supported by their family.

Avoid criticising. Criticism usually does not lead to constructive change. None of us likes to be criticised and many of us tend to ignore criticism. If you must say something, be sure your criticism is valid. If you do not live close, are you sure you completely understand the problem?

Recognise that the primary care-giver must make the final decisions.   Although you can offer help and advice, the relative who provides care day after day must be the one to decide whether, for instance, she can use outside help and whether she can continue to provide care.

Take on the job of finding help.   Care-givers are often so overwhelmed that they cannot seek a sitter, a day care centre, better medical care, supportive equipment or help for themselves. Just finding respite can entail many telephone calls. Take on this job and be gentle and supportive as you persuade your relative to use respite.

Be informed.   You will help most if you understand the disease as well as what the care-giver is experiencing. Excellent books are available on these topics. Attend family support group meetings in your community. You may meet other long-distance family members, and you can learn from primary care-givers what *their* long-distance relatives did that helped most. Avoid the temptation to ignore the problem. Dementing diseases are so devastating that the whole family must pull together.

Call the ill person's physician and others who have assessed him. If he is willing, ask direct questions. (See Chapter 2.) If you have concerns about the diagnosis, the adequacy of the assessment or the likely course of the disease, ask the professionals who know the person.

Take on the tasks the confused person used to do.   Balance the chequebook, take the car to the garage, bring over a home-cooked meal.

Give the care-giver time off.   Care for your relative for a weekend, a week or for a few days, so that the primary care-giver can get away. Many Alzheimer's Disease Society groups will teach you the basics of caregiving before you undertake this. Not only will it be valuable for the care-giver to get away, it will also bring you and the care-giver closer together. Although moving an ill person to another home can be upsetting, especially early in a dementing illness, it might serve as a 'holiday' for the ill person as well as the care-giver. Do things that are therapeutic and fun for the ill person: take walks, go out to dinner, play with the cat together or go window shopping.

Obtain help if you cannot provide it yourself.   In many communities, you can obtain sitter care and adult day care. You can also pay someone to do the shopping or to mend the car.

Care-giving and your job

Many care-givers are juggling the care of a person with dementia and a full or part-time job. The double demands of caring and holding down a job can be overwhelming. Some care-givers have to take time off from work each time there is a problem with the ill person. Sometimes, when there is no other choice, care-givers must leave the confused person alone, even if this is really not safe. Even care-givers who use a good day care centre or a reliable sitter, face extra demands and problems. For example, when the person with dementia is awake and active at night, the care-giver loses sleep.

If you are thinking about leaving your job to provide full-time care, consider the options carefully. Many care-givers have found that they were more stressed and more depressed after giving up a job. Full-time care-giving may mean that you must tolerate the person's annoying behaviour all the time. You may also feel more isolated and confined than previously. Leaving your job usually means a significant loss of income. It may mean putting your career on hold and not remaining up to date in your profession. Returning to work after several years of care-giving can be difficult. Will there be a vacancy? Will you have lost seniority or benefits?

Before you make a decision, discuss your options with your employer. Can you arrange more flexible hours? Can you share the job? Is a paid or unpaid leave of absence possible? Some loving daughters find that a good residential or nursing home is a wiser choice for both themselves and their ill parent.

Your children

Having children at home can create special problems. They, too, have a relationship with the sick person, and they have complex feelings – which they may not express – about his illness. Parents often worry about the effect that being with an impaired person will have on children. It is hard to know what to tell a child about a parent's or grandparent's 'odd' behaviour. Sometimes parents worry that children will learn undesirable behaviour from people with dementing illnesses.

Children are usually aware of what is going on. They are excellent observers and, even when things are carefully concealed from them, often sense that something is wrong. Fortunately, children are marvellously resilient. Even small children can benefit from an honest explanation of what is happening to the person with a dementing illness – in language they can understand. This helps to allay their fears. Reassure the child that the illness is not 'catching' like chicken pox, and that neither children nor parents are likely to get it. Tell the child directly that nothing he did 'caused' this illness. Sometimes children secretly feel to blame for the things that happen in their family.

> *One father put a pile of dried beans on the table. He took little pieces of the pile away as he gave his young son the following explanation of his grandfather's illness: 'Grandpa has an illness that makes him act like he does. It isn't catching. None of us is going to get like Grandpa. It's like having a broken leg, only little pieces of Grandpa's brain are broken. He won't get any better. This little piece of Grandpa's brain is broken, so he can't remember what you just told him; this little piece is broken, so he forgets how to use his cutlery at the table; this little piece is broken, so he gets angry too readily. But this part, which is for loving, Grandpa still has left.*

It is usually best to involve children actively in what is happening in the family and even to find ways in which they can help. Small children frequently relate well to impaired, confused people, and can establish special and loving relationships with them. Try to create an atmosphere in which the child can ask you questions and express his feelings openly. Remember that children also feel sadness and grief, but they may be able to enjoy the childlike ways of an impaired person without feeling sad. The more comfortable you feel in your understanding of the illness, the more easily you will be able to explain it to your child.

Children may need help knowing what to tell playmates who tease them about a 'funny' parent or grandparent.

It is unlikely that children will mimic the undesirable behaviour of a person with a dementing illness for long, if, when it occurs, you don't make an issue out of it, and if the child is receiving enough love and attention. Clearly explain (probably several times) to the child that his parent or grandparent has a disease. He cannot help what he does but the child can, and is expected to, control his behaviour.

Young people may be frightened by strange, unexplained behaviour. Sometimes they worry that something they did or might do will make the person worse. It is important to talk about these concerns and to reassure the young person.

One family with children ranging from ten to sixteen shared with us the following thoughts based on their own experience:

- Don't assume that you know what a youngster is thinking.
- What's going on in a child's head is not what we think! Anyone who has been spent time with children can think of examples.
- Children, even small children, also feel pity, sadness and sympathy.

- If we had it to do all over again, we would talk more with the children.
- The effects of this illness linger long after the confused person has gone to a hospital or nursing home. Get together with the children afterwards and continue to discuss things.
- Make an effort to involve all of the children equally in the person's care. Children can find it hard to be depended on or they can feel left out. Sharing in care gives them a sense of responsibility.
- The parent closest to the impaired person needs to be aware of the children, and the impact of her grief and distress on them. Sometimes a person can be so overwhelmed by her own troubles that she forgets the children. Her behaviour can be as hard on the children as the illness itself.

Perhaps the biggest problem arising when there are children at home is that the parent's time and energies are divided between that person and the children – with never enough for both. In order to cope with this double load, you will need every bit of help available – the assistance of the rest of the family, the resources of the community, and time – for you to replenish your own emotional and physical energies. You may find yourself torn between neglecting the children and neglecting a 'childish' or demanding person with a dementing illness.

As the person's condition worsens, so may your dilemma. The declining person may need more and more care, and may be so disruptive that children cannot feel comfortable at home. You may not have the physical or emotional energy to meet the needs of children or adolescents *and* the sick person. Children growing up in such a situation may suffer as a result of the person's illness.

You may make the painful decision to place the impaired person in a hospital, if a place is available, or in a nursing home in order to create a better home environment for the children. If you face such a decision, you and your children need to discuss what is to be done, talking over what the various alternatives will mean to each member of the family. 'We will have less money for luxuries, but we wouldn't have Dad shouting all night.' 'We would move and have to change schools, but I could bring friends home.'

The support of your doctor, clergyman or a counsellor is helpful at such times. Families often find it easier to make decisions when they know they are not alone.

Teenagers

Adolescents may be embarrassed by 'odd' behaviour, reluctant to bring friends home, resentful of the demands made on you by the confused person, or hurt by the confused person's failure to remember them. Adolescents can also be extraordinarily compassionate, supportive, responsible and altruistic. They often have an unspoiled sense of humanitarianism and kindness which is refreshing and helpful. Certainly they will have mixed feelings. Like you, they may experience the grief of seeing someone they love change drastically at the same time as feeling resentful or embarrassed. Mixed feelings lead to mixed reactions that are often puzzling to other family members.

The adolescent years can be hard for young people, whether there are problems at home or not. However, many adults, looking back, recognise that sharing in family problems helped them to become mature adults.

Ensure that your adolescent understands the nature of the disease and what is happening. Be honest with him about what is going on. Explanations, given gently, help a lot. Children seldom benefit from mistaken attempts to shelter them. Involve the adolescent in family discussions and in conferences with health professionals, so that he, too, understands what is happening.

Spend time away from the impaired person, when you are not exhausted or cross, in order to maintain a good relationship with your adolescent and to hear about his interests. Remember that he has a life apart from the illness and the situation at home. Try to find space for his teenage friends away from the impaired person.

Remember that you may be less patient or more emotional because of the extra demands placed upon you. Again, breaks for you may help you to be more patient with your children.

When a grandparent moves into your home, it is important that both he and your children know who sets the rules and who disciplines the children. When the grandparent is forgetful, it is important that your children know what is expected of them to avoid conflicts like, 'Grandmother says I can't go out on dates' 'Granddad says I have to turn off the TV.'

When the ill person has adolescent children, these young people lose a parent at a critical time in their own lives. At the same time, they must cope with the illness and its never-ending problems. They can also feel that they are losing the remaining parent if that person is distracted by grief and fully occupied by care-giving.

In this situation you face almost insurmountable burdens. You must arrange for enough help to allow you to maintain your own mental and physical health, and to continue to assist your children. Since adolescents often are more comfortable with an outsider than a parent, ask a relative, teacher or church member to assume the role of 'special friend'. A few Alzheimer's Disease Society groups offer support for young people. (See also Chapter 14.)

Family members tell us that they experience many feelings as they care for a person with a chronic, dementing illness. They feel sad, discouraged and alone. They feel angry, guilty or hopeless. They feel tired or depressed. In the face of the reality of a chronic illness, emotional distress is appropriate and understandable. Sometimes families of people with dementing illnesses find themselves overwhelmed by their feelings.

Human feelings are complex and they vary from person to person. In this chapter we have tried to avoid oversimplifying feelings or offering simplistic solutions. Our goal is to remind you that it is not unusual to experience many feelings.

Emotional reactions

People have different ways of handling their emotions. Some people experience each feeling intensely, others do not. Sometimes people think that certain feelings are unacceptable – that they should not have certain feelings or that, if they do, no one could possibly understand them. Sometimes they feel alone with their feelings.

Sometimes people have mixed feelings. One might both love and dislike the same person, or want to keep a family member at home and put her in a hospital or nursing home, all at the same time. Having mixed feelings might not seem logical, but it is common. Often people do not realise that they have mixed feelings.

Sometimes people are afraid of strong emotions, perhaps because such feelings are uncomfortable, perhaps because they are afraid they might do something rash or perhaps because they are concerned about how others will view them. These and other responses to our feelings are not unusual. In fact, most of us will have similar responses at one time or another.

We do not believe there is a 'right' way to handle emotions. We think that recognising how you feel and having some understanding of why you feel the way you do is important, because your feelings affect your judgement. Unrecognised or unacknowledged feelings can influence the decisions a person makes in ways that he does not understand or realise. You can acknowledge and recognise your feelings – to yourself and to others – but you have a choice of when, where and whether to express your feelings or to act on them.

People sometimes worry that not expressing feelings causes stress related diseases. Suppose you know that you are often angry with the behaviour of a person with a dementing illness, but you decide not to shout at her because it only makes her behaviour worse. Will you develop ulcers, migraines or hypertension? Researchers disagree about the relationship between feelings and diseases. At present, the causes of diseases such as ulcers, migraines and hypertension are unknown. It has not been our observation that these conditions are more common among families who care for people with dementing illnesses. We do believe, however, that as families appreciate that the irritating behaviour of a confused person is a symptom of her disease, they feel less frustrated and angry and they can care better for the confused person.

As you read this section, remember that each person and each family is different. You may not experience these feelings but we have discussed them in order to help those family members who *do* feel angry or discouraged, tired or sad, etc. Rather than reading the whole of this section, you may prefer to consult it when you feel a particular passage might be helpful.

Anger

It is understandable for you to feel frustrated and angry: angry that this has happened to you, angry that you have to be the care-giver, angry with others who don't seem to be helping, angry with the impaired person for her irritating behaviour, angry that you are trapped in this situation.

Some people with dementing illnesses develop behaviour patterns that are extremely irritating and that can seem impossible to live with. You will understandably feel angry and may sometimes react by shouting or arguing.

Mrs Palling felt that she must not get angry with her husband. They had had a good marriage and she knew that he could not help himself now that he was ill. She says, 'We went to dinner at my son and daughter-in-law's house. I have never felt comfortable with my daughter-in-law, anyway, and I don't think she understands about Joe. As soon as we got inside the door, Joe looked around and said, "Let's go home." I tried to explain to him that we were staying for dinner and all he would say is, "I've never liked it here. Let's go home."

'We sat down to dinner and everyone was tense. Joe wouldn't talk to anyone and he wouldn't take his hat off. As soon as dinner was over, he wanted to go home. My daughter-in-law went into the kitchen, and shut the door and started banging the dishes. My son made me go into the study with him and all the time

Joe *was shouting, "Let's get out of here before she poisons us."*

   '*My son says I'm letting Dad ruin my life, that there is no reason for Dad to act that way, that it isn't sickness, it's that he's become spiteful in his old age. He says I have to do something.*

   '*So we got in the car to go home and all the way home Joe shouted at me about my driving, which he always does. As soon as we got home, he started asking me what time it was. I said, "Joe, please be quiet. Go and watch television." And he said, "Why don't you ever talk to me?" Then I started yelling at him and I yelled and yelled.*'

Episodes like this can exasperate even the most patient person. It seems as if they always occur when we are most tired.

   The things that are most irritating sometimes seem trivial – but trivial matters mount up, day after day.

Mrs Jackson states, 'I had never got along with my mother that well, and since she's come to live with us, it's been terrible. In the middle of the night she gets up and starts packing.

   '*I get up and tell her, "It's the middle of the night, Mother," and I try to explain to her that she lives here now, but I'm thinking if I don't get some sleep I won't be any good at work tomorrow.*

   '*She says she has to go home, and I say she lives here, and every night a fight starts at two o'clock in the morning.*'

A person with a dementing illness may be able to do some things very well and yet appear unwilling to carry out other, seemingly identical tasks. When you feel that the sick person can do more or is just 'acting up' to upset you, it can be infuriating. For example:

Mrs Graham says, 'She can load the dishwasher and set the table at my sister's house, but at my house she either refuses to do it or she makes a terrible mess. Now I know it's because I work and she knows I come home tired.'

Often the person who has the greatest responsibility for the impaired person feels that other members of the family don't help enough, are critical, or don't come to visit. A great deal of anger can build up around these feelings.

   You may be irritated with doctors and other professionals at times. Sometimes your anger toward them is legitimate. At other times you may know that they are doing the best they can, yet you still feel angry with them.

People with a religious faith may question how God could allow this to happen to them. They may feel that it is a terrible sin to be angry with God or they may fear that they have lost their faith. Such feelings can deprive them of the strength and reassurance faith offers at the time when they need it most. To struggle with such questions is part of the experience of faith.

Said a minister, 'I wonder how God could do this to me. I haven't been perfect, but I've done the best I could. And I love my wife. But then I think I have no right to question God. For me that is the hardest part. I think I must be a very weak person to question God.'

Never let a person make you feel guilty about your anger with God. Much has been written about such feelings. C. S. Lewis's book, *A Grief Observed*, eloquently describes his own struggle with these questions. Reading this and other books, and talking honestly to your minister, priest or rabbi can be comforting.

Remember, it is only human to be angry when faced with the burdens and losses caused by a dementing illness.

Expressing your anger to the sick person often makes her behaviour worse. Her illness may make it impossible for her to respond to your anger in a rational way. You may find that her behaviour improves when you find other ways of managing both your frustrations and the problems themselves.

The first step in dealing with anger is to know what you can reasonably expect from a person with a dementing illness, and to understand what is happening to the brain to cause irritating behaviour. If you are not sure whether the person can change her behaviour, find out from your doctor or other professional staff. For example:

An occupational therapist discovered that Mrs Graham's sister had an old dishwasher that her mother had operated before she became ill. Mrs Graham had a new dishwasher that her mother could not learn to use because her brain impairment made it impossible for her to learn even simple new skills.

It may be possible to change the person's irritating behaviour by changing the environment or the daily routine. However, just knowing that unpleasant behaviour is the result of the disease that the person cannot help can be reassuring.

It is often helpful to think about the difference between being angry with the person's behaviour and being angry with the person herself.

She is ill and often cannot prevent her behaviour. Certainly the behaviour can be infuriating, but it is not aimed at you personally.

A dementing illness might make it impossible for a person to be deliberately offensive because she has lost the ability to take purposeful action. Mrs Palling's husband was not deliberately insulting his family. His behaviour was the result of his illness.

It often helps to know that other families and professional care-givers have the same problems.

Says Mrs Kemp, 'I didn't want to send my husband to the day hospital, but I did it.

'It helped me so much to find out that his constant questions made trained professionals angry too. It wasn't just me.'

Many families find that discussing their experiences with other families helps them to feel less frustrated and upset.

Sometimes it is helpful to find other outlets for your frustrations: talking to someone about it, cleaning out cupboards, or chopping wood – whatever ways you have used in the past to cope with your frustrations. A vigorous exercise programme, a long walk or taking a few minutes to relax totally may be helpful for you.

Embarrassment

Sometimes the behaviour of a person with a dementing illness is embarrassing and strangers often do not understand what is happening.

Says Mrs McGregor, 'I say my husband has Alzheimer's disease. "Old timer's disease?" they say. 'No, Alzheimer's disease!' I say, and I spell it. If my husband had a brain tumour they would understand. How I wish he didn't have a disease nobody has ever heard of.

Says one husband, 'Going through the supermarket, she keeps taking things down off the shelves like a toddler, and people stare.'

Says a daughter, 'Every time we try to give Mother a bath she opens the window and shouts for help. What are we to tell the neighbours?'

Such experiences are embarrassing, although much of your embarrassment may fade as you share your experiences with other families. In such groups, families often find they can laugh over things like this.

Explaining to neighbours usually helps gain their understanding. You might like to give them 'handouts' about dementing diseases. There is another reason why this is important. Although dementing diseases are common, many people still think 'senility' is the natural result of ageing. By explaining the illness to your neighbours you are helping to dispel ignorance and misunderstanding. Your neighbours may well know someone else with one of these diseases who needs treatment.

Occasionally, some insensitive person will ask, 'Why does he act like that?' or 'Whatever is wrong with her?' Sometimes it may be most effective to say 'Why ever do you ask?'

> *One courageous husband says, 'I still take my wife out to dinner. I don't like to cook and she likes to go out. I ignore other people's glances. This is something we always enjoyed doing together and we still do!'*

Some families prefer to keep their problems 'in the family'. This may work best for some people, but friends and neighbours usually know a problem exists and can be more helpful and supportive if you've explained the problem to them. Dementing illnesses are so overwhelming that it is almost impossible to manage alone. There should be no stigma attached to having a dementia.

Helplessness

It is not uncommon for family members to feel helpless, weak or demoralised in the face of a chronic dementing illness. These feelings often grow worse if you cannot find a doctor or other professional who seems to understand dementing illnesses. We have noticed that families and the people with dementing illnesses possess resources within themselves on which they can draw in order to overcome feelings of helplessness. Although you may not be able to cure the disease, you are far from helpless. There are many ways of improving life for both the forgetful person and the family. Here are some suggestions:

- Things often seem worse when you look at everything at once. Instead, focus on small things that you *can* change.
- Take one day at a time.

- Be informed about the disease. Read and talk about ways others manage.
- Talk to other families who face similar problems.
- Become involved in exchanging information, supporting research and reaching others.
- Discuss your feelings with your doctor, social worker or clergyman.

Guilt

It is quite common for family members to feel guilty: about the way they treated the person in the past; about being embarrassed by the person's 'odd' behaviour; about losing their temper with an impaired person; about not wanting this responsibility; about considering placing the person in a nursing home; and for many other reasons, some trivial, some important. For example:

> *'My mother's illness ruined my marriage and I can't forgive her for it.'*

> *'I lost my temper with Dick and slapped him. Yet I know he is ill and can't help himself.'*

You may feel guilty about spending time with your friends away from the person you love, especially when the person is your spouse and you have been accustomed to doing most things together.

You may feel vaguely guilty without knowing why. Sometimes people feel that the person with a dementing illness makes them feel guilty. 'Promise me you will never put me in a nursing home' or 'You wouldn't treat me that way if you loved me' are things the confused person may say that can make you feel guilty.

You may feel guilty about things you must do that take independence away from the person. Stopping a person from driving or from living alone is a difficult decision for a family member to take. Caring for a person with dementia often makes people feel guilty because it forces them to make decisions for someone who was previously fully able to make decisions for herself.

Sometimes we feel guilty when a person close to us, whom we have always disliked, develops a dementing disease.

> *'I've never liked my mother and now she has this terrible disease. If only I had been closer to her when I could.'*

Families sometimes ask if something they did or failed to do caused the illness. Sometimes the care-giver feels responsible when the person deteriorates. You may feel that if only you had taken more time with her or kept her more active she would not have become worse. You may feel that a hospital admission for a surgical operation or for medical reasons 'caused' this condition.

The trouble with feelings of guilt is that, when they are not recognised for what they are, they can keep you from making clear-headed decisions about the future, and from doing what is right for the impaired person and the rest of the family. Once such feelings are recognised, they are not surprising or hard to manage.

The first step is to admit that feelings of guilt *are* a problem. They become a problem when they affect your decisions. If you are being influenced by guilt feelings, you must make a decision. Are you going to go around in a circle with one foot caught in the trap of guilt, or are you going to say, 'What is done is done' and proceed from there? Often, when we look realistically at a situation, there is no way of remedying the fact that you never liked your mother or that you slapped an impaired person for example. However, guilt feelings tend to keep us looking for ways of remedying the past instead of allowing us to accept the fact that you can stop trying to make up for your guilt feelings and can make decisions and plans based on what is best now. For example:

Mrs Dempsey had never liked her mother. As soon as she could, she had moved away from home and telephoned her mother only on special occasions. When her mother developed a dementing illness, she brought her mother to live with her. The confused woman disrupted the family, kept everyone up at night, upset the children and left Mrs Dempsey exhausted. When the doctor recommended that her mother should enter a nursing home, Mrs Dempsey only became more upset. She could not bring herself to put her mother in a nursing home, even though this clearly would have been better for everyone.

When the feelings of guilt in such a relationship are not acknowledged, they can be destructive. Perhaps being faced with a chronic illness is a good time to be honest with yourself about not liking someone. You can then choose whether to give a person care and respect without being influenced by your feeling of dislike. We have little control over whom we like or love, but we do have control over how we act towards them. When Mrs Dempsey was able to face the fact that she did not like her mother and that she felt guilty about that, she was able to go ahead and arrange for her mother to receive residential home care.

When the person with a dementing illness says things like 'Promise you won't put me in a nursing home', it is helpful to remember that sometimes the person with a dementing illness *cannot* make responsible decisions and that *you* must make the decisions, acting not on the basis of guilt but on the basis of your responsibility.

Not all feelings of guilt arise over major issues or keep you from making good decisions. Sometimes you may feel guilty about little things – being cross with the confused person or snapping at her when you are tired. Saying, 'I'm sorry' often clears the air and makes you both feel better. Often the confused person, because she is forgetful, will have forgotten the incident long before you have.

If you worry that you have caused the illness or made it worse, it is helpful to learn all you can about the disease and to talk over the person's illness with her doctor.

In general, Alzheimer's disease is a progressive illness. Neither you nor your doctor can prevent this progression. It may not be possible to halt or reverse a multi-infarct dementia either. Keeping a person active will not stop the progress of such a disease, but it can help the person use her remaining abilities.

A person's condition may first become apparent after an illness or hospital admission, but often, upon close examination, the initial stages of the illness may have occurred months or years earlier. At present, earlier identification of Alzheimer's disease does not help to slow or reverse its progression.

If you don't feel happy about doing things for yourself and by yourself, remember that it is important for your life to have meaning and fulfilment outside of the care of the confused person. Rest and the companionship of friends will do much to help you maintain a positive outlook.

When guilt feelings are preventing you from making clear-headed decisions, you may find it helpful to talk the whole matter over with an understanding counsellor, a minister or with other families. Realising that most people experience the same emotions helps to put nagging feelings of guilt into perspective. If you still feel immobilised by guilt, this may be a symptom of depression. Depression in care-givers and what to do about it is discussed later in this chapter.

Laughter, love and joy

A dementing illness does not suddenly end a person's capacity to experience love or joy, nor does it end her ability to laugh. And although your life may often seem filled with fatigue, frustration or grief, your capacity for these emotions is not diminished either. Happiness may seem out of place in the face of trouble, but in fact it crops up unexpectedly. The words of a song written by Sister Miriam Theresa Winter of the Medical Mission Sisters, reflect this:

> I saw raindrops on my window
> Joy is like the rain.
> Laughter runs across my pain,
> slips away and comes again.
> Joy is like the rain.

Laughter might be called a gift to help our sanity in the face of trouble. There is no reason to feel badly if you laugh about the mistakes a confused person makes. She may share the laughter, even if she is not sure of the joke.

Fortunately, love is not dependent upon intellectual abilities. Focus on the ways you and others still share expressions of affection with the impaired person.

Grief

As the person's illness progresses and the person changes, you may experience the loss of a companion and a relationship that was important to you. You may grieve for the 'way she used to be'. You may find yourself feeling sad or discouraged. Sometimes little things may sadden you or prompt you to cry. You may feel that tearfulness or sadness is welling up inside you. Often such feelings come and go, so that you alternate between feeling sad and feeling hopeful. Feelings of sadness are often mixed with feelings of depression or fatigue. Such feelings are a normal part of grieving.

We usually think of grief as an emotional experience that follows a death. However, grief is in fact an emotional response to loss and so is a normal experience for people who love a person with a chronic illness.

Grief associated with a death may be overwhelming at first and gradually lessen. Grief associated with a chronic illness, however, seems to go on and on. Your feelings may shift back and forth between hope that the person will get better, and anger and sadness over an irreversible condition. Just when you think you have 'adjusted', the person may change and you will start to grieve again. Whether it follows a death or whether it results from being with a person with a dementing illness, grief is a feeling associated with losing a person who was important to you.

Families often say that their own sadness at losing a loved one is increased because they must watch the suffering of the person as her illness progresses.

Says Mrs Owens, 'Sometimes I wish he would die so it would be over. It seems as if he is dying a bit at a time, day after day. When something new happens I think I can't stand it. Then I get used to it and something else happens. And I keep hoping – for a new doctor, a new treatment, maybe a miracle. It seems as though I'm on an emotional treadmill going around and around and it's slowly wearing me down.'

There are certain changes that come with a chronic dementing illness which seem especially hard to bear. Particular characteristics symbolise a person for us: 'He was always the one who made decisions' or 'She was always such a friendly person'. When these characteristics change, feelings of sadness may be precipitated which are sometimes not understood by people distanced from the situation. For example, when a person is unable to talk or understand clearly, her family may feel acutely the loss of her companionship.

Another problem is that the grief that follows a death is understood and accepted by society, while the grief that comes with a chronic illness is often misunderstood by friends and neighbours, especially when the ill person looks well. Your loss is not visible. 'Be grateful you still have your husband' or 'Keep a stiff upper lip', people may say.

There are no easy remedies for grief. Perhaps you will find, as others have, that it is eased somewhat when it is shared with other people who are also living with the unique tragedy of a dementing illness. You may feel that you should keep feelings of sadness and grief to yourself, and not burden others with your troubles. However, sharing these feelings can be comforting and give you the strength you need to continue to care for a declining person.

Depression

Depression is a feeling of sadness and discouragement. It is often difficult to distinguish between depression and grief, or between depression and anger, or depression and worry. Families of the chronically ill often feel sad, depressed, discouraged or low, day after day, week after week. Sometimes they feel apathetic or listless. Depressed people may also feel anxious, nervous or irritable. Sometimes they don't have much appetite and have trouble sleeping. The experience of being depressed is painful; we feel miserable and wish for relief from our sad feelings.

A chronic dementing illness takes its toll on our emotions and provides a real reason for feeling low. Sometimes counselling helps reduce the depression you experience, but counselling cannot cure the situation that has made you depressed; it can only help you deal with it. Many families find that it helps to share experiences and emotions with other families in support groups. Others find that it helps to get away from the impaired person and to pursue hobbies or spend time with people whose company they enjoy. When you are unable to get enough rest, your fatigue may make your feelings of discouragement worse. Obtaining assistance, so allowing you to rest, may help, but the feelings of discouragement and depression may still remain – understandably.

For a few people, depression goes beyond – or is different from – the understandable feelings of discouragement caused by this illness. In such a case it is important to consult a doctor. He can help significantly with this sort of depression. If any or several of the things listed on page 235 are happening to you or to someone else in the family, it is important to find a doctor who can help you or who can refer you to a counsellor.

Care-givers sometimes use alcohol, tranquillisers or sleeping pills to keep themselves going. However, alcohol or medication may increase your fatigue and depression, and sap what little energy you have left. If you find this happening to you, you are not alone: many other care-givers have done the same, but it is important for you to *seek help now*. (See also Chapter 13.)

Isolation; feeling alone

Sometimes a family member feels that he is facing a situation alone. 'Despair', one husband said to us. 'Write about that feeling of being alone with this.' You may feel very much alone when the one person with whom you could share everything has changed. You may feel that you must face the illness all alone.

This is a miserable feeling. We are all individuals and no one else can truly understand what we are going through. The feeling of being alone is not uncommon when people are facing a dementing illness. Remaining involved with others – your family, your friends, other people with ill relatives – can help you feel less alone. Sharing experiences with them will help you to realise that others experience similar feelings. While you may feel that you can never replace the relationship you had with the confused person, you will gradually find that friends and family are offering love and support.

Worry

Who doesn't worry? We could fill many pages with examples of family worries, but you already know them. They are real worries, serious concerns. Worry combines with depression and fatigue, and is a fact of life for many families. Each person has his own way of coping: some people seem to shrug off serious problems while others seem to fret interminably over trivia. Most of us fall somewhere in between. Most of us have also discovered that the kind of worrying we do when we lie awake at night does not solve the problem but it does make us tired. Some of this kind of worrying is often inevitable, but if you find yourself doing it often, you may want to look for other ways of managing your problems.

A woman who faces some real and terrible possibilities in her life tries this approach: 'I ask myself what is the worst thing that could happen. We could run out of money and lose our home. But I know people wouldn't let us starve or go homeless. It seems as though I don't worry as much once I've faced what the worst could be.'

Being hopeful and being realistic

As you struggle with a dementing disease, you may find yourself sometimes following up every possible hope for a cure, and at other times feeling discouraged and defeated. You may find yourself unable to accept the bad news the doctors have given you. Instead, you may seek second, third and even more medical opinions at great expense to yourself and the sick person. You may find yourself refusing to believe that anything is wrong. You may even find yourself giggling or acting in a silly manner when you really don't have anything to laugh about. Such feelings are normal and are usually a part of our mind's efforts to come to terms with a distressing event.

Sometimes, of course, ignoring the problem can endanger the sick person (for example, if she is driving or living alone when she cannot do so safely). Seeking many medical opinions can be futile, exhausting, and expensive, but sometimes seeking a second opinion may be wise. You can ask for a second opinion through the NHS, but you may not necessarily be able to receive one.

This experience of a mixture of hope and discouragement is common to many families. The problem is complicated when professionals give conflicting information about dementing illnesses.

Most families find reasonable peace in a compromise between hope and realism. How do you know what to do?

Realise that we may be a long way from a major research break-through, or we may be close. Miracles do happen, and yet not often.

Ask yourself if your going from doctor to doctor or if your reaction is making things more difficult or even risky for the confused person. If you are ignoring her impairment is she endangering herself by driving, cooking or continuing to live alone?

Put the sick person in the care of a doctor whom you trust. Make sure that this physician is knowledgeable about dementing illnesses and keeps himself abreast of current research. Avoid quack 'cures'.

Keep informed about the progress of legitimate research. Join the Alzheimer's Disease Society to keep abreast of new knowledge.

Mistreating the confused person

'Sometimes I couldn't stand it. My wife would get to me so, always on at me about something, and the same thing over and over. Then I would tie her into her chair and go out for a walk. I felt terrible about it, but I couldn't stand it.'

'My mother would scratch at herself in one spot until it bled. The doctor said we had to stop it. I tried everything until one day I guess I snapped: I grabbed her and shook her, and I screamed at her. She just looked at me and began to cry.'

'I never hit my wife, but I would get so mad at her, it was like I would get spiteful: I would tell her I was going to put her in a nursing home if she didn't behave. It would make her cry. I know she couldn't help what she did and I don't know why I did that.'

Care-giving is difficult, and frustration is understandable: care-givers endure overwhelming burdens. Perhaps you have found yourself hitting or slapping or screaming at the person you care for. Perhaps you have promised yourself it will never happen again, but somehow it does.

In itself, losing your temper is not terrible; it is a warning that you need help with your burden. Anger is common in care-givers. Yelling at the ill person is also common but should be taken as a warning sign that your frustration is building. However, hitting, shoving, shaking or tying down a person is a sign that you have lost control and need help. Even if this has happened only once, it is a danger signal. You may need regular time away from the person. You may need someone you can talk to, someone who can help you talk about your frustrations. You may need to turn the tasks of full-time care over to someone else, perhaps a nursing home. If you lose your temper and do things you wish you had not, then you *must* ask for the help you need. To continue in silent isolation *is* mistreating the confused person.

Call the nearest branch of the Alzheimer's Disease Society or the Carers' National Association. Most of the people who answer telephones or lead support groups in these groups have heard many such problems or been through them themselves. Most will understand and they will help you find sitters or other outside help. (See Chapter 13.)

Not everyone has the capability to be a full-time care-giver. If the person who needs care is someone whom you did not like or who mistreated you, you may have mixed feelings about care-giving. Sometimes the most responsible thing you can do is to recognise that someone else should provide the day-to-day physical care.

Physical reactions

Fatigue

Fatigue often accompanies depression. It is difficult to know which comes first. People who care for a person with a dementing illness are often tired simply because they aren't getting enough rest. However, being tired adds to the feelings of depression. At the same time, being depressed may make you feel more tired. Always feeling tired is a problem for many people who care for a person with a dementing illness.

Do what you can in little ways to relieve your exhaustion. For example:

Mrs Levin says, 'He gets up in the night and puts his hat on and sits on the sofa. I used to wear myself out trying to get him back to bed. Now I just let him sit there. If he wants to wear his hat with his pyjamas, it's OK. I don't worry about it. I used to think I had to clean my windows twice a year and my kitchen floor every week. Now I don't. I have to spend my energy on other things.'

It is important for your health that the person sleeps at night or is at least safe if she is awake. (This problem is discussed in more detail in Chapter 7.) If you are regularly up at night and still caring for the person all day, your body is paying a price in exhaustion, and you will not be able to keep up such a routine indefinitely. You may not always get enough rest, but, it is important to know your own limits. We have made suggestions throughout this book about finding ways of avoiding complete exhaustion.

Illness

Illness is a camp follower of depression and fatigue. It often seems that people who are discouraged and tired fall ill more frequently than others. And people who aren't feeling well are more tired and discouraged. When someone else is dependent on you for care, your illness can become a serious problem. Who takes care of the confused person when you have the flu? You, probably. You may feel that you have no choice but to carry on and hope you don't wear out.

Our bodies and our minds are not separate entities; neither one is the slave of the other. Both parts together make a whole person, and that whole person can become less vulnerable – but not invulnerable – to disease.

Do what you can to reduce fatigue, and ensure that you get enough rest. Eat a well-balanced diet. Take enough exercise.

Arrange a holiday or to take some time away from your duties as care-giver.

Avoid abusing yourself with alcohol, drugs or overeating. Ask your GP to check you routinely for hidden problems such as high blood pressure or anaemia, and chronic infections.

Few of us do all that we could to maintain good health, even when we have no other serious problems. When you are caring for a chronically ill person, there is often not enough time, energy or money to go around, and it is *you* that most often goes without. However, for your sake, and, very importantly, for the sick person's sake, you must do what you can to maintain your health.

Sexuality

It can seem insensitive to think about your own sexuality when there are so many pressing worries – a chronic illness, financial concerns, and so forth. However, people have a lifelong need to be loved and touched, and sexuality is a part of our adulthood. It deserves to be considered. Sometimes sex becomes a problem when a person suffers from a dementing illness, but it remains one of the good things a couple can still enjoy. This section is for those couples for whom it has become a problem. Do not read this *expecting* a problem to develop.

If your spouse is impaired

Despite the so-called sexual revolution, most people, including many doctors, are uncomfortable talking about sex, especially when it involves older or handicapped people. This embarrassment, combined with misconceptions about human sexuality, can leave the spouse or companion of a person with a dementing illness alone in silence. Often articles on sex are no help. It is sometimes difficult to discuss the subject with one's friends, and, if one *is* brave enough to ask the doctor, he may quickly change the subject.

At the same time, sexual problems, like many other problems, are often easier to face when they can be acknowledged and talked over with an understanding person.

The spouse of a brain-impaired person may find it impossible to enjoy a sexual relationship when so many other aspects of the relationship have changed so drastically. For many people, their sexual relationship can only be good when the whole relationship is good. You may be unable to make love with a person with whom you can no longer enjoy sharing conversation, for example. It may not seem 'right' to enjoy sex with a person who has changed so much.

When you are feeling overwhelmed by the tasks of caring for a sick person, or when you are tired and depressed, you may be totally uninterested in sex. Sometimes the person with the dementing illness is depressed or moody and loses interest in sex. If this happens early, before the correct diagnosis has been made, it can be misinterpreted as trouble in the relationship.

Sometimes the sexual behaviour of a person with a brain disorder may change in ways that are hard for her partner to accept or manage. When the impaired person cannot remember things for more than a few minutes, she may still be able to make love, and want to make love, but will almost immediately forget when it is over, leaving her spouse or partner heartbroken and alone. A few such experiences can make you want to abandon this aspect of life for ever.

Sometimes the person you have cared for all day may say, 'Who are you? What are you doing in my bed?', which can be heartbreaking.

Memory loss sometimes causes a formerly gentle and considerate person to forget the happy preliminaries to sex. This, too, can be discouraging for the partner.

Occasionally a brain injury or brain disease will cause a person to become sexually demanding. It can be devastating to a spouse when a person who needs so much care in other ways makes frequent demands for sex. This problem is rare, but it is difficult to treat when it does occur. Medication is seldom helpful except in sedating the ill person. If the problem persists, you should think about placement in a residential or nursing home. When the sexual behaviour of a person with a dementing illness changes, this very likely relates to the brain injury or brain damage and is something the person cannot help, rather than being a purposeful affront to your relationship.

Often what people miss most is not the act of sexual intercourse but the touching, holding and affection between two people. Sometimes, for practical reasons, the well spouse chooses to sleep in a separate room, and sometimes a formerly affectionate person will no longer accept affection when he becomes ill.

Mr Bishop says, 'We always used to touch each other in our sleep. Now if I put an arm across her she jerks away.'

What can you do about problems of sexuality? Like many of the other problems, there are no easy answers.

It is important for you to understand from your spouse's doctor the nature of her brain damage and how it affects this and all other aspects of behaviour. If you seek help with this problem, ensure that the counsellor is qualified. Since sexuality is such a sensitive issue, some counsellors are uncomfortable discussing it or they give inappropriate advice. The counsellor should have experience addressing the sexual concerns of handicapped people and should clearly understand the nature of a dementing illness. He should also be aware of his own feelings about sexual activity in elderly or handicapped people. There are many excellent counsellors who have talked about sexuality with families and who will not be shocked or surprised at what you say. There are also some insensitive people posing as sex counsellors whom you will want to avoid. SPOD (Sexual and Personal Relationships of the Disabled), 286 Camden Road, London N7 (tel: 071 607 8851/2) can advise on these matters.

If your impaired parent lives with you

So far, we have discussed the problems of the spouse of a person with a dementing illness. However, if your ill parent has come to live with you, the sexual aspect of your marriage can be badly disrupted, and this can affect other areas of your relationship. You may be too tired to make love, or you may have stopped going out together in the evening and thus lost the romance that precedes love making. Your confused parent may wander around the house at night, banging things, knocking on your door or shouting. Alternatively, the least little noise may rouse the parent you tried so hard to get to sleep. Love making can turn into hurried sex when you are too tired to care or it can cease altogether.

Relationships are enriched by shared activities: talking together, working together, facing trouble together, making love together. A strong relationship can survive issues being put aside for a while, but not for ever. It is important to find the time and energy to sustain a good relationship and find ways of creating the romance and privacy you need at times when neither of you is exhausted.

The future

It is important to plan for the future. The future will bring changes for the person with a dementing illness and many of these changes will be less painful if you are prepared for them.

Some husbands and wives discuss the future while both of them are well. If you can do this, you will feel more comfortable continuing by yourself, knowing what your partner wished for you. If she wishes to do so, it may be possible for the forgetful person to talk about her future. Planning how she will dispose of her possessions sometimes helps a person to feel that this is *her* life and that she has some control over it. Other people will not want to think about these things and should not be pressurised into doing so.

Members of the family may also want to discuss what the future will bring, perhaps one topic at a time. Sometimes thinking about the future is too painful for some members of the family. If this happens, you may have to plan alone.

Here are some of the things you will want to consider. (We have discussed each of these concerns elsewhere in this book.)

- What will the ill person be like as his illness progresses and as he becomes increasingly physically disabled?
- What kind of care will he need?
- How much will you honestly be able to continue to give to this person?
- At what point will your own emotional resources be exhausted?
- What other responsibilities do you have that must be considered?
- Do you have a spouse, children or a job that also demands your time and energies?
- What effect will this added burden have on your marriage, on growing children, or on your career?
- Where can you turn for help? How much help will the rest of the family give you?
- What financial resources are available for this person's care? What will be left for you to live on after you have met the expenses of care? It is important to make financial plans for the future even if you and

the ill person have only a limited income. The care of a severely ill person can be expensive (see Chapter 15).

- What legal provisions have been made for the person's care?
- Will the physical environment make it difficult for you to care for an invalid?
- Do you live in a house with stairs that the person will eventually be unable to manage? Do you live in a big house that may be difficult to maintain? Do you live a long way from the shops? Do you live in an area where crime is a problem?

As time passes, you, the care-giver, may change. In some ways you may not be the same person you were before this illness. You may have given up friends and hobbies, or you may have changed your philosophy or your ideas in the process of learning to accept this chronic illness. What will your future be like? What should you do to prepare for it?

You as a spouse alone

This was a difficult section of this book for us to write. We know that husbands and wives think about their futures but we have no 'right' answers to give you. Each person is unique. What is right for one person is not right for another, and only you can make those decisions. However, there are several factors you will want to consider.

Your status changes. Sometimes a spouse feels that she is neither part of a couple (because they cannot still do things together, still talk together, or still rely on each other in the same ways) nor a widow.

Couples sometimes find that friends drift away from them. This is a particularly difficult problem for the well partner. 'Couple' friends often drift away simply because the friendship, based on the relationship between four people, has now changed. Establishing new friendships can be difficult when you can no longer include your spouse. You may not want to make new friends alone.

You may face a future without the ill person. Statistics indicate that a dementing illness shortens the life of the victim. It is probable that she will die before you, or that she will become so ill that she needs hospital or nursing home care. It is important that when the time comes and you are alone, you have friends and interests of your own.

A husband described trying to write an account of what it is like to live with a person suffering from a dementing illness. He said, 'I realised that I was telling the story of my own deterioration. I gave up my job to take care of her, then I had no time for my hobbies, and gradually we stopped seeing our friends.'

As the illness progresses, and the person needs more and more care, you may find yourself giving up more and more of your own life in order to care for her. Friends drift away, there is no time for hobbies and you find yourself alone with an invalid.

What then happens to you after she has become so ill that she must be placed in a nursing home or hospital, or after she dies? Will you have 'deteriorated', become isolated, without other interests, lonely, used up? You need your friends and your hobbies throughout the long illness to give support and a change of pace from the job of care-giver, but you are going to need them even more once you are on your own.

Even though placing a person in a nursing home means that others will provide the day-to-day care and that you will have more free time, you may find that you feel as burdened and distressed after the person's placement as you did before. Place reasonable limits on the amount of time you spend at the nursing home, be prepared for an adjustment period, and make plans to resume interests and contact with friends (see Chapter 16).

The problems of being alone but not single are real. Usually the marital relationship between husband and wife changes as the dementia progresses. For many care-givers, however, the relationship continues to have meaning. For others it means establishing a new relationship with another person.

> One husband said, 'I will always take care of her, but I've started going out with other women again. She is no longer the person I married.'
>
> A wife says, 'It was a terribly difficult decision. For me, the guilt was the hardest part.'
>
> Another husband said, 'For me, caring for her, keeping my promise, is most important. It is true that she is not the same, but this too is a part of our marriage. I try to see it as a challenge.'

Sometimes a person falls in love again while he is still caring for his spouse. If this happens to you, you face difficult decisions about your own beliefs and values. Perhaps you will want to talk this over with other people close to you. Perhaps the 'right' decision is the decision that is 'right' for you. Family members often find that their children and in-laws are very supportive.

Not all marriages have been happy. When a marriage was so unhappy that a spouse was already considering divorce, the illness can make the decision more difficult. A good counsellor can help you sort out your mixed feelings.

In any event, should you be faced with questions about new relationships, divorce or remarriage, you are not alone. Many others have also faced, and overcome, these hurdles.

When the person you have cared for dies

People often have mixed feelings when the person they've been caring for dies. You may feel glad that the ill person's suffering and your responsibilities are over, but sad at the same time. There is no 'right' way to feel after the death of someone with a dementia. Some people have shed their tears long ago and feel mostly relief. Others are overwhelmed by grief.

Talking about your feelings with someone you trust can be helpful. Sometimes saying things out loud helps clarify your feelings and thoughts. If you find your feelings changing over time, remember that this, too, is normal.

When much of your time and emotional energy were focused on the person's care, often for many years, you may find yourself at a loose end after the death. You may have lost touch with friends, or given up your job or your hobbies. No longer carrying the responsibility you have had for so long may bring feelings of both relief and sadness.

One wife said tearfully, 'I don't have to tell anyone how they can reach me when I'm away.'

13 Caring for yourself

The impaired person's well-being depends directly on your well-being. *It is essential to find ways of caring for yourself so that you do not exhaust your own emotional and physicals resources.*

When you care for a person who has a dementing illness, you may feel sad, discouraged, frustrated or trapped. You may be tired or over-burdened. While there are many reasons for feeling fatigued, the most common is not getting enough rest. You may put aside your own needs for rest, friends and time alone in order to care for the sick person. If you have multiple responsibilities – family, job, children – your own needs have probably been neglected.

Even if you are not caring for the person full time, you may have little time for yourself. You may be going to the care home after work several days a week or spending the weekend providing care so the full-time care-giver can get some rest. Whatever your direct care responsibilities may be, you probably feel anxious, saddened and frustrated.

Throughout this book we have offered suggestions for ways of modifying annoying behaviour. While such modification will help considerably, it is often not possible to eliminate some forms of behaviour and they may continue to annoy. In order to continue to cope, you will need to get enough rest and to get away from the ill person from time to time.

This book has emphasised that behaviour problems are caused by the brain damage. Neither you nor the confused person can prevent such problems. However, your *mood* can affect the ill person's behaviour. When you are rushed, tense or irritable, the ill person may sense your feelings. He may become more anxious or more irritable, move more slowly, or adopt an annoying behaviour. When you are rested and feel better, the person may manage better and feel better too.

It is not unusual for family members to feel alone in their struggle with a chronic illness. Friends drift away and it may not be possible to meet people with similar problems. You may not be so mobile and life narrows down to a tight circle of lonely misery. Feelings of sadness and grief seem more painful when you also feel alone with your problem.

For all these reasons you need to take care of yourself. You need enough rest, time away from the sick person, and friends to enjoy, to share problems with, and to laugh with. In addition, you may find you need to cope with your feelings of discouragement or to sort out disagreements within the family. You may decide that it will help you to join forces with other families in order to exchange concerns, to make new friends and to advocate better resources for people with dementing illnesses.

Take time off

'If only I could get away from Alzheimer's disease,' Mrs Murray said. 'If only I could go somewhere where I didn't have to think about Alzheimer's disease for a little while.'

It is absolutely essential, both for you and for the person with a dementing illness, that you have regular time to 'get away' from twenty-four hour care of the chronically sick person. You must have some time to rest and to be able to do things just for yourself. This might involve sitting down uninterrupted to watch TV or it might be sleeping through the night. It may mean going out once a week, or taking a holiday. We cannot overemphasise the importance of this. The continued care of a person with a dementing illness can be exhausting and emotionally draining. It is quite possible to collapse under the load.

It is important that you have other people to talk to, to help you and to share your problems. We know that it can be difficult to find ways of caring for yourself. You may not have understanding friends, your family may not be willing to help, and it may seem impossible to get time away from the impaired person. He may refuse to stay with anyone else, or you may not be able to afford help. Finding ways of meeting your own needs often takes effort and ingenuity. However, it is so important that it must be done.

If resources to give you time off are difficult to find, perhaps you can piece together a respite plan. For example:

Mr Cooke was under considerable stress as he was caring for his wife seven days a week. He thought there was no help available until he discussed the problem first with his GP and then with a social worker. The latter arranged for Mrs Cooke to attend an Age Concern day centre one day a week and for a Crossroads Care Attendant to take over caring for Mrs Cooke every Friday afternoon.

You may have to compromise and accept a plan that is not as good as you would like. Also, the care others give may not be the same as the care you try to give, and the confused person may be upset by the changes. Family members may complain about being asked to help. Paying for care may mean small financial sacrifices. For example there is often a charge for transport to day centres or respite care at home. But be persistent in your search for help, and be willing to make compromises.

Taking time off, away from the care of the confused person, is one of the single most important things that you can do to make it possible for you to continue to care for someone with a dementing illness.

> *Mrs Murray went on, 'We had planned for a long time to go to France when he retired. When I knew he would never be able to go, I went alone. I left him with my son. I was scared to go alone, so I went with a tour group. He would have wanted me to, and when I came back I was rested, ready to face whatever came next.'*

Give yourself a present

Could you do with a 'lift' once in a while? An occasional self-indulgence is another way of helping yourself cope. Some people may buy themselves 'presents': a magazine or a new dress; listen to a record; stand outside and watch the sunset; order a favourite restaurant meal as a take-away.

Friends

Friends are often marvellously comforting, supportive and helpful. The support of good friends will do much to keep you going through the hardest times. Remember that it is important for you to continue to have friends and social contacts. Try not to feel guilty about maintaining or establishing friendships on your own.

Sometimes friends and neighbours find it hard to accept that a person is ill when he *looks* fine, and sometimes people shy away from 'mental' illness. Many people do not know how to behave with a person who is forgetful or whose behaviour changes. You may want to explain that this is an organic disease that causes gradual deterioration of the mind. The person cannot help his behaviour and he is not 'crazy' or 'psychotic'. There is no evidence that the disease is contagious. It is a disease condition and not the inevitable result of old age.

Even if the person can talk quite reasonably, and a casual observer cannot see any sign of mental deterioration, he may still not remember names or be able to follow conversations. It is important to explain to friends that forgetfulness is not bad manners but something the person cannot avoid.

It can be painful to tell old friends what is happening, especially those who do not live nearby and have not seen the gradual changes a dementing disease causes. Some families have solved this problem by composing a Christmas letter in which they lovingly and honestly share this illness with distant friends.

Avoid isolation

What can you do if you find yourself becoming isolated? It takes energy and effort to make new friends at a time when you may be feeling tired and discouraged. But this is so important that you must make the necessary effort. Start by finding one small resource for yourself. This will give you the guidance and energy to find others. Call your nearest Alzheimer's Disease Society or Carers National Association Branch or start a group if there isn't one in your area. Renew ties with your church or other religious group. Your minister, priest or rabbi can offer you comfort and support. Friendships within the church can develop, and some churches have resources to provide practical help for you.

As you find time for yourself away from the person you are caring for, use that time to do things with other people: pursue a hobby or attend discussion groups. New friends are most easily made when you are involved in shared activities.

We know that it can be difficult to find the time or energy to do anything beyond caring for the impaired person. Some activities can be put to one side while you are burdened with care, but it is important not to completely discontinue them. When you are no longer required to care for this person, you will need friends and activities.

> '*I used to be a leading member of the Women's Institute but can no longer attend regularly. I still make the occasional cake for bazaars and keep in touch . . . later I hope to become a more active member.*'

> '*I play the violin. I can't play with the quartet any more, but I keep in touch with them and I still practise a little. When I have more time, there will be a place for me in the local symphony orchestra.*'

Some spouses have deliberately sought out new activities.

> '*My wife became unwell just about the same time as I retired. All I was doing was taking care of her. I thought I should get some exercise, so I joined*

a senior citizens' exercise group. I take my wife to the day centre on the day I go to that group.'

Find additional help if you need it.

Mrs Scott says, 'I worry that I am drinking too much. John and I used to have a drink when he got home in the evening. Now, of course, he doesn't drink, but I find I have to have that sherry and another one at bedtime.'

Fatigue, discouragement, anger, grief, despair, guilt and ambivalence are all normal feelings that may come with caring for a chronically ill person. Such feelings may seem overwhelming and almost constant, and the burden you carry can be staggering. Sometimes one's coping skills are overwhelmed and things can drift out of control. You may want to seek professional help if this happens.

Recognise the warning signs

Each individual is different and each person has his own way of responding to problems. A healthy response for one person may be unhealthy for another. Ask yourself the following questions:

- Do I feel so sad or depressed that I am not functioning as I should?
- Am I often lying awake at night worrying?
- Am I losing weight?
- Do I feel overwhelmed most of the time?
- Do I feel terribly isolated and alone with my problem?

While depression and discouragement are common feelings for families of people with chronic diseases, if you are often lying awake at night worrying, if you are losing weight, or if you feel isolated, alone with your problem, or overwhelmed, you may need some help to be able to manage your feelings.

Am I drinking too much?

Definitions of alcohol abuse vary widely. The amount of alcohol that is too much for one person may not be too much for another. Ask yourself is my drinking interfering with how I function with my family, my job or in other ways? If it is, you are drinking too much. Do you ever drink too much to be able to care properly for the sick person? Are others, your co-workers, for example, having to 'cover' for you? Alcoholics Anonymous (listed in the telephone directory) is a good self-help organisation. Often the group will help you solve practical problems like transportation and finding a 'sitter' so that you can attend meetings. Call them, explain your special circumstances and ask for their assistance.

Am I using pills to get me through each day?

Tranquillisers and sleeping pills should be used only under the careful supervision of a doctor and only for a short time. If you are already using tranquillisers or sleeping pills on a regular basis, ask your doctor to help you give them up. Some medication can cause drug dependency. Abrupt withdrawal can be life threatening and must be supervised by a doctor.

Let's imagine that you are abusing alcohol or medication. You have joined the ranks of thousands of other ordinary people. Your problem may have arisen from the stress caused by caring for someone with a dementing illness. There is no reason to be ashamed. There *is* a reason to obtain help *now*.

Am I drinking too much coffee each day?

While not nearly as serious as dependency on stimulant drugs such as amphetamines, excessive caffeine use can be hard on your body and can reduce your ability to manage stress. (Caffeine is also found in tea and most soft drinks.)

Am I screaming or crying too much?

Do I often lose my temper with the impaired person? Do I hit him? Do I find myself more angry and frustrated after I talk with my friends or family about these problems? Do I find that I am irritable with a lot of people – friends, my family, the doctors, my co-workers – not just one or two people in my life?

How much screaming or crying is too much? One person may feel that any crying is too much, while another feels that crying is a good way of 'getting things out of my system'. You probably know already if your moods are exceeding what is normal for you.

Anger and frustration are normal responses to caring for a person whose behaviour is difficult. However, when your anger begins to spill over into other relationships or when you take out your anger on the impaired person, it may be helpful to find ways of managing your frustrations so that it does not drive people away from you or make the impaired person's behaviour worse.

Am I thinking about suicide?

Mr Cameron said, 'There was a time when I considered giving my wife an overdose, and then killing myself.'

The thought of suicide can come when a person is feeling overwhelmed, helpless and alone. When someone feels that he cannot escape an impossible situation or feels that he has lost the things that make life worth living, he may consider suicide. Suicide may be considered if someone feels that the situation he faces is hopeless, that there is nothing either he or anyone else can do. The present can seem intolerable, and the future bleak, dark, empty and meaningless.

One family member who attempted suicide said, 'Looking back, I don't know why I felt that way. Things have been hard, but I'm glad I didn't die. My perceptions must have been all mixed up.'

This consideration – that one's perception is that things are hopeless – is important. If you are feeling this way, it is imperative to find another person (a counsellor or social worker) whose perception of the situation may be different and with whom you can talk.

Counselling

It may be that all you need is more time away from a seemingly demanding, difficult person or more help in caring for him. But perhaps you see no way of finding more help or more time for yourself. Perhaps you feel trapped by your situation. Talking problems over with a trained person is one good way of helping you to feel less pressurised. You and he can sort out the problems you face one step at a time. Since he is not as involved in the problem as you are, he may be able to see workable alternatives that haven't occurred to you. At the same time you will know that you have a lifeline in this person that you can turn to when you feel desperate. Family or friends can be of help as well, but if they are too close to the situation they may not be able to see things objectively.

Should you find a counsellor? Do you need 'help'? Most people are not 'sick', 'crazy' or 'neurotic'. Most people are healthy individuals who sometimes have trouble coping with real problems. They may feel overwhelmed or discouraged, or find that they are thinking in circles. Such a person may find that talking over feelings and problems helps to clarify them.

Ask yourself, do I feel that I am out of control of my situation or at the end of my tether? Is my body telling me I am under too much stress? Do I often feel panicky, nervous, or frightened? Would it help just to talk the whole thing over with someone who understands? If the answer to some of these questions is yes, it may be that you are carrying too heavy a burden and that it would be helpful to seek counselling.

We believe that most people most of the time do not need counselling. However, we know that counselling is sometimes a great help to families struggling with a dementing illness. Such help may come from discussion groups, the clergy, an objective friend, or a social worker, nurse, psychologist or doctor.

The first step in seeking outside help is often the hardest. One's reasoning sometimes goes round in circles.

'I can't get out of the house because I can't get a sitter. He's terrible to anyone in the house but me. I can't have counselling because I can't leave the house and a counsellor couldn't help me with that anyway.'

This kind of circular thinking is partly the product of your situation and partly the way you, in your discouragement, see the problem. A good counsellor can help you objectively separate the problem into more manageable parts, and, together, you can begin to make changes one step at a time.

Sometimes people feel that it is a sign of weakness or inadequacy to go to a counsellor. When coping with the burden of a dementing illness, you need all the help you can get, and this is not a reflection on your strength.

People sometimes avoid counselling because they think that the therapist will delve into their childhood and 'analyse' them. However, many therapists begin by helping you in a matter-of-fact way to cope with 'here and now' concerns. Find out in advance what approach the therapist you select prefers. If you decide to seek counselling, your choice may be influenced by who is available and who is knowledgeable about dementing illnesses.

Psychiatrists are doctors and they are able to prescribe drugs to treat mental illness. They have a good understanding of the physical problems that accompany psychological problems. Psychologists, social workers, psychiatric nurses, the clergy and some other professionals can also have excellent therapeutic or counselling skills. If they do, they may be a good choice. You will need to select a person whose services you can afford, who is knowledgeable about dementing illnesses, and with whom you feel comfortable.

You have a responsibility to discuss with the counsellor any concerns you might have about your relationship with him. If you have a private counsellor and are worried about your bill, if you don't like his approach, or if you wonder if he is telling your family what you have said, *ask* him.

There are several ways of finding a counsellor. If you have an established relationship with a GP with whom you feel comfortable, ask if he can counsel you or can refer you to someone he feels is a good counsellor. Ask a health visitor. If you have friends who have had counselling, ask them if they liked the person they consulted. If there is an active carers' group in your area, ask if there is someone other members have consulted. Ask your GP if you can see a specialist. Contact the British Association for Counselling who keep nationwide lists of counselling contact points.

Not all counsellors are equally good, nor are they all knowledgeable about dementia. Select a counsellor as carefully as you would any other professional service and find out what his qualifications are. If, after a period of time, you do not think the counsellor is helping you, discuss this with him and then consider trying a different therapist.

Joining with other carers: a step beyond

Many carers feel alone with the dementing illness, unable to find doctors, other professionals, or friends who understand, and unable to find information. To meet this need for communication, carers and support groups in many areas have established volunteer organisations. These groups are involved in helping each other, sharing solutions to management problems, exchanging information, supporting needed legislation and research, and educating the community. These organisations welcome members who are concerned about all of the dementing illnesses, of which Alzheimer's disease is the most common. Over and over, all around the country, carers tell us how important it is to know others who are faced with these problems. The number of carers' support groups is growing rapidly. These groups offer friendship, information about the diseases, and information about resources and doctors in your area, and they give their members the opportunity to exchange ideas about how to cope.

While there is a number of independent local carers' groups, many have been set up in association with, or are supported by, national organisations which can put you in touch with local contacts and groups. The Alzheimer's Disease Society specialises in the needs of carers looking after people with all kinds of dementia. The Carers' National Association caters for carers of all sorts of dependants, including dementia sufferers.

Most groups have someone who will listen supportively to your concerns, and who has been a care-giver or has worked with care-givers. That person may be available over the telephone or in person. You do not usually need an appointment for a telephone conversation and there is no charge. Often you can reach someone quickly during office hours. Such people are usually not trained professionals. They cannot offer therapy or prescribe medications. However, if you need assistance beyond their expertise, they can often refer you to someone who has worked with families in a similar situation.

Some Age Concern groups run carers' support groups. Many groups provide mutual support in the shape of a forum for the discussion of common problems, and also practical help such as sitting services and advice.

Some organisations publish newsletters that may be helpful even if you live too far away to attend meetings. Newsletters give ideas on how to cope, notices of changes in the law and insurance coverage, and updates on research.

The national addresses of all these organisations are listed in Appendix II. Joining such organisations can help you fight for legislative attention to be focused on the needs of families and patients.

Support groups

'I did not really want to go to a group, but my mother was driving me crazy and so finally I went. The speaker talked about enduring power of attorney. Until then I didn't realise I had to get one to take care of my mother's property. Then over coffee I was talking to three other women. One of them told how her mother was driving her crazy hiding the silverware in the cupboard. She said one day she suddenly realised it didn't matter where they kept the silverware.

Until then I thought I was the only one dealing with things like that. I told them about my mother and these other women understood.'

'There are usually more women than men in groups, you know. I didn't want to go to a hen party, but there was this other fellow there whose mother-in law lives with them, and he really understood what I am going through. Going to that support group saved my marriage.'

Thousands of family members have had the same experiences. People in support groups *understand*. Many support groups meet once a month, but schedules vary. They may be led by a professional or by family members.

You will find all sorts of people in support groups: bankers and building workers, men and women, adults and children, spouses, long-distance carers, and professionals who work with people with dementia.

The dementing diseases strike people of all groups and races, and their families are struggling with grief, exhaustion, behaviour problems and limited public services. Families of all races are doing all they can to care for their loved ones.

Excuses

When we are overwhelmed and tired, we find excuses for not joining a support group. We don't have the energy and we don't feel able to face a room full of strangers. Here are some answers to those excuses shared by families.

I'm not a group type of person

The families we know say, 'Go anyway', even if this is the only group you ever attend. These diseases are so terrible and last so long that our usual methods of coping are not sufficient. We all can use suggestions on how to cope. Just hearing how someone else deals with similar problems can renew your energy.

I can't leave my patient

Fatigue can lead to inertia. It is easier just to stay at home rather than
find a sitter or to put up with the objections of the ill person. Ask the
Alzheimer's Disease Society if they can help you find a sitter or ask a
friend or relative to stay with the person for a few hours. If the confused
person objects, ask the sitter to visit a few times while you are there.
(See pages 147–148.) You may just have to ignore the sick person's
objections.

I can't talk to strangers

The members of support groups have faced similar problems and won't
remain strangers long. If you are shy, just listen to begin with.

I can't drive at night

Ask the group leader if someone can pick you up. Although problems
like these are real concerns, letting them keep you from getting the
support you need indicates your depression and fatigue. There are ways
around these problems if you are determined.

Sometimes a particular support group is not right for you. For example,
if all the other members live with their impaired relative and yours is in
a nursing home, you may feel that you don't fit in. Many areas have
several support groups. Visit another group, or attend a meeting and ask
around for a group that has concerns similar to yours.
   Support groups aren't for everyone. Some people have no need of the
extra support these groups provide. Others find it more comfortable to
talk individually with a knowledgeable person. Before you decide that
support groups are not for you, we urge you to try one.

Advocacy

Until the late 1970s, when the movement to publicise Alzheimer's disease and related disorders began, families were truly alone with their

burden. They did not know about each other, there were no local support group and helplines, there were no books from which to seek guidance, and few professionals had heard of dementia.

Since then, Alzheimer's disease research centres have been established at some universities and medical schools, and the most significant advance has been the widespread recognition of Alzheimer's disease and similar disorders. Your friends and relatives have probably heard of them, and many professionals in various health-related fields have attended courses about the dementing illnesses.

However, much remains to be done. There has only been enough money forthcoming to support a small number of the worthwhile research projects that seek funding. Diagnosis and follow-up care are not as comprehensive as they should be. Most families are still unable to obtain adequate day or respite care, or help at home, and in many areas the Alzheimer's Disease Society branches, helplines and support groups are understaffed, with most of the work being provided by a few hard-working volunteers. Nursing home care may fall short of what is required by people with dementia. Many staff will learn little about the daily management of dementia, and state funding for residential and nursing home placement is inadequate to cover the cost of care in many parts of the country.

Families often tell us that giving support is a way to fight back against this terrible disease. Perhaps you will want to get involved too. Here are some ways in which you might contribute:

- Participate in research projects. (See Chapter 18.)
- Answer telephones or assist with office work.
- Volunteer your skills. Can you balance the books for a small, volunteer-run day programme? Can you repair the plumbing for a struggling care-giver?
- Lead a support group. Often the best group leaders are those who have been care-givers.
- Locate and reach out to other care-givers who need support. If you have ties to minority groups, you might contact others and let them know that they are not alone.
- Participate in fund raising. Even small amounts of money can make a difference. Effective fundraising requires many skills and several good books are available on the subject.
- Teach your local elected officials and agency leaders about dementia.

Setting up an organisation or support group

If no group exists near you, consider forming one yourself. Start by finding three or four other families and perhaps a helpful professional (social worker or community psychiatric nurse). It is not hard to find other families. Word of mouth will probably produce three or four. Local ministers, nursing homes, district nurses and branches of Age Concern can put you in touch with others.

Your group can write for information from other groups and informally exchange ideas. The national organisations already mentioned may be able to help you form a carers' group. Here, however, are some ideas:

1 At the first meeting, establish specific time limits for meetings and stick to them. Meetings that run late may become a burden. For the same reason, if refreshments are served, agree to keep them simple.
2 Set simple, specific objectives for each meeting. These could be 'informal discussion of problems' or 'electing officers', but objectives will help the group to focus on a target.
3 Avoid tackling too much at a time. A few concrete and attainable goals are less likely to overwhelm people already under pressure from their private lives.
4 Be informed. Find out what other groups are doing.
5 Discuss members' responsibility to maintain confidentiality about personal information shared in the group.
6 Different people have different ways of reacting to a crisis. Make it clear from the start that members should not be judgemental.
7 Agree to give each person time to talk, so that no one person dominates the conversation.

Family members who are caring for a sick person at home may have little remaining energy for the work involved in organising a group. However, families whose loved one has entered a care home or has died may be able to participate and will be an invaluable resource. Also, professionals who work with elderly people may wish to join the group and lend their skills. Local community psychiatric services, voluntary organisations, Social Services Departments and churches may be willing to sponsor a group. They may also employ staff with organisational expertise.

Sharing groups

Many organisations and hospitals run established discussion groups for carers. These are small sharing groups led by a trained therapist.

Families often find these groups helpful. Such groups can be set up by anyone with skills in group therapy.

Peer support groups

Support groups sometimes operate without professional guidance. Such groups should have goals of mutual encouragement and not be used as therapy groups. They should consist of four to ten people. One way of organising the leadership is to meet in a different home each time. The discussion leader for that meeting is the host, thus rotating leadership through the members of the group. It is often helpful for members to make a commitment to regular participation for a certain set number of meetings. At the first meeting, discuss items 1, 5, 6 and 7 listed on page 244. In addition, remember that a peer support group is not a therapy group; it is designed for mutual exchange and support. Give each person present an opportunity to talk. One or two people should not monopolise the discussion. Good group members avoid giving each other advice. Instead, they listen with interest and concern, and give information.

Throughout this book we have emphasised the need for resources to help you. However, the unfortunate fact is that resources you need may not be available. Doctors and other professionals may not be well informed about dementing illnesses, and funding for patient care and research may be insufficient.

Only when the general public and the policy makers recognise that dementias are diseases and become aware of the needs of the patients and families, will new resources and adequate funding be made available. You may want to do what you can to campaign for the development of new or better resources, or for a change in unjust policies. You may want to help educate those who are uninformed about dementia. Here are some ways of making your efforts most effective:

1 Discuss your opinions with your MP and local councillors and ask what you can do to support change. Give them your specific concerns in writing.
2 Form a pressure group with other carers of people with dementing illnesses. Contact the Alzheimer's Disease Society and the Carers' National Association.
3 Give written information or bibliographies concerning these problems to the people, including doctors, with whom you have contact.

This chapter is written especially for the young people who live with or know a person with a dementing illness.

It is important to understand what is wrong with the person and why she acts as she does. When you understand why the person does certain things, it is easier not to be angry with her. Also, it is important to understand that she acts as she does because she is ill, not because she wants to or because of you. The person has a disease that destroys part of the brain. When a large number of brain cells are lost, the brain can no longer work as it should. That is why the person forgets names, is clumsy or is unable to talk properly. Parts of the brain that knew how to do these things have been damaged so the person cannot control her actions. She cannot help herself.

Sometimes these people get upset over little things. That is because the brain can no longer understand what is going on (even when you explain it to the person). Sometimes people with dementing illnesses don't look ill or act in a strange way, but they may criticise you or correct you too much. The person may not be able to help this because her illness makes her forget things.

You may worry about what will happen to the person or about whether something you do might make her worse, especially when you are not sure what is happening. Most likely nothing you can do will make the person worse. You can make her temporarily more upset, but this does not make her condition worse.

If you worry about things, ask questions. Read other parts of this book. You may want to go back to it from time to time. Read any other material you can find on these diseases also. Ask your parents or the doctor treating the person what you want to know. You will get the best results if you raise the subject when there are not a lot of other things going on and when adults are not too tired. However, sometimes adults try to keep bad news from young people, so keep asking.

When you read or talk about these diseases, what you find out may be discouraging. You may find out that the person will not get better and you may react by feeling bad about the whole thing. If there are things you really don't want to know, don't feel that you are expected to ask about them. Many people have mixed feelings. You may feel sorry for the sick person but also angry that she has to live in your house. Your moods may change a lot too. Sometimes you may put the whole thing out of your mind and not even be able to think about it. Most of these reactions are the normal result of facing problems.

Even in the best circumstances, living with an illness like this is hard. Here are some of the problems that young people have shared with us.

> '*No privacy: Granddad walks into my room whenever he wants.*'
>
> '*Having to be quiet. Not being able to play the stereo. As soon as I come in the door, I have to be quiet or Granddad gets excited.*'
>
> '*The way he eats makes me feel sick.*'
>
> '*I can't bring my friends over because they upset Granddad. Also, I don't want to bring them over because he acts in such strange ways.*'
>
> '*Having to give up my room.*'
>
> '*Everybody depends on me more. I have to take a lot of responsibility.*'
>
> '*Everybody is so busy with Granddad and so tired, we never do anything enjoyable as a family anymore.*'
>
> '*I'm afraid of what he will do.*'
>
> '*I'm afraid he will die.*'
>
> '*I just feel discouraged all the time.*'
>
> '*My parents become angry with me more than they used to.*'

You may have some of the same problems, like having to be quiet or having to give up your room. Some things are easier when you understand what is wrong with the person. You can't cope with some things alone and you may need to get an adult to help you. Sometimes it is helpful to pick out the one thing that bothers you the most and ask your family to help you change that. Together, you can often find compromises that will help. For example, you might be able to put a lock on your door or buy earphones for your stereo. If you have given up your room, perhaps you and your friends can find a place in the garage or garden shed where you can get away from the impaired person.

Some young people tell us that it is not the impaired person's behaviour that is the worst problem, but rather the behaviour of their parents, or of the person's husband or wife.

> '*I don't mind Granddad, but Grandmother moved in too, and she wants me to do everything just like she did when she was young.*'

> '*It isn't Granddad, it's my mother always fighting with my grandmother.*'

These may be real problems for you. The person who is your grandparent is also the wife or husband of a sick person and is probably upset. Even when a person doesn't get upset, she may be feeling sad or unhappy, and this may make that person cross, impatient or hard to live with. Probably the best you can do is to be understanding, since you know that grief and worry are the cause of the trouble. When a grandparent is setting strict standards for you or nagging you, ask your parents to tell you how they want you to manage the situation. If things get too difficult, find an adult who is not tired and upset – perhaps somebody outside your family – to whom you can talk.

Most of what we have written above is intended for young people living with an impaired grandparent. However, such an illness sometimes strikes one's own parents. If your father or mother is ill, life is probably much more difficult. We hope this book will help you, but no book can solve the problems that you are experiencing in *your* house with *your* family.

It is important for you and your unimpaired parent to talk about what is happening and about the problems you are having. In addition, it may be helpful for you, your unimpaired parent and any other children in the family to find someone with whom you can all talk from time to time. If your parent is unable to seek help, you may have to ask the doctor or your teachers to help you. Children with a parent who has a dementing illness should not have to cope by themselves.

Belonging to a scout troop, a youth club, an athletics team or some other group such as an evening class, will give you a chance to get away from the troubles at home and allow you to concentrate on having fun with other young people.

Things are not all bad when a parent has a dementing illness. Young people often have useful ideas about how to solve problems and your unimpaired parent will value your understanding during this difficult time. You and she will be able to look back with pride on the way you have coped together.

It is important to remember, when you are caught in a situation you cannot control, that you *do* have control over how you react to it. *You* decide how a situation affects your life.

If your marks at school fall, or if you are arguing with your parents a lot, being unco-operative or just trying to ignore the situation, you need to talk the problem over with someone. Often you can talk things over with your parents, with other adult friends or with teachers. Some people are easy to talk to and some are not. Sometimes a counsellor is a good person to talk to. If you cannot talk to your parents, your teachers can usually help you find a counsellor. Some people feel funny about talking to a counsellor, but there is no need to feel that having counselling means that there is something 'wrong' with you. Here are some of the things that happen when you talk to a good counsellor or someone else who is a good listener:

- You can 'let off steam'.
- You can ask for the counsellor to be there when you talk to your parents so that you don't fight with them.
- You can find out what your parents are thinking.
- You can explain your side of the problem.
- You can ask about things that worry you, such as whether the impaired person will die.

None of the above may solve the problem, but they will make living with the problem easier.

You might like to contact the National Association of Young People's Counselling and Advisory Services, Magazine Business Centre, 11 Newarke St, Leicester, LE1 5SS.

15   Financial and legal issues

To discuss in detail the financial and legal issues that may arise from the care of a person with a dementing illness is beyond the purpose and scope of this book. However, we have outlined some of the key factors for you to consider. You may need to seek professional financial and legal advice.

Making a financial assessment

Providing care for the person with a chronic illness can be costly. In addition, the older person may be living on a fixed income and inflation can be expected to continue to eat into that income. It is important to assess both available financial resources and potentially increasing costs of care, and to make plans for the impaired person's future. If you are a spouse, your own financial future may well be affected by the decisions and plans you make now. Many factors must be considered, including the nature of the illness and your individual expectations.

You will need to look first at the sick person's own assets and financial resources. Consider occupational and state pensions, savings accounts, property, cars, and any other potential sources of income or capital.

You should find out what help could be forthcoming from the state in the way of benefits and grants (including those for adaptations to the home). Help may also be available for the practical care of the impaired person. Command over resources of your own will give flexibility in any decisions you need to make, but help from the state can augment the person's income, and the use of welfare services may mean that less income is required to pay for some aspects of care.

Begin by assessing the potential costs of care, both now and as the person becomes more severely impaired, and assess her available resources. *Whether the ill person has little income or whether she is affluent, it is important to plan ahead for her financial future.*

The costs of care in a residential or nursing home are discussed in Chapter 16. You should always consider that your family member may need this form of care and you *must* read this section and plan ahead. Planning ahead can save you a great deal of anguish in the future.

Potential expenses

Lost income

- Will the impaired person have to give up her job?
- Will someone who would otherwise be employed have to stay at home to care for the person?
- Will her pension be affected?
- How much of her income is fixed and therefore subject to the vagaries of inflation?

Housing costs

- Will you or the impaired person have to move to a home that is on the ground floor, closer to services or easier to maintain?
- Will you have to move a parent into your home? Will you have to redecorate a room for her?
- Will you have to make modifications to your home (new locks, grab rails, safety devices, wheelchair ramps)?
- Will the wear and tear upon the home be greater?
- Will the impaired person have to enter sheltered housing, a nursing home or a long-stay hospital?

Medical costs

Will you need

- private medical care?
- visiting nurses?
- doctors?
- occupational therapists or physiotherapists?
- medication?

- appliances (hospital bed, special chair, wheelchair, bath aids and other adaptations)?
- disposable care supplies (continence aids, petroleum jelly, tissues, cotton swabs, etc.)?

Cost of help or respite care

Will you need

- someone to help in the home?
- someone to stay with the person?
- someone to help with care?
- day care?
- intermittent residential care?

Food costs

Will there be the additional cost of having meals prepared or of eating out?

Transportation costs

Will you need

- someone to drive if you cannot?
- taxis?

Legal fees

The costs involved in drawing up legal documents such as a will or in giving you the power to arrange the impaired person's affairs should be listed.

Miscellaneous costs

These may include the purchase of easy-care clothing, incontinence supplies, and various devices for safety or convenience, as well as the use of services such as a laundry.

Residential and nursing home costs

In addition to basic costs, you may be charged for continence pads, laundry, medication, disposable supplies, therapies, chiropody and hair care.

Resources from the state

Many benefits are available from the state, and in each case detailed requirements for eligibility may change from year to year. In particular there are benefits which are affected by the different ages at which men and women can first receive the State Pension (these may change in the future). It is therefore essential to consult the latest edition of the leaflets mentioned throughout this section. A book such as *Your Rights*, from Age Concern will give you a straightforward starting point for further consideration, as it describes all the main pensions and benefits that are available; or you may wish to consult the more detailed Disability Rights Handbook produced by the Disability Alliance. Social Security also provide a free phone service on 0800 66 557 (England, Scotland and Wales), 0800 616 757 (Northern Ireland).

State Pension

A State Retirement Pension is paid to those who have paid sufficient National Insurance contributions in their own right, or to wives whose entitlement comes through their husbands' contributions. It cannot be paid before the age of 65 for a man and 60 for a woman in her own right, although a husband could receive a dependant spouse's allowance if she is below that age and he is over 65. If the impaired person leaves work early, the local Social Security Benefits Agency office will be able to tell her how much her pension will be when she reaches retirement age. An older person may already be receiving the State Pension.

Disability Working Allowance

Sometimes a younger person will want to continue working but may have to change her job and only be able to earn a low income. If she is working at least 16 hours a week and has been receiving one or more of certain disability benefits, she may be eligible for the Disability Working Allowance. This is a means tested benefit and will take into account her income and savings as well as her family responsibilities. It was introduced in April 1992 and is described in Social Security leaflet DS 703 (Disability Working Allowance).

Sickness or Invalidity Benefit

If the impaired person is below State Pension age, and is unable to continue work, there may be an entitlement to Statutory Sick Pay or to a sickness benefit for 28 weeks. After that there is normally entitlement to Invalidity Benefit which can be paid up to the age of 70 (men) and 65 (women). For more information, see Social Security leaflet NI244 (Statutory Sick Pay), NI16 (Sickness Benefit) and NI16a (Invalidity Benefit). If a person first became incapable more than five years before State Pension age, there may be an additional entitlement to an Invalidity Allowance.

Severe Disablement Allowance

For those who are not entitled to Invalidity Benefit, there is a Severe Disablement Allowance which is available for people who are under 65. This allowance is only available to people who are normally resident in the United Kingdom, as are other benefits which are not means tested but which relate to the degree of disability. To receive this allowance the person must have been incapable of work for a certain period of time and, if they were over 20 when the incapacity began, they must be assessed as being over 80% disabled or must be drawing another benefit such as the Disability Living Allowance 'Care Component' at one of the two higher levels. Such benefits are described below.

Disability Living Allowance

The Disability Living Allowance 'Care Component' is for people who need help with personal care or require supervision because they might be a danger to themselves or to others. This benefit is for those who become disabled before 65 and claim the benefit before they are 66 and there are three levels of payment. The highest rate is for people who need continual supervision or frequent help with their normal bodily functions, such as eating, going to the toilet or washing during the day, and prolonged or repeated attention at night. The middle rate is for those who only need attention by day or by night, and the lower rate is for those who only need help for a significant portion of the day, perhaps to prepare and cook a meal, or to get in and out of bed. For people who become impaired after age 65 there is an Attendance Allowance, but this is only available at the two higher rates.

Both allowances are paid regardless of whether a person receives help from someone else. What matters is that they need such help – not that they are actually receiving it. The allowance does not have to be spent on buying care although you may find the local authority may take this into consideration when assessing the level of charges for social services.

Further information about these benefits can be obtained from leaflet DS 704 (Disabled Living Allowance) and DS 702 (Attendance Allowance).

If the impaired person has a mobility handicap, she may be eligible for the 'mobility component' of the Disability Living Allowance. This is available for people who become unable or virtually unable to walk before their 65th birthday. It can be claimed until the age of 66. There are two levels of payment. The higher rate is for those who are unable to walk or have great difficulty in walking because of a physical disability, are blind and deaf, or who are mentally impaired with severe behaviourial problems. If a person can walk but needs someone with her for guidance or supervision, she may qualify for the lower rate.

Although the mobility component is given to people who need help getting around, it can be spent however the person chooses. Because the Disability Living Allowance was only introduced in 1992 you may be more familiar with the old term for this element of the benefit which was the Mobility Allowance.

Additional help is available for severely disabled people through an independent means tested fund financed by the state, but this may end in April 1993. For more information, write to the Independent Living Fund, PO Box 183 Nottingham NG8 3RD.

Invalid Care Allowance

If the person is being cared for by someone who cannot work because he or she spends at least 35 hours a week caring, the carer may be able to claim the Invalid Care Allowance. It is available to anyone whether married or single who is over 16 and under 65. The benefit is explained in leaflet NI 212 (Invalid Care Allowance). When the carer has to stop work, contributions to the basic State Pension can be protected under Home Responsibilities Protection which is explained in leaflet NP 27, 'Looking after someone at home? How to protect your pension.'

Income support

If the impaired person's income is insufficient to cover basic living costs, additional help towards living and housing costs may be forthcoming from Income Support. This is a means tested benefit which takes into account the savings and income of the person and her spouse (including a partner of the opposite sex). People who are still repaying a mortgage or a loan for repairs and improvements, may have their interest payments taken into consideration. Others may be paying ground rent or service charges which can also be included.

Income Support will top-up weekly income to levels set annually by the government. Its level will depend on the age and degree of disability of the person and her spouse. The older and more disabled she is, the higher the amount she will be considered to need. The highest payment is known as the Severe Disability Premium. It is available for single disabled people who live alone and receive an Attendance Allowance or the Disabled Living Allowance Care Component at one of the two higher levels, but who are not cared for by someone receiving an Invalid Care Allowance. If two people living together are both severely disabled, they can receive the Premium, providing no one, or only one person, is receiving the Invalid Care Allowance in order to look after them.

There is also help through Income Support for carers in similar financial circumstances by means of a Carer's Premium which is available to people entitled to the Invalid Care Allowance.

For further information about Income Support, see Social Security guide IS1. If the impaired person is living with you, she may still be eligible for Income Support but her presence may affect any Housing Benefit you claim.

The Social Fund

Help can also be obtained from the Social Fund which gives lump sum payments to meet exceptional circumstances. These are only available to people with a very low level of savings and most are loans. However, one element is a grant – the Community Care Grant – which can be used to enable an impaired person to remain in the community, for instance by providing a grant for minor house repairs or by paying for removal costs to more suitable accommodation. These grants are all discretionary, but there is also a statutory right to a grant for the basic cost of a simple funeral if the person responsible for the cost has a low income and the deceased person had insufficient savings to cover the cost. Social Security guide SB 16 and leaflet SFL 2 give detailed information about the Social Fund.

Housing Benefit

Assistance towards housing costs can also be achieved through the Housing Benefit scheme which covers rent for private, housing association or council tenants. It is means tested, calculated on the same basis as Income Support, but the savings limit is higher and the benefit is available to people on higher income. This means that someone who is ineligible for Income Support may be able to obtain Housing Benefit. Social Security leaflet RR1 describes the Housing Benefit system and further advice should be sought from your London Borough, Metropolitan Borough or District Council.

Council charges

There is also help towards paying for local council services in the form of the Community Charge Benefit which is calculated and administered in the same way. This will continue to operate in some form when the Community Charge is abolished and replaced by a council tax. Ask at your local council office for information. Your council will also explain about the exemption from the Community Charge for people who are severely mentally impaired, which includes people with dementia. The government has given an assurance that families which include a person in receipt of an exemption from the Community Charge will not be disadvantaged when the new council tax comes into effect.

Resources of the impaired person's spouse, children and other relatives.

There are no legal requirements for children and other relatives to give financial support, but there are laws relating to the financial responsibility of the spouse. If the impaired person is left without income, or with insufficient income for her needs, the Social Security Benefits Agency will examine the income of the spouse, or of a partner of the opposite sex, in calculating any means tested benefit.

In some cases (such as with State Pensions), a divorced wife may be entitled to benefits from a former husband. It is important to be familiar with laws that may affect an unimpaired spouse if it is likely that impaired spouse may eventually need expensive care. Advance planning may protect the spouse financially. This is important for families of modest means as well as for more affluent families.

Laws regarding the financial rights and responsibilities of family members, particularly when they apply to residential and nursing home care, are complex (see Chapter 16). Not all social workers, tax accountants or lawyers understand them. The Alzheimer's Disease Society or Age Concern may be able to advise or refer you to professionals with expertise in this area. In addition, families have feelings of obligation to each other. With obligation come dilemmas:

'Dad put me through college. Now it's my turn.'

'I want to help my mother, but I also have a son to put through college. What do I do?'

'I know Mum would be better off if I could buy an electric wheelchair for her, but my husband's job depends on the van and right now the engine has to be rebuilt. I don't know what to do.'

These are difficult questions and families often disagree over how money should be spent. Because public support for families is limited, these diseases can be financially devastating, particularly for the well spouse. (See also Chapter 11.)

Resources from a private pension

When a person is forced to leave work before retirement age, there may be income from an occupational pension. It will be necessary to consult with the employer, personnel officer or trade union to see what rights the pension fund will give.

Sometimes the person will have a collection of occupational pensions if she has changed employers and you will need to contact more than one pension fund. Anyone who has difficulty in doing so can approach the Occupational Pensions Advisory Service who may be able to trace the fund for you. They are at 11 Belgrave Road, London SW1 (tel: 071-233 8080). The person may have also been paying additional voluntary contributions into her pension through another company. Usually her employer will be able to tell you the name of the company. Sometimes, perhaps because the person was self-employed, her only pension is in a personal scheme. If she does not have an occupational pension, you should discuss together whether she has tried to plan her future in this way.

Resources from insurance

If a private health insurance policy is held, it may cover active medical treatment, but health insurance policies often exclude payment for dementing or chronic illnesses. You need to know exactly what the insurance covers. Find out what life insurance policies the person has and whether these can be a resource. Some insurance policies waive the premiums if the insured person becomes disabled. This is a saving for her.

Where to look for the forgetful person's resources

Sometimes an impaired person forgets what financial resources she has or what debts she owes. People may be private about their resources or disorganised in recording them. Sometimes suspiciousness is a part of the illness and the individual hides what she has. Families may not know what resources could be used to provide for a person's care. Finding out what resources a person has can be difficult, especially when documents are in disarray or are hidden.

Debts usually emerge on their own, often in the post. Most businesses will be understanding if a debt or bill is not paid on time. When you do find a bill, ring the company concerned, explain the circumstances, and arrange with them how and when the bill is to be paid. If the confused person is mislaying post, you may be able to have it held for you at the post office.

Assets may be harder to find. Review recent post. Look in the obvious places such as a desk, an office, clothing and other places where papers are kept. Look under the bed, in shoe boxes, in pockets, in old purses, in kettles or other kitchen items, under rugs and in jewellery boxes.

There are many kinds of assets:

Bank accounts   Look for bank books, banks statements, cheque books, savings books, passbooks, statements of interest paid, and details of joint accounts held with others. Most banks will not release information about accounts, loans or investments to anyone whose name is not on the account. However, they may give limited information (such as whether there is an account in an individual's name) if you send a letter to the bank from your doctor or lawyer explaining the nature of the person's disability and the reason for your request. Banks will release information about the amount in an account or about current transactions only to a properly authorised person. However, often you can piece together what you need to know from the papers you find.

Share certificates, bonds, savings certificates and accounts, building society accounts   Look for the actual bonds, passbooks, notices of payments due, notices of dividends paid, earnings claimed on income tax and details of regular amounts paid out from bank account receipts. Also look for cancelled cheques, correspondence or receipts from a broker. Look for records of purchases and sales.

Insurance policies (life insurance, health insurance).   These are among the most frequently overlooked assets. Life insurance and health insurance policies may pay out lump sums or other benefits. Look for premium notices, policies and for cancelled cheques that give you the name of the insurer. Contact him for full information about the policy. Some insurers will release this information upon receipt of a letter from a doctor or solicitor. Others will need proof of your legal right to information.

Safe deposit boxes   Look for a key, bill or receipt. You will need a court order to open the box.

Property (houses, land, businesses, rented property, joint ownership or partial ownership of the above)   Look for regular payments into or from a current account, gains or losses declared on income tax, keys, fire insurance premiums (on houses, businesses and other property). The insurance agent may be able to help you. Ownership of property is a matter of public record. The Land Registry may be able to help you locate properties, if you are a properly authorised person.

Retirement Pensions or disability benefits   These are also often overlooked. Look for evidence of existing pensions or benefits. Special benefits may be available from past employment, union membership and military service. Check into retirement or disability benefits from all past employers. Look for an old curriculum vitae which will list previous jobs. Look for benefit letters.

Income tax   Look for evidence of an under-payment. The Inland Revenue will help with queries on income tax if the person enquiring has a Power of Attorney or powers under the Court of Protection.

Collections, gold, jewellery, cash, loose gems, cars, antiques, art, boats, camera equipment, furniture and other negotiable property.   In addition to looking for such items, look for valuable items listed on property insurance policies. Some of these items are small enough to be easily hidden. Others may be on view but can be so familiar as to be overlooked.

Wills   If the individual has made a will, it should list her assets. Wills, if not hidden, are often kept in a safe deposit box, recorded by the court, or kept by a solicitor.

Trust accounts   Look for statements of interest paid and personal loans. Look for withdrawals, payments correspondence and details of maintenance payments. (Occasionally divorce settlements provide for payment of maintenance should the wife become disabled.)

Foreign bank accounts   Look for statements of interest paid and bank statements.

Inheritance   Find out whether the impaired person is someone else's heir.

Funeral arrangements   Look for evidence of a prepaid funeral or of payment for a cemetery plot.

Legal matters

The time may come when a person with a dementing illness cannot continue to take legal or financial responsibility for herself. This may mean that she can no longer balance her cheque book or that she has forgotten what financial assets or debts she has. It may mean that she is unable to decide responsibly what to do with property or to give permission for needed medical care.

Often these abilities are not lost all at once. A person who is unable to manage her cheque book may still be able to make a will or to accept medical care. However, as her impairment increases, she may gradually reach the point where she cannot make any decisions for herself, and someone will have to assume legal responsibility for her.

The most efficient way of preparing for this eventual disability (which could happen to any of us) is for the person to make plans for herself before she becomes unable to make her own decisions. A person should make a will when she is still considered legally competent to do so. This is called testamentary capacity. It means that the person knows, without prompting, that she is making a will, the names of and her relationship to the people who will receive her property, and the nature and extent of the property.

A person who is still able to manage her own affairs may sign a Power of Attorney, which gives a spouse, child or any other person who has reached legal age, authority to manage her legal affairs. A Power of Attorney can give broad authority to the specified person or it can be limited. A Limited Power of Attorney only gives the person authority to do specific things (sell a house or review income tax records, for example).

Since a Power of Attorney authorises someone to act on another person's behalf, the person giving such power should ensure that the one selected will, in fact, act in her best interests and in accordance with her wishes.

Enduring Power of Attorney

An ordinary Power of Attorney becomes invalid once the impaired person is unable to handle her affairs. However, since 1986, it has been possible to create an Enduring Power of Attorney. The person giving such a power, known as the donor, can either appoint someone to manage her financial affairs at once and to continue to act as Attorney when she becomes mentally incapable, or to act as an Attorney for her only when she becomes mentally incapable. To take out such a Power, the person must be mentally capable of understanding what the Enduring Power is and what it is intended to do.

Enduring Power of Attorney forms may be purchased from a law stationers, but we believe it is important to discuss the whole matter with a solicitor. He will then need to discuss with the confused person how best to protect herself and what type of powers should be transferred. He will need to feel sure that it will be the confused person and not you who is making the decision.

If you do need the services of a solicitor, ask a friend or family member to recommend one. Alternatively, you can call the Law Society, 113 Chancery Lane, London WC1 (tel: 071-242 1222), and they can give you the names of solicitors near you. Lists should also be available from your local library. Find out from the solicitor if he practices the sort of law you need and is knowledgeable about it. Misunderstandings can be avoided by discussing with him what he charges and what services he can offer for that fee.

If you have been given an Enduring Power of Attorney, you have the same responsibility as any Attorney. Once the person begins to lose mental capacity to manage for herself, the Enduring Power must be registered with the Court of Protection (see page 264). This will be your decision. No medical evidence is required, but it is important not to take over the person's affairs unnecessarily and you may feel happier to consult the person's doctor before making the decision.

Before registering with the Court, you must notify the person, and at least three of her nearest relatives in a given order of priority; so that, if they wish, they can object if they feel that something is wrong. If there are objections, you will be notified and the Court will convene a hearing to consider whether the objections are valid.

Once the Power is registered, you will have full authority to act as Attorney. If you need to take certain actions which were not specified in the Enduring Power, the Court can give authority. It will not supervise your actions but has the power to do so if there are allegations of abuse against you.

Further information about Enduring Power of Attorney can be obtained from the Enquiries and Applications Branch of the Public Trust Office, Stewart House, London WC2 6HD (tel: 071-269 7300).

By making a will and granting an Enduring Power of Attorney while she is still able to do so, the person who feels her memory may be beginning to fail can be sure that if her condition worses her life will continue the way she intended, and her property will be distributed as she wished, rather than in a way imposed by a court. The person may continue to manage her own affairs or part of them, until such time as a designated person must take over.

Someone who holds a Power of Attorney is legally responsible to act in the other person's best interests, but once in a while someone abuses this responsibility. The risk of abuse is small in an ordinary Power of

Attorney, but an Enduring Power transfers greater responsibility and requires greater trust. A person who wants to plan ahead for her eventual disability must consider this decision carefully.

Families sometimes find it difficult to face these things when the person still seems quite able. Sometimes a confused person resists these steps. Unfortunately, waiting until the person cannot be consulted makes it more difficult and sometimes impossible to manage her affairs without applying for legal authority to do so.

Court of Protection

Should the person become so mentally impaired that she cannot complete an Enduring Power of Attorney, then the legal authority to manage her affairs must be obtained through the Court of Protection who can make an order appointing someone to act on behalf of the person who is called the 'patient', to receive the income and administer the property under the direction of the Court. Such a person is called a Receiver and is often a relative or close friend. Application for this should be made to the Probation Division of the Public Trust Office.

If there is no relation or friend able or willing to act, or if there is a family disagreement, or if the person's affairs are very complicated, a professional adviser such as a solicitor or accountant may be appointed. In exceptional cases, where there is no one suitable or willing to act as Receiver, the Court can appoint the Public Trustee, who is head of the Public Trust Office, as the Receiver. In certain cases, the appointment of a Receiver may not be necessary, the matter being dealt with by a simple short procedure order authorising the relative or friend to use the person's means sensibly without a Receiver having been appointed.

Application to the Court may be made by any person (but preferably by a near relative) either by instructing the solicitor to carry through the application, in which case the solicitor will prepare the necessary forms, or, alternatively, by making application yourself with the assistance of the Personal Application Branch of the Court. Unless the estate is very small, fees are payable to cover the cost of administration, but the Court can postpone or waive fees in cases of hardship.

Before granting an application, the Court will need to be satisfied, after considering medical evidence, that the person is incapable of managing and administering her property and affairs by reason of mental disorder. You will therefore have to supply the medical evidence and also a reference for yourself on your suitability to act as Receiver. The person will be notified by the Court of your application and you must inform all other relatives who are either equally or more closely related than you are to the patient. Challenges can be made, in which case you should be informed. You can attend the hearing when the decision is made on receivership, but it is unusual to do so.

If appointed as the Receiver, you will be required to present the Court with an annual account of all receipts and payments made. You will normally be required to take out a security bond to ensure that, if affairs are mishandled, the person is reimbursed.

Leaflets are available from the Court on its procedures, as is a booklet on the duties and responsibilities of a Receiver.

Other ways of handling money

In many cases, neither a Power of Attorney nor powers under the Court of Protection are sought. It may be possible to provide for the impaired person's needs out of income which can be utilised by simpler procedures. For example while the person still understands what she is doing, Social Security benefits can be managed by an agent. In such a case, the holder of the pension book signs on the front of the order form and on the back it states that a named person can collect the account and sign the order form. Where this is happening regularly, the Department of Social Security Benefits Agency may issue a card stating that the named person is authorised to collect the money on behalf of the book holder. The agent is authorised to collect the money, but not to spend it or to keep it without being told to do so by the claimant.

If the person you are caring for cannot make a valid appointment of an agent because she is unable to understand why she is appointing an agent and the power she is donating, you should apply for her benefits and pensions to be managed by an appointee on her behalf. (See form BF56 from the Social Security Benefits Agency office.) The appointee can make claims, receive payments and spend the money on the claimant's requirements. In such a case, the Social Security Benefits Agency staff should first make enquiries to satisfy themselves that the person is mentally incapable of handling her affairs, that someone has not already been appointed by the Court of Protection as a Receiver, and that the proposed appointee takes an active interest in the claimant's welfare and is a suitable person for this task. In practice, these enquiries are not always carried out.

Some occupational pensions are handled in the same manner. Inquiries should be made to the employer, personnel officer or trade union for further information since there is a variety of ways in which companies will deal with this situation. It is possible for tax refunds and some monies from life assurance policies to be paid to the next of kin of people who are mentally incapable of managing their own affairs. In certain circumstances, banks and building societies may allow withdrawals for the benefit of the account holder. Where families think ahead, they may wish to consider a joint account which would allow the carer to continue to withdraw money or if it is too late to do this, you can become an authorised agent. This is likely to require medical certification. The situation should be discussed with the manager of the local branch.

When in doubt, the Enquiries and Applications Branch of the Public Trust Office will always advise on whether it will become necessary to apply to the Court. However, if the income is sufficient, there may be no need to use capital assets such as savings which can remain lodged in a safe place. But when circumstances change radically, it may be necessary to seek legal powers of action. For instance, the home may need to be sold for the person's benefit.

If the home is owned jointly by a husband and wife, and one of them becomes impaired, the unimpaired spouse will need an Enduring Power of Attorney or power gained through the Court of Protection in order to sell the home.

The ways in which a person's affairs can be managed are more fully described in *Managing Other People's Money* by Penny Letts and published by Age Concern.

Non-financial decisions

There are many decisions, not covered by any legal authority, which will need to be made by others if a person is no longer capable of making them herself. Consent to medical treatment, or a decision to move the person into a residential care or nursing home may be the most common you encounter. This is why it is so important, while the person is still capable, to consider what she would like to happen in a variety of circumstances, to discuss these with her family and to prepare a written note of her wishes. Although a family member is not legally bound to carry out these wishes, it will give the person confidence to know that she has made her wishes explicit.

Sometimes a disabled person is unable to care for her daily needs and must have hospital or nursing home care. She may refuse to consent to this or may be unable to make the decisions involved in such a move. Often the hospital or nursing home will accept the consent of the next of kin, a husband or wife, or son or daughter. Sometimes, however, application may have to be made to the hospital managers under Sections 2,3 and 4 of the 1983 Mental Health Act by either the nearest relative or an approved social worker, supported by two medical recommendations that the person should be compulsorily admitted to hospital. Application might also be made to the local authority for guardianship by the same procedure under Sections 7 and 8 of the Act, which will require the person to live at a certain place, attend for medical treatment, or allow access where the patient is residing for treatment. There may be circumstances in which the Mental Health Act is deemed not to apply and yet you feel she is not caring for herself, or letting others care for her, or not living in healthy conditions. You would then need to approach the local Social Services Department to see whether a social worker could persuade her to accept help or move. In the last resort, Public Health Physicians have the power under Section 47 of the 1948 National Assistance Act to apply to the magistrate for an order to forcibly place her in a hospital or other place of safety where she can have the necessary care and attention.

One particular concern your relative may have is about suffering from an incurable illness and how she would be treated if she was unable to make her wishes known. She may, for example, wish to refuse certain forms of treatment aimed at the preservation of the person's life. Specifying how a terminally ill patient wishes to be treated is known as an advance directive or 'living will' and there are now forms available for this purpose. They can be obtained from the Voluntary Euthanasia Society – EXIT, 13 Prince of Wales Terrace, London W8 5PG (tel: 071-937 7220). Such directives have no legal authority, but can inform the family and doctors of the person's wishes.

Because only a patient's *financial* affairs can be handled by another person with legal authority, in 1991 the Law Commission published a consultative paper, *Mentally Incapacitated Adults and Decision Making: An Overview*. (The Law Commission is the public body charged with researching aspects of law reform.) Its recommendations, when eventually presented to the government, may lead to a major change in the law. This is how the Enduring Powers of Attorney were introduced. Some people believe that there should be a more general power, such as a form of guardianship, which should cover both financial and other personal matters. There may therefore be a change in the future in how you can be authorised to make decisions for a demented person.

As the disease progresses, it may become more difficult for you to care for a person at home. Taking care of a person with a dementing illness can be a 24-hour-a-day job and may require the skills of professionally trained people. At some point, the family may be unable to continue providing all the care that is needed.

Placing your family member in a care home can be a difficult decision to make and it often takes time. Families usually try other solutions first. However, a time may come when looking for a place in a care home is the most responsible decision the family can make.

You may feel great sadness and grief at having to accept the inevitable decline of a spouse, parent or sibling. You are likely to have mixed feelings. You may experience a sense of relief that a decision has finally been made and that part of the care will be assumed by others, yet feel guilty for wanting someone else to take over these real burdens. You may also feel angry that no other choices are available.

The decision to place your relative in long stay care is not one to be taken lightly. Such a step may be seen by your relative as a final loss of independence, even though this might not actually be the case. For both the well-being of the elderly person, and for your own peace of mind, it is therefore important to be sure that this is the right move.

Thinking about long-stay care

Remember that with good support it is possible for some very confused elderly people to remain in their own homes. The range of support services which may be available have already been described in Chapter 10. There are some imaginative schemes which provide care for dementing people in the early hours of the morning, late at night and at intervals in between. It is therefore worth checking to see whether there is any provision which you have overlooked which may enable your relative to 'stay put'. Do not be afraid to admit your lack of knowledge and to ask for help. Research among care-givers of demented relatives has consistently shown an alarmingly high level of ignorance about existing support as no one, including general practitioners, has thought to give them the necessary information.

However, the needs of confused elderly people and their care-givers may not be met by often overstretched services. It may not be possible to design a care package which can meet the precise needs of the person who is very confused and perhaps also physically frail, incontinent and generally difficult to look after. The appropriateness and extent of support services is thus one important factor to consider when deciding whether the person should enter long-stay care.

Other indications that long-stay care is necessary could include:

- *A deterioration in the physical and mental health of your elderly dependant.* You may find that you can cope with dementia, but the onset of incontinence or the habit of constant and repetitive questioning may prove to be the last straw.
- *Not being able to prevent your relative wandering from home and getting lost.* This is particularly worrying at night.
- *Your own health suffering as a result of the strain of caring.* If you become ill, you are unable to care properly for your elderly dependant or for any other dependants such as a spouse or children.
- *The health and well-being of other members of the family suffering.* They may feel, rightly or wrongly, that you are neglecting them, or they may be disturbed by constant sleepless nights. This could be important, for example, when children are studying for exams.
- *Your being unable to manage financially to continue to care for your family member at home.* You may need to go out to work to support yourself, making it impossible for satisfactory care arrangements to be made.

There may be other considerations to bear in mind, particularly as each family's circumstances are different. If you think about things calmly you can confidently proceed on the basis that what you have decided is right for you, your dependant and your family.

Just as when seeking day or home care, care-givers often wait too long before placing a family member in a care home. Both you and the ill person may find it easier if you plan for a placement before you are exhausted, and while he still has the ability to adjust to a new setting.

Making the decision

If the stage has been reached when you feel you can no longer continue caring, try and take a break to allow yourself time to reflect on the situation. A relative or close friend might come and stay in your home to look after your dependant while you go away for a few days. It is important for you to consider matters carefully and to consult widely. Involve the impaired person as much as possible and ask him what he thinks. This will make him less likely to resist any changes which you see as unavoidable. People with dementia may fear change and they may function less effectively in unfamiliar surroundings. That is why it may be helpful if your relative has visited a home with you several times before he goes there to live permanently or if he has attended a day centre which is run in that home. If, however, your relative is so confused that he cannot understand, you may find it less distressing if you make the arrangements on your own.

The views of other members of the family should also be sought. If you have brothers and sisters, they may feel they have a right to be consulted on your father's future. They may wish to take over the caring role. They may have some ideas about how to deal with the present situation. It is not unusual for family members to disagree about a parent going into a care home. Some members of the family may want the impaired person to remain at home while others feel the time has come for him to enter a home.

There may be financial implications which, unfortunately, can often cause deep resentment within families as some members see their 'inheritance' disappearing as residential home fees are paid. It is important for all interested parties to have their say in the matter. Everyone should have access to the full facts and a chance to ask questions, so it may be easiest to call a 'family conference'. If the family is in full agreement, so much the better, but if at the end of the day there is disagreement on how to proceed and nobody else is prepared to look after the dementing relative, you will have to make your own decision about what to do, confident in the knowledge that you have consulted everyone affected.

Friends can be a great support so it may be helpful and comforting to discuss the situation with them. They may know about homes if they have looked after an elderly parent. The value of carers' support groups is discussed elsewhere in this book and if you belong to one it is obviously appropriate to discuss questions about long-stay care with other members of the group. The Carers National Association and the Alzheimer's Disease Society will give you the names and addresses of their local contacts who may be able to advise you.

In addition to discussing the matter with other members of the family, you should seek advice from the GP, a social worker or, perhaps, the community psychiatric nurse, community nurse, geriatrician or psychogeriatrician. Some may be better informed than others about what may be available locally, so it can be useful to seek a range of views. Remember that when you are contemplating long-stay care for your relative, it is important to have his medical needs properly assessed by either a doctor or a specialist. There is more about this on page 283.

As with so many things, the need to 'be prepared' applies to finding long-stay care. In many areas there are shortages of such accommodation, and once you have taken the decision it can be very frustrating to find there are no places available and that you face a long waiting-list. Hindsight is of little comfort, so if you think you may be likely to need long-stay care for your relative, you should gather as much information as possible well in advance of the need arising.

However, sometimes there is very little time to make preparations. Many elderly people enter hospitals or homes in emergency or crisis situations, perhaps following a fall, medical complication, or an unexpected breakdown in the system of care. Such emergency admissions can be very bewildering, disruptive and alarming for a confused elderly person. You will want to do everything you can to help to ease the impact of such a move – for instance, by making sure that the new care-givers understand the habits and preferences of your relative.

Types of long-stay care

Confused elderly people can be cared for in several different forms of long-stay care, rather suggesting that no one type of care is necessarily the most appropriate. While, in theory, distinctions may be drawn between the different forms of care, in practice these differences are often blurred, and people with similar care needs can be found in all types of home.

There are three main categories of long-stay care for confused elderly people:

- *residential care homes*, which are run by local authorities, voluntary and non-profit making agencies, private organisations and housing associations;
- *nursing homes* which, with the exception of a few NHS nursing homes, are run by private, voluntary and non-profit making organisations and housing associations;
- *long-stay hospital* provision which may be in geriatric or psychogeriatric beds in an NHS unit.

A further form of care which often seems attractive, perhaps because it seems less 'institutional' to caring relatives, is *sheltered housing*. This is self-contained accommodation which gives people their own front door. Often there is a warden on site who has the job of keeping a watchful eye on residents. The warden is not expected to provide care or nursing treatment but will alert other agencies when help is needed. Most sheltered housing schemes have alarm systems which the resident can operate in emergency situations.

People living in sheltered housing may receive services such as meals-on-wheels, home care or district nursing. However, they are generally expected to look after themselves and to be fairly independent. For this reason, sheltered accommodation is not really an option for confused elderly people who might not, for example, be able to operate an alarm or alert the warden, or who may become disoriented by the move from their former home. Unless there is a special (or 'very') sheltered housing complex catering for confused and dementing elderly people in your locality, sheltered housing is not really worth exploring in any depth.

Care in homes arranged by the local authority

Local authorities (Counties, Metropolitan Boroughs and London Boroughs) have a duty under Part III of the National Assistance Act 1948 to provide accommodation for people who need it by virtue of age or infirmity and for whom it is not otherwise available. This Act was amended by the 1990 NHS and Community Care Act to include people who need care by reason of 'illness', rather than 'infirmity'. This part of the Act is scheduled to take effect from April 1993.

Traditionally, local authorities have mainly provided such care in their own 'Part III' homes, so named after Part III of the 1948 Act. It is up to each local authority to decide how many homes and places it provides, which means that there have always been great differences in the amount of care available from authority to authority.

The community care system described in Chapter 10 will bring changes to the way local authorities arrange the provision of Part III care. Some authorities will continue mainly to use their own homes. However, many authorities are reducing the number of care homes which they run. Some are transferring homes to the management of trusts, housing associations or voluntary bodies.

From April 1993, local authorities will be responsible for purchasing or providing care on behalf of people whom they assess as needing it. People who apply to the local authority for help with care will be assessed for their care needs. Their financial circumstances will also be assessed to determine how much they should pay. The local authority will decide what kind of care it is able to arrange, and how much of the cost of care the person will have to pay.

This system will seem quite different from the old one, under which local authorities' involvement in arranging residential care was mainly restricted to their own homes. After 1993, some of the residential care which local authorities arrange will be in their own homes, but they will also have contracts with independent nursing and residential care homes to provide a certain number of care places.

If you are thinking about care arranged by the local authority, you should contact your local Social Services Department to ask for an assessment of your relative's needs. Make sure that *your* needs are also understood. You can find the Social Services Department in your telephone directory under the name of your County, or Metropolitan or London

Borough. The local Citizens Advice Bureau or Age Concern should also be able to advise you.

In many areas there are waiting-lists for places in homes run by the local authority. It is possible after 1993 that there will be waiting-lists for places in homes arranged through contract by the local authority. Your relative's or your GP may be willing to add support to his case; it is likely that he or she has been consulted as part of the assessment procedure. If you feel you have an urgent need which has not been taken into account in the assessment, you could try to gain the support of your local councillor. You can also have your situation examined again by making a complaint through the complaints procedure which the Social Services Department must operate. If the person is placed on a waiting-list, remember to check every few months to see if places are available.

It is not clear at the time of writing how much choice of home you will have after 1993, if you are looking to the local authority to arrange care. Local authorities will have different arrangements for contracted places. Some will have made arrangements in advance for a certain number of places in various care homes. They may be able to make only a limited number of special arrangements for people whose needs cannot be met by these large contracts. Other authorities, however, will be endeavouring to meet people's special needs with an individual contract in each case. You will have to find out what arrangements your relative's local authority has made.

In any case, it is likely that when a place becomes available you will need to make a decision within a few days. If you are not familiar with the home, arrange to visit it. The assessment should, as far as possible, have matched the chosen home to the person's needs. If you are unhappy about the choice, see if you can discuss this with the people concerned. It should be possible for him to have a trial stay in the home, and this should be requested.

Standards of care in Part III homes vary, just as they do in homes run by independent providers. There has been much progress in improving the quality of care for elderly mentally confused people, but such progress has not occurred in every home. In some areas there are staff shortages, and many local authorities and independent providers face shortages of money for improving care in homes. It is important to note that the Inspection Units created in 1991 inspect local authority homes as well as those run by private and voluntary organisations. This should mean, over time, that all homes in an area conform to the same standards of care.

Private and voluntary homes

Private homes are run for profit by private organisations and individual proprietors. They may be part of a large chain, or quite small operations, run and managed by the owners.

Voluntary homes are non-profit making and are run by charities and religious organisations. Sometimes such homes are open only to particular groups, to followers of a certain religious faith or denomination, or to people with special needs, illnesses or other common characteristics. Some voluntary homes may, for example, cater just for retired teachers, lawyers, actors or ex-members of the armed forces. Residents and their relatives may feel reassured by the fact that a voluntary home is being sponsored by a recognised charity to which redress may be sought if there is ever cause for complaint.

Care homes vary greatly in size. They may be quite small, perhaps taking no more than 8–12 residents, but some are much larger. Depending on where you live, you may find that homes have waiting-lists. In addition, homes can choose to whom they offer accommodation. Many shy away from what they see as a difficult and demanding client group, although there are some which specialise in providing care to people with dementing illnesses.

Any home not directly run by the local authority and providing personal care for four or more elderly and dependent people is required by the Registered Homes Act 1984 to register with, and be inspected at least twice a year by, the local authority's Inspection Unit. It is a punishable offence to operate an unregistered home. Registration should only be granted if the people owning and running the home are suitable, if adequate services and facilities are provided, and if the building is suitable. The local authority will specify on the certificate of registration the number and type of residents a home may accommodate, and each local authority has its own definition of what is 'adequate' in terms of services and facilities. By law, residential homes are required to display the certificate of registration 'in a conspicuous place' and to maintain certain records. Regulations are being introduced in the 1990s under the Registered Homes (Amendment) Act 1991 to formalise a simplified registration procedure for 'small homes' – those caring for three or fewer residents.

Residential homes do not provide nursing care but are expected to provide a level of care which is equivalent to that which might be given by a competent and caring relative who is able to respond to both physical and emotional needs. This need not prevent a confused person being cared for in a residential home – he may not need nursing – and in any case he would still be able to receive general practitioner services and community nursing as though he were in his own home. If a person needs continuous nursing, a nursing home would be the appropriate place. It is illegal for a residential home to act as a nursing home.

Applications for places in private and voluntary homes should usually be made to the home in question which will provide you with details of charges and conditions. If you know of a home which you like or one which has been recommended by friends, so much the better. Often, however, members of the public are unsure of how to find a private home. All private and voluntary homes are required to register and so each local authority will have a list of registered residential homes in its area. Social workers should be able to provide you with a list, and while they cannot recommend a particular home, they may be able to advise you on the ability of certain homes to meet the needs of your relative.

Your local Age Concern or Citizens Advice Bureau may be able to give you some advice, and there are some national charities which help people seeking homes. Visits are made to private homes in the Greater London area by the charity Counsel and Care, which will provide general advice on seeking care home accommodation. Elderly Accommodation Counsel is a charity which maintains a database of homes and which can provide lists for different parts of the country, showing prices and the type of people cared for. Age Concern England also produces a regularly updated fact sheet called 'Finding Residential and Nursing Home Accommodation.' This fact sheet lists helpful organisations and summarises what you need to think about and look for when considering residential or nursing home care.

Nursing homes

There are few NHS nursing homes. While some nursing homes are provided by voluntary organisations and housing associations, the majority are run by private proprietors or organisations. As their title suggests, nursing homes provide nursing care by qualified nurses to people suffering from sickness, injury or infirmity. It is the provision of nursing, as opposed to simply care, which makes them different from residential homes.

Any home providing nursing care has to be registered with the District Health Authority and inspected by it at least twice a year. By law, the person in charge must be either a registered medical practitioner or a qualified nurse, and there should be adequate staff on duty to allow each patient efficient nursing care from suitably qualified staff 24 hours a day. The certificate of registration, which must be displayed in a conspicuous place, will state the maximum number of people for whom the nursing home can care. The District Health Authority will also issue a notice specifying the required qualifications of the nursing staff in the light of the number and type of patients in the home.

Personal recommendation from people with relatives in a private nursing home is the best way of finding a suitable home for your dependant. Failing that, you could contact the Registration Officer of your local District Health Authority, who should be able to provide you with a list of homes in the area. The local Social Services Department, Community Health Council, local Age Concern, Citizens Advice Bureau or Council of Voluntary Service may also be able to provide you with a list or advise you. Counsel and Care visits and provides information on homes in the Greater London area, and the Registered Nursing Home Association publishes a national directory of its members, thereby providing the addresses of a number of homes throughout the country. Elderly Accommodation Counsel and the Independent Healthcare Association can also provide information.

Dual registered homes

The category of 'dual registered home' was created in the Registered Homes Act 1984. These homes provide residential and nursing home care in the same building, or set of buildings. This means that people receiving residential care in such a home do not have to move if they become sufficiently dependent to need nursing care. The home is registered as a residential home *and* as a nursing home, and so provides the two sorts of care, in a resident's own room, in separate parts of the home or in distinct wings.

Even though the whole of the home will be dual registered, the home is still required to state the maximum number of people for whom each type of care will be provided. Each part of the dual registered home will be subject to the same regulations, controls and inspections as a residential or nursing home, as outlined above. There are relatively few dual registered homes.

Which home is best?

It is important to choose the 'right' home if you possibly can. The points which follow apply to all homes, whether residential, nursing, statutory, voluntary or private.

Problems in finding a home, or the need to make a quick decision, can make it very tempting to accept the first place which has an empty bed. This should be resisted if possible. If you have time, try to look at several homes. Vacancies in private homes are quite common in some areas, although it can be difficult finding homes which care for people with dementia. Financial considerations will also be important. Later in this chapter we look at financial issues, but it is important here to emphasise that a place in a home shouldn't be accepted unless you are sure that the arrangements for paying the fees are acceptable to you and any others involved. It is also important to remember that you may not have the authority to take decisions about your relative's financial affairs if you do not have an Enduring Power of Attorney or an appointment as a Receiver through the Court of Protection. There is much more about this in Chapter 15.

Ideally, you should always visit a home, have a good look round and ask questions. Take a friend or another member of the family with you. They may be less emotionally involved than you and able to help you to think through your decision. Try to visit more than once if there is time. On the second visit you will notice things which you missed before. Many families say that the things you notice when you first enter a home may not be the things that matter as time goes on. Allow plenty of time to visit, talk to alert residents and the staff, and try to picture how your relative will fit in.

When Mr Armitage first visited The Haven Residential Care Home he was favourably impressed. He liked the spacious entrance hall and the long clean corridors with residents' names on the doors. Staff members were in fresh uniforms, and the rooms were sunny and well-lit. However, after visiting his father several times at the home, Mr Armitage noticed that no residents used the entrance hall which had first so impressed him. It now seemed more important that the care assistants were friendly to his father, and helped him promptly to use the toilet when he needed it.

Mr Armitage's father had always enjoyed mealtimes. Mr Armitage wished the home had spent more money on a cook and less on the attractive entrance hall, as his father was depressed by the bland, lukewarm food. There was also a rule that everyone had to be in their rooms by 8.30 pm and awake by 7 am, which was not at all in line with his father's habits before he entered the home.

When you meet the manager of the home, you should feel free to ask questions about the home's registration and about financial procedures. Don't take anything for granted. If there are things which you don't understand, ask. Make sure that there is a written contract, and that you have seen it and had time to consider it before your relative is actually in the home. Many homes do not offer a written contract. This is now not in line with recognised good practice. However, many contracts contain clauses which you may not like, and you should read them carefully. You should take professional advice if the contract contains a clause requiring you to be responsible for the fees. Unless the relative is your spouse, you have no legal obligation to do this. However, if you refuse to sign such an undertaking, the home could choose not to offer the place to your relative.

You may wish to discuss the following matters before you sign any papers:

- Will your relative receive a refund of advance payments if he leaves the home? Is a payment in advance required before the trial period has been completed?
- How will payments be made, and how will regular accounts be presented?
- Does the written agreement show the care which will be provided within the fees, and make clear what will be charged for as 'extra'? Note particularly if there are charges for television, telephone, laundry, personal care supplies, incontinence supplies, chiropody or physiotherapy.
- How does the home ensure the security of your relative's personal money?
- Under what circumstances can the home ask your relative to leave? How much notice must they give you?
- What happens if residents require more or less care than they currently have? Might they have to leave? What arrangements are made for funerals, and for payment if the resident dies?

If the manager is reluctant to answer these questions, this may be an indication of how you will be treated after the person has entered the home.

The home should have a brochure outlining the care provided, the philosophy of the home, and the charges. Make sure, however, that the reality of the home matches the description in the brochure.

You will know the sorts of things which please and upset you and the person, and which are important to you both, so find out if these individual needs will be met. There will be an endless list of questions you will probably want to ask, and each person's needs and preferences differ, but here are some questions which you might consider:

Daily living

- Does the home encourage its residents to do as much as possible for themselves, and to make choices about as many aspects of their daily lives as they can?
- Do residents have the choice of single or shared rooms? If they share,

do they (or you) have a say about whom they share with?
- Are residents encouraged to bring personal possessions with them – pictures, plants, furniture?
- What are the meals like? Are special diets catered for? Can visitors come at mealtimes? Try to visit the home at a mealtime. Does the food look appetising? Are meals adequate? Are snacks available?
- Are residents with dementia served in a small, quiet area, or in a large, noisy dining-room? Are care workers or nurse assistants helping people who cannot feed themselves? Are people with swallowing problems closely supervised?
- Are the arrangements for getting up and going to bed acceptable to you and your relative? Are residents routinely sedated at night?

Visiting

- Are there free visiting hours, and can residents speak to their visitors in private? May children visit?
- Is the home close enough to allow you to visit frequently? Is there enough parking and public transport? Will you feel comfortable visiting the home?

Activities

- What provision does the home make for taking residents out – on outings, to the shops, to places of worship or to entertainments? Do clergy visit regularly?
- What physical activities are available for residents? Is there supervised daily exercise? Even people who are in a wheelchair or confined to bed need exercise, and those who can walk should be doing so. Exercise may reduce the restlessness of people with dementing illnesses.
- What other activities are there? Are residents encouraged to continue their hobbies? Do the activities offered seem dignified and adult? Will they interest your relative?
- Can residents help with the day-to-day activities of the home – cleaning, cooking, gardening, looking after pets?

Health care

- Do residents have a choice of GP? If the home has its own doctor, how frequently does he or she attend patients in the home? Can you meet with this doctor if you have concerns?
- Are toilets available in all parts of the home, fully equipped with handles and other helpful equipment?
- How is incontinence managed? For instance, individualised toileting is preferred over catheters for people who are able to get to the toilet. Look around. Do you see more than a few people who have catheter bags hanging from their wheelchairs or beds?
- Ask the manager if any residents have pressure sores.
- Can wheelchairs go everywhere within the home, and easily in and out? Is there a lift?

Cleanliness and safety

- Is the home clean? Look at bathrooms and toilets, and at the kitchen.
- Is there a strong smell of urine? This may indicate either poor patient care or poor housekeeping. Occasional odours are difficult to avoid.
- Are bathrooms and other areas equipped with grab rails, handrails, non-skid floors and other devices for residents' safety?
- What provisions are made for the safety of people who wander or become agitated? Do staff members have the time to spend with someone who becomes upset? Are doors secure? Is the lighting good (but not glaring), is the furniture sturdy and the temperature comfortable? Is the home reasonably quiet?
- What provisions have been made for fire safety? Will these protect your relative in the event of a fire?
- Ask how the home balances the protection of residents from risk with the need to encourage as much independence as possible. Are the home's policies in this respect acceptable to you?
- Does the home have a written policy on the use of restraints? Look around. Are people sitting in furniture from which they cannot 'escape'? Restraints should not be used unless all other measures to control the person have failed and they are necessary to protect him from harm. Experienced staff members can usually manage wandering and agitation without restraints. No one should ever be left unsupervised in a restraint for any period of time.

Staff

- Does the home employ enough staff to assist your relative individually or to wait while he slowly does some things for himself? How many people must each assistant take care of? Does this seem reasonable, given the severity of the residents' impairments? What level of staffing is there at nights and at weekends? Do the staff seem hurried?
- Do the staff understand dementing illnesses and how to care for people like your relative?
- Do staff seem happy and friendly? Contented staff are less likely to take out their personal frustrations on the residents. Ask staff members how staff turnover rates compare with those at other homes in the area. This can be a good clue to the level of staff satisfaction.
- How much training is available for care workers or nurse assistants? Have they had special training in care of people with dementia? If they have not had training, how willing are they to accept information from you on how to manage your relative?
- What specialist training has the home's manager had? Is the home involved in staff development through the National Vocational Qualifications (NVQ) scheme?
- People with dementia are sensitive to the way they are treated. Observe how the staff treat residents. Do they address them as adults or as if they were children? Do they stop and pay attention to residents who approach them? Do they greet people before attending to them? Do they seem sensitive to needs for privacy and dignity?

Care and services

- Does the home have care plans for its residents? Are you welcome to help draw up a care plan for your relative?
- What information does the home want to know about your relative? Does the home want to know about your relative's likes and dislikes, habits, how you manage behaviour, what abilities the person still has? These things are essential for good care.
- What is the home's policy on administering medication? Does the home ensure that the medication of residents is regularly reviewed?

The surroundings

- Is the home pleasant to be in and well lit? Are residents' personal possessions on view in their rooms? Pleasant surroundings and kind, patient staff are important to a confused person. Also, you need to feel comfortable when you come to visit.
- Do you think that your relative will feel comfortable here? There are 'homey' homes that have worn furniture but seem more like home to some people. Other people will feel more comfortable in a newer home. Is it too noisy and confusing or too quiet and boring? Is there more than one lounge, and somewhere quiet without a television?
- Glare, noise and dim light all add to the difficulties experienced by a person with dementia. If these things bother you, chances are they will also create unnecessary stress for a person with dementia.
- Does the home encourage residents to say how they feel about living there, and provide written information for residents and/or their families about how to discuss a problem or make a complaint?

All these questions relate to the quality of life in the home. There are a number of publications which give detailed guidance on different aspects of quality in homes. These are listed in Appendix III.

Many homes allow residents to have a trial stay for a few days or for several weeks and it is wise to take advantage of this provision if your circumstances allow. The actual experience of your relative living in a particular home will enable you to judge how happy you both are with its arrangements. You will probably find that it will not take you long to 'get the feel' of the place and know if it will provide a satisfactory standard of care. Hopefully it will.

When you are evaluating a home, remember that other care-givers may do things differently from you. You may need to accept the differences. Also, remember that the forgetful, confused person may give you an inaccurate report of what is happening. Nevertheless, you remain responsible for monitoring the quality of care.

If you are able to place your family member in a good care home, you may notice that he does better than he did at home. Families sometimes have mixed feelings about this. While they are pleased to see their family member doing well, they are sad that they could not bring about this change at home. Keep in mind that it is easier for professional staff to create a therapeutic programme. They can leave the resident at the end of a shift and they are not doing the care-giving alone! When the person is doing well in a home and you are free of the other demands of care, you have more time and energy for giving him the love and the sense of family that no one else can give. This will also be true if he is in a hospital.

Long-stay hospital care

As we have seen, the decision to place someone in a home is not an easy one. For some people with dementing illnesses, a hospital may be more appropriate than a residential or nursing home. This could be for a number of different reasons: there may be no homes in the area which can care for the person; it may not be possible to finance care in a home; the person's condition or behaviour may be such that he would be better off in a hospital, with the full range of medical care and supervision available to him.

There are no hard and fast rules about who should be in a hospital long-stay bed and who should be in a care home. In many areas the health authority has reduced the number of long-stay beds, so, in practice, care is only available in nursing or residential homes. This can present serious problems for people who cannot pay for such care. However, in other areas, health authorities have worked hard to develop a system in which people with dementia are fully assessed, and to match choices about placement as closely as possible to their care needs. In such areas there is likely to be a choice of small NHS units near to where the person lives, or care homes, which may be paid for by the person's own resources, or, if he qualifies, through state help.

For many people with dementia, the route to a care home or place in a hospital is through an admission to hospital, either because of an acute medical problem, such as a fall, or for assessment. The person will be referred by the family doctor to a specialist.

There are several kinds of specialists who may see your relative. A geriatrician specialises in the general diseases of elderly people. A psychogeriatrician specialises in mental illness in old age, or a general psychiatrist may be involved. The specialist will make quite a detailed assessment of the person's condition. If possible, you should go along to support him, and to ask and answer questions.

The aim of the assessment is to make an accurate diagnosis of what is wrong and to see whether your relative's condition can be improved. The consultant may decide that quite lengthy treatment or permanent long-stay hospital care is needed. However, in many cases the hospital will treat your relative's immediate problem, and then it will be suggested that he does not need hospital care but should be looked after in a residential or nursing home. Or the hospital may propose that you continue to look after him at home.

It will be important at this time for you to be clear about your own needs, your own ability to continue caring, and your relative's ability to fund the cost of care in a care home. In England, a Department of Health Circular (HC(89)5) was issued to health authorities in 1989 setting out the procedures which should take place at the time of hospital discharge. The circular states that relatives' and carers' views should be taken into account when planning discharge; furthermore, it states that no NHS patient should be discharged to a private nursing home against his wishes where he or a relative will be responsible for the fees. The Patient's Charter states that hospitals should follow the guidance in this circular.

It is important to remember that a hospital has no authority to discharge a patient to a care home, unless someone is willing to take contractual responsibility for the fees, or unless the health authority itself will pay the full fees. A patient should not be discharged home if it is clear that he is not capable of looking after himself, or if the care-giver can no longer cope with care.

Families often report that they can be placed under a lot of pressure to take their relative home, or to find a care home. The duty of health authorities to provide continuing nursing care is not entirely clear, but at the time of hospital discharge, patients and their relatives can exercise some choice when the doctors have said that continuing nursing care is required. On the other hand, it is much more difficult to obtain long-term care in the NHS when the patient is at home and the health authority says it has no appropriate facilities. In such cases, the care-giver may have no alternative but to carry on caring if care in an independent home cannot be afforded.

If it is decided that the person does need long-stay hospital care, you will probably feel a combination of different emotions, often sadness, grief and guilt. These feelings are quite usual but you should talk about them with your family, friends, a social worker, your doctors or a relatives' support group. You can be assured that hospital care is what he needs. Moreover, you should try and prepare him for going into hospital. You may have several days or weeks to do so while a bed is being found or while he is in the assessment ward. During that time, find out what possessions and clothes should be taken into the hospital and check that they are clearly labelled with his name. Also, if you can, spend some time explaining to him what is going to happen, that it is for the best, and that you, the family and friends will visit him in hospital.

The type of hospital and ward in which he will be placed will vary from area to area, depending on the type of service provided and what is available. He may be cared for in a geriatric or psychogeriatric ward of a general hospital, in a dementia unit, or in a ward for mentally ill elderly people in a psychiatric hospital. If the person suffers from a severe degree of dementia and shows extreme behavioural disorders, he is likely to be placed under the care of a psychogeriatrician in a psychiatric hospital. If he is mildly to moderately confused, with other medical problems, immobility and/or is doubly incontinent, he may be placed in a geriatric ward with elderly patients who although frail are quite alert.

In some districts long-stay care is not located in the same hospital as the assessment and rehabilitation wards. Unfortunately, it is also all too often the case that long-stay care is located in old, Victorian buildings which may seem unfriendly and imposing. In many areas, outmoded and dilapidated buildings are being replaced with new purpose-built units. In other areas, however, health authorities are closing old units without ensuring that appropriate replacements are available. In such cases, relatives of people with dementing illnesses are very concerned about what might happen in the future, should their relative require long-stay NHS care. You might like to see what plans have been made in your area for continuing care by obtaining a copy of the local authority's community care plan, and the separate health authority plan, if there is one.

It is also important to remember that more important than the buildings, is the quality of the care provided. Most hospital staff are committed people who work in very difficult, sometimes understaffed, conditions. Occasionally things can go wrong and when you see this happening draw it to the attention of the hospital administration so that it will not happen again. Hospital administrators should welcome comments on the services provided.

The standard of care provided in long-stay units is improving all the time, and there is some very imaginative and exciting work being carried out with confused elderly patients. Some schemes involve volunteers from the local community who, working alongside hospital staff, spend much time improving the quality of the patients' lives. While the patient's dementia cannot be reversed, with careful support the decline can sometimes be arrested or slowed down. Do not look upon the long-stay hospital care as the end of the road for the person; view it positively as the most appropriate form of care available. You will also find that since you no longer have the responsibility and stress of caring for him, you can now relate more favourably to him and be in a position to recall the happier times you have shared together.

Charges and financial implications

There is no charge for anyone who lives in a National Health Service hospital (including NHS nursing homes) but those who stay may have State Pensions and benefits reduced or stopped. For example, the position at the time of writing is that State Retirement Pension is reduced after six weeks, with a further reduction after 52 weeks. Income Support and other income-related benefits may also be affected after six weeks in hospital, while Attendance Allowance will stop after a maximum of four weeks in hospital. Social Security leaflet NI9 will give details of the deductions currently made.

For anyone who has more income than basic pensions it costs less to live in a NHS hospital than a residential or nursing home.

Most people will not have sufficient income to enable them to pay for care in a home indefinitely; it is important therefore to look at the financial aspects of the situation well in advance.

State help with care home fees

In April 1993, a new system of public financing of care in homes is planned to take effect. Until then, people are assessed by local authorities under one set of rules for their ability to pay for Part III care, while people needing help with the fees in private and voluntary sector homes turn to the Department of Social Security to apply for special levels of Income Support if their savings are below £8,000.

Because the system is scheduled to change in 1993, you will need to seek good advice about how the old and the new systems work. Anyone who was already living in a private or voluntary home *before* the date when the new system took effect, will continue under the old Income Support scheme. (This means that they should claim under that scheme even if they started off paying for themselves, but their savings have run down to the level where Income Support can be claimed – currently £8,000.) People in local authority Part III homes, however, will have their resources reassessed under the new scheme, which should work out to their advantage in almost all cases. We can't stress too much how important it is for you to obtain good advice about paying for care. It is too often the case that decisions, based on inadequate or inaccurate information, turn out to have disastrous financial consequences. Age Concern produces detailed factsheets which explain all the assessment systems in considerable detail. These are regularly updated and can be obtained free on receipt of a large, stamped addressed envelope.

From 1993 the person who needs care in a home will use a combination of funds to pay for that care. These will include the retirement and any private pension, and savings. If the pensions and savings are below Income Support level (See page 256) the person will be eligible to apply for a special Residential Allowance which will be added to Income Support as a contribution to the housing costs of care in homes.

Where the local authority is making arrangements for care, it will pay the full cost of a care home place, charging the resident according to his income and savings, in line with national rules, and leaving the resident with a nationally defined sum for personal expenses. Where relatives add to what the local authority agrees to pay, perhaps to pay for a more expensive home, their contribution will be fully taken into account.

These assessment procedures will be complicated, and they are not fully decided at the time of writing this book. In any case, such procedures change from time to time, and you must acquaint yourself with the system before making any decisions about where the person should be placed.

One important thing to remember is that people paying for themselves in a care home may be eligible for the care component of the Disability Living Allowance, if they are under the age of 65, or Attendance Allowance if they are over this age. There is more information about these benefits in Chapter 15.

Moving to a home or hospital

Once a home has been found and financial arrangements have been made, the next step is the actual transfer to the home. We have discussed helping the impaired person to adjust to home or day care on p. 182. Many of the same points apply when a person moves to a residential or nursing home, or to hospital.

Tell the person where he is going if you think there is any chance he will understand. Take familiar items that he is fond of with him (pictures, mementos, a rug or a radio). If possible, he should help select these. Even a person who is upset or severely impaired needs to feel that this is his life and he is still important.

You may have to close your ears to the person's accusations if he blames you for the move. If he repeatedly becomes upset when the home is mentioned, it is not helpful, we feel, to keep mentioning it. You may need to continue matter-of-factly with arrangements. Try to avoid dishonest explanations such as, 'We are going for a ride' or 'you are going for a visit'. This can make the person's subsequent adjustment in the home or hospital more difficult.

Many people with dementia will make a better adjustment to the move if the family visits frequently in the early weeks. People vary: some residents need time on their own before they begin to join in new activities. If the person has trouble settling in, ask yourself whether your own tension and anxiety are making it more difficult for him to relax in the new surroundings. Avoid a home that asks you to stay away until the person gets used to his surroundings. This only increases his feeling of being lost. You may find that, during visits, the person may greet you with accusations or beg you to take him home with you. Remember that these may be the only words he can find to express his understandable anxiety and unhappiness. Offer reassurance and affection and avoid being drawn into arguments. After the first weeks, you can taper your visiting to fewer hours. Find a schedule that supports the resident while allowing you to regain your own resources.

Some families have written down information about the person for the staff. Does the person take a bath in the morning or at night? Does he go to bed early or late? Who are the people in his life whom he may ask for? What do certain words or behaviours mean? How do you respond to things he often does? What will comfort him? What will trigger outbursts?

You may not find a home you really like, or you may feel that the staff are not giving the person the kind of care he should receive. However, you may have no alternative but to leave the person in that home. The manager of an excellent home suggests that you avoid complaints and do all that you can to establish a friendly relationship with the staff. This may mean a compromise on your part, but may well encourage their co-operation.

If you are moving the person to the home from a hospital, you may have had little or no time to search for a home and to plan an orderly transition. You may be exhausted by all that has had to be done in a few hours or days. If this happens, at least try to go with the person to the home and to have some familiar things waiting there for him.

Adjusting to a new life

The change to living in a home or hospital means major adjustments for the impaired person. Making these adjustments takes time and energy for staff, residents and family, and it can be a painful process. Remember that the move need not mean the end of family relationships. As time goes on, your relationship with the impaired person may improve. Your relative can continue to be part of the family even though he has moved into a setting that better meets his needs. However, we know that the difficult part of the adjustment is the feelings you and the person may experience about it.

Visiting

It is important to your relative for you to visit. Even if he does not recognise you or does not seem to want you there, your regular visits help at some level to sustain his awareness that he is valued and is a part of a family. Sometimes people beg to be taken home or cry when you leave. It is tempting to avoid such scenes by visiting less often, but usually the benefits to everyone from the visit far outweigh the upset that comes at the end. Feeling grief and anger at being in a home or hospital is understandable.

You may be distressed by the atmosphere of the home or by the other people you see there. Relatives find it painful to see a loved one so impaired. Because dementing illnesses interfere with communication and comprehension, families can have difficulty thinking of things to do when they visit. In the following section we describe things that families tell us make visiting easier.

You can help your relative orientate himself in his new home. While you are visiting, explain again why he is there (for example, say, 'You are too ill to stay at home'). Review the daily routines of the home; make a schedule for him if he can read it. Help him find the bathroom, toilet, dining-room, television and telephone. Help him find his things in the cupboard. Think of a way to identify the door of his room as his. Decorate his room or living area with his possessions. If you have a dog or a cat which your relative liked when he lived with you, ask the hospital or care staff if you can bring it into the home.

Tell him exactly when you will visit next and write this down so that he can use it to remind himself. Some families write a letter to the resident mentioning highlights of the most recent visit and the time of the next. The staff can read the letter to the resident between visits to reassure him that you do come frequently. Encourage other members of the family, and friends, to visit, but first explain what they are likely to see. Try to continue to involve the person in family outings. If he is not acutely ill, take him for rides, shopping, home for dinner or overnight, or to worship. But first discuss such ideas with the appropriate staff and before you tell your relative. Such activities may not be beneficial. His routine may be disrupted too much and he may become very distressed when he returns to the hospital or home. On the other hand he may benefit from a change of environment and a short break. Even if he resists going back, he may eventually come to accept this routine, and he will benefit from the knowledge that he is still part of the family. Occasionally it continues to be difficult to persuade the person to return. In this instance it is better to visit him at the home.

Help the person to remain part of special family events such as birthdays and holidays. Even if he is depressed or confused, he usually should still be informed of sad events.

Telephone calls between visits help a forgetful person to keep in touch and remind him that he is not forgotten. Don't expect him to be able to remember to call you.

Take an old photograph album, an old hat from the loft, or some other item that may trigger memories of the past, and urge the person to talk about things he remembers from long ago. If he always tells you the same story, accept this. It is your listening to him and your presence that communicate that you still care.

Talk about the family, neighbours and gossip. Remind him of family birthdays and anniversaries, and give news of grandchildren, nieces and nephews. Even if the person is not fully aware, he can enjoy the act of

listening and talking. Being together is important to both of you. Confused people may not be interested in some topics, such as current events.
If the person seems restless, try changing subjects; do not insist on
bringing him up to date on information.

Be sympathetic about his complaints. Listening to the things he complains about tells him that you care. He may make the same complaint
over and over because he forgets that he has told you. Listen anyway;
it is your empathy that he needs. Investigate his complaint thoughtfully,
however, before you complain to the staff or act on it. Remember that
his perception of things may be inaccurate, although there may be an
element of truth in the complaint.

Sing old, familiar songs. Don't be surprised if other residents drift by
to listen or participate. Music is a wonderful way of sharing. Nobody
will mind if your singing isn't very good. Take along tape recordings of
the family or children.

Make a personal history scrapbook telling the story of the person's
life – where he grew up, when he married, his children, his job, hobbies,
and so on. Write in large letters. Illustrate it with photographs, clippings,
bits of fabric, medals, etc. Making the scrapbook can occupy both of
you for several visits. Reviewing it may help him recall his past. Even if
he does not remember, he may be reassured that he has a past.

Make a personal history box. Put in items that will trigger memories;
treasured keepsakes, antique kitchen or farm tools that will be familiar
to the person, assorted screws and bolts for a handyman or spools of
thread for a seamstress. Look for items with interesting colours, weights,
textures and sizes. The person may enjoy sorting and touching the things
in this box. You and the staff can use it to trigger memories. Include a
card that gives information about the items: 'This is an old-fashioned
apple corer like the one Mother used when she made apple purée for
her five children.' 'Dad wore these dancing shoes until he was seventy.'

Avoid too much excitement. Your arrival, news and conversation may
over-excite the impaired person and could precipitate a catastrophic
reaction.

Do things that show that you are interested in his new home. Walk
around it together, talk to his room-mate, or to other residents and staff.
Remind him to smell the flowers and see the birds when you walk around
outside.

Help him to care for himself. Eat a meal together, do his hair, rub his
back, hold hands, help him to take some exercise. Bring a treat that you
can eat together while you are there. Avoid bringing food the staff must
store. If the person has difficulty eating, you may want to visit at mealtimes and help to feed him. If other confused or upset residents interrupt
your visit, you may be able to tell them gently but clearly not to talk
with you now. If necessary, ask where there is a more private place for
you to visit. Sometimes visits go more smoothly if you include one or
two other residents in a simple activity.

If the person enjoys it and if it does not precipitate a catastrophic reaction, take along children (one at a time) or a pet (ask the staff in advance). Seeing the people in a home is usually helpful for young children. You can prepare the child by talking about the things she might see, such as catheters or intravenous tubes, and explaining that they help such people to maintain their bodily functions.

Sometimes a person is so ill that he cannot talk or recognise you or respond to you. It is hard to know what to say to such a person. Try holding hands, rubbing the person's back, or singing. One clergyman said this about his visits:

'I've grown in these visits. I am so used to doing, doing, doing and there is nothing I can do for these people. I've learned to just sit, to just share being and not to feel I have to do or talk or entertain.'

Sharing family life and loving a person who is in an institution and who is in the late stages of a dementing illness is not easy, but perhaps you will find your own meaning in doing so, as this man has.

When problems occur in the home or hospital

Sometimes serious problems about patient care do arise.

Mr Rosen says, 'My father has Alzheimer's disease and we had to put him in a nursing home. He got terribly ill and was transferred to a hospital, where they said his condition was made worse because he was dehydrated. Apparently the home failed to give him enough fluid. I feel as if I am guilty of not checking up on this and I feel that I can't send him back to a home that neglects him.'

As you know, people with dementing illnesses can be difficult to care for, especially in the late stages of the disease. If Mr Rosen complains to the nursing home staff, he may only make them angry. If he tries to move his father, he may find there are no other better homes available locally, or that none of them will accept a person with Alzheimer's disease or who is dependent on state funding.

We hope you will not encounter problems like this. If you do, first take time to consider what kind of care you can reasonably expect. You should expect the person to be kept as well as possible, to be well fed and hydrated, to be protected from obvious risks, and to be clean and comfortable. Concurrent illness should be recognised and patients watched for drug reactions and interactions.

However, sometimes the care home can be 'wrong if they do and wrong if they don't'. It is often not possible to treat completely every condition or solve every problem. For example, allowing a person to walk independently may be good for his heart, fitness and self-confidence, but may result in a fall. Asking the staff about the risks and benefits of the care they are providing can help you to decide what risks you are willing to accept.

Staff problems are a frequent cause of inadequacy in care. A home or hospital may not be able to give the kind of individual care that you could give at home. However, if there are not enough staff members to keep residents clean, comfortable and fed, and their medical needs monitored, then something is wrong.

Talk over your concerns honestly but calmly with the proprietor or manager of a home, or a social worker or unit manager in a hospital; offer them the information you have about the care of people with dementia. How do they respond? Do they thank you for talking to them and say they will take care of the problem, or do they make excuses and brush you off? If a doctor or other professional is aware of the problem, ask for that person's support in correcting the situation.

> *Mr Rosen said, 'The doctor at the hospital was so helpful. He called the nursing home and talked to them, explained that people with dementia can easily become dehydrated and should be watched.'*

If this does not solve the problem, contact the Registration Officer of the District Health Authority or the local authority about your concerns. You may need to seek other support in helping to improve standards of care in a home. Perhaps you could join with other relatives of people in the home or hospital, and work together to improve the care provided.

In America, it is against the law to discharge a person from a home because the family has made a complaint. It is also against the law to mistreat a patient whose family has complained. There is no such law in England, and families sometimes find that their complaints seem to fall on deaf ears. Others are frightened to complain about care in a home or hospital, for fear that their relative may be badly treated as a result. If this is a problem for you, consider whether the situation could be any worse – perhaps by complaining you will actually improve things for him, and for all the other people being cared for in the home or hospital as well.

Sexual issues in residential homes, nursing homes and hospital

Some confused people in residential homes, nursing homes and hospitals undress themselves in public, masturbate or make advances to staff or other residents. Sexual behaviour in these long-term care facilities differs in significant ways from such behaviour at home; it is no longer a private matter, but in one way or another has an impact on staff, on other residents and on the families of residents, and it raises the ethical issue of whether a person who is impaired can or should retain the right to make sexual decisions for himself.

While our culture seems to be saturated with talk about sex, it is the sexuality of the young and beautiful that is being discussed. Most of us are uncomfortable considering the sexuality of the old, the unattractive, the handicapped or the demented. Hospital, and residential and nursing home staff also often feel uncomfortable. If the staff report inappropriate behaviour to you, remember that much of the behaviour that at first seems sexual is really caused by disorientation and confusion. You and the staff can work together to help the person know where he is, where he can use the toilet, and where he can undress. Often all that is needed is to say, 'It isn't time to go to bed yet. We'll put your pyjamas on later.' Distractions such as offering a glass of fruit squash or a cup of tea are helpful.

Confused persons may become close friends with another resident, often without a sexual relationship. Friendship is a universal need that does not stop when one becomes demented. Occasionally one hears stories about people getting into bed with other residents. This is not hard to understand when we consider that most of us have shared a bed with someone for many years and have enjoyed the closeness which this sharing brings. The confused person may not realise where he is or whom he is with. He may not realise he is not in his own bed. He may feel that he is with his spouse. Remember that living in a home or hospital can be lonely, and there may not be much opportunity for the confused person to be held and loved. How you respond to such an incident depends on your attitudes and values and on the response of the staff.

Some residents will masturbate. Staff mostly ignore such behaviour which is usually done in private. If it occurs in public, the person should be quietly returned to his room or taken back to his bedside.

Flirting is a common and socially acceptable behaviour for men and women. In a home, a person may flirt to reinforce old social roles. It makes a person feel younger and more attractive. Tragically, the dementia may cause the person to do this clumsily, making offensive remarks or inappropriate gestures.

When the staff are trained to remind the person matter-of-factly and kindly that this behaviour is not acceptable, and to redirect him to another activity or location, it seldom remains a problem. Residents can be provided with other opportunities to re-experience their social roles.

Your own adjustment

You also will experience changes in your life when a family member moves to a home or hospital. If the person lived with you, and especially if he is your spouse, the adjustment may be difficult. You may be tired from the effort of arranging for the placement and, on top of your fatigue, you may feel sad at the changes that have taken place. The move to a home or hospital may intensify your feelings of grief and loss. You may have mixed feelings of relief and sorrow, guilt and anger. Guilt can arise because you are no longer caring, and because you remember quarrels and outbursts of temper which may have arisen in the past. You might regret that you are no longer caring, despite the fact that to do so would be an impossible task. You may feel angry at the lack of services which meant that you were unable to look after your relative at home. You may grieve an apparently lost relationship.

At the same time, it is a relief not to have to carry the burden of care, to be able to sleep or read uninterrupted. Still, you probably wish things were different and that you could have continued to care for this person yourself.

Families often tell us that in the first few days they feel lost. Without the usual demands of caring for an impaired person, they cannot decide what do with themselves. At first, you may not be able to sleep through the night or relax enough to watch television. If these problems continue for a long time, you should discuss them with your doctor, a social worker or possibly with a carers' support group. Many carers continue to attend a group after their dependant has gone into a home or hospital. It can help them to adjust to their new life and, at the same time, they can offer support to others who may just be taking up a caring role.

The visits to your relative may be trying, especially if the home or hospital is some distance away. The visits may be depressing. Sometimes confused people are temporarily worse until they adjust to a new setting, and this can upset you. Sometimes, too, the other people in the home are depressing to see.

Care home and hospital staff are geared to providing care for many people and you may not feel that your loved one is receiving the individual care that you would like. Other things about the home or the staff may upset you. It's not unusual for family members to feel angry with the staff from time to time. If you are upset with the home or the staff, you have a right to discuss your concerns with them, to be given answers, and to receive an assurance that the person's care or status in the home will not be jeopardised by your doing this.

If there is a social worker at the home or hospital, she may help you to work out your concerns. If there is not, discuss your concerns in a calm, matter-of-fact way with the administrator or the manager.

Often things are better after the move, especially when they have been difficult at home. Since other people are responsible for daily care, you are not always tired, and as you can get away from the person's irritating behaviour, you may be able to relax and enjoy your relationship for the first time in a long while.

If other family members do not visit, it may be because they find it very hard to face visiting, or don't know what to talk about. If someone in your family reacts this way, try to understand that this may be their way of grieving and you may not be able to change them.

Sometimes family members spend many hours at the home, helping with the patient. Only you can decide how much time you should spend visiting. Ask yourself if part of your reason for being there has to do with your loneliness and grief, and whether it might be better if you spent less time there so that the resident can adjust to the new home.

Time does pass and gradually the acute phase of adjustment also passes. As time goes on, you will settle into a routine of visits. It is natural for you gradually to build a life apart from the person who has changed so much.

The staff of the hospital or home will also enjoy your visits. They like to see other people taking an interest in the patients and residents. Use your visits as an opportunity to talk to the staff and tell them about your relative and his past. This information is welcomed since, if the person is very demented, it enables them to relate to him more as an individual who has lived an interesting life, perhaps once held an important job, visited unusual places or whatever else he may have achieved – and everyone has achieved or contributed something to life. If the nursing and care staff can think of your relative in these terms they will be better able to provide him with the sort of care and attention which you quite rightly think he deserves. The staff will derive greater satisfaction from this, the person will be better off and you will find the long-stay care which he is receiving less institutional and much more acceptable.

Sometimes the brain does not work as it should. Such problems may be called retardation, dyslexia, dementia or psychosis. They may be caused by an injury to the brain, a genetic condition, chemicals in the environment which are damaging to the brain, or many other things. In this chapter we explain how dementia differs from other problems of the brain and describe some of the most common causes of dementia.

Dementia

Doctors and scientists group the different things that can go wrong with the brain by their symptoms. Just as fever, coughing, vomiting and dizziness are symptoms of several different diseases, memory loss, confusion, personality change and problems with speaking are also symptoms of several diseases.

Dementia is the medical term for a group of symptoms. It describes a global decline in intellectual ability sufficiently severe to interfere with a person's daily functioning, which occurs in a person who is awake and alert (not drowsy, intoxicated, or unable to pay attention). This decline in intellectual functioning means a loss of several kinds of mental processes that may include mathematical ability, vocabulary, abstract thinking, judgement, speaking or co-ordination. It may include changes in personality. 'Not feeling quite as sharp as you used to' does not mean that one is developing a dementia. The person's ability must decline from what was normal for her. This is different from mental retardation, in which a person has been impaired since infancy.

These symptoms of dementia can be caused by many diseases. Some of the diseases are treatable; some are not. In some, the dementia can be stopped, in some it can be reversed and in others the primary condition cannot be changed. Some of these diseases are rare. Other diseases are not rare, but the people who have them do not usually become demented. Do not assume that a dementia is the inevitable result of having these diseases. A *partial* list of the conditions that can cause dementia follows:

Metabolic disorders

- thyroid, parathyroid, or adrenal gland dysfunction
- liver or kidney dysfunction
- certain vitamin deficiencies, such as Vitamin B12 deficiency

Structural problems of the brain

- normal pressure hydrocephalus (abnormal flow of spinal fluid)
- brain tumours
- subdural haematoma (bleeding beneath the skull which results in collections of blood which press on the brain)
- trauma (injuries to the brain)
- hypoxia and anoxia (insufficient oxygen)

Infections

- tuberculosis
- syphilis
- fungal, bacterial, and viral infections of the brain, such as meningitis or encephalitis
- acquired immune deficiency syndrome (AIDS)

Toxins (poisons)

- carbon monoxide
- drugs
- metal poisoning
- alcohol (scientists disagree about whether alcohol can cause dementia)

Degenerative diseases (causes generally unknown)

- Alzheimer's disease
- Friedreich's ataxia
- Huntington's disease
- Parkinson's disease
- Pick's disease
- progressive supranuclear palsy
- Wilson's disease
- multiple sclerosis

Vascular (blood vessel) disease

- stroke or multi-infarct disease
- Binswanger's disease

Auto-immune diseases

- temporal arteritis
- lupus erythematosus

Psychiatric diseases

- depression
- schizophrenia

Korsakoff's syndrome causes an impairment only in memory and not in other mental functions. It looks like a dementing illness but, because it affects only one area of mental function, it is not a true dementia. Most research indicates that about 50 per cent of the cases of dementia are caused by Alzheimer's disease, 20 per cent are caused by multi-infarct disease, and 20 per cent are caused by a combination of Alzheimer's disease and multi-infarct disease. About 10 per cent of the cases of dementia are caused by one or other of all the remaining conditions.

Alzheimer's disease

Alzheimer's disease was first described by a German physician, Alois Alzheimer, in 1907, and the condition was named after him. The disease Alzheimer originally described occurred in a woman in her fifties and was called *presenile dementia*. Neurologists now agree that the dementia that occurs in the elderly is the same as, or similar to, the presenile condition. It is usually called senile dementia of the Alzheimer type (SDAT), dementia of the Alzheimer type (DAT) or Alzheimer's disease (AD).

The symptoms of the disease are usually a gradual, though sometimes almost imperceptible, decline in many areas of intellectual abilities, and an accompanying physical decline. Early in the illness, only memory may be noticeably impaired. The person is more than a little forgetful. She may have difficulty learning new skills or with tasks that require abstract reasoning or calculation, such as maths. She may have trouble with her job or she may not enjoy reading as much as she used to. Her personality may change or she may become depressed.

Later, impairment in both language and motor abilities is seen. At first, the person will be unable to find the right word for things or will use the wrong word, but she will gradually become unable to express herself. She will also have increasing trouble understanding explanations. She may give up reading or stop watching television. She may have increasing difficulty carrying out tasks that were once easy for her. Her handwriting may change or she may walk with a stoop, or shuffle, or become clumsy. She may get lost easily, forget that she has turned on the cooker, misunderstand what is going on or show poor judgement. She may display changes in her personality or uncharacteristic outbursts of anger. She will be unable to plan responsibly for herself. Families often do not notice the beginnings of language and motor problems, but as the disease progresses all of these symptoms will become apparent.

Late in the illness, the person becomes severely impaired, incontinent, unable to walk or prone to falling frequently. She may be unable to say more than one or two words, and may not recognise anyone, or only one or two people. She will need nursing care from you or from professionals. She will be physically disabled as well as intellectually impaired.

Alzheimer's disease usually leads to death in about seven to ten years, but it can progress more quickly (three to four years) or more slowly (as much as fifteen years). Occasionally Alzheimer's disease progresses slowly for years and then more rapidly. The relatively stable periods are sometimes called 'plateaus'. Typically the disease is slowly but relentlessly progressive. Under a microscope, changes can be seen in the structure of the brain of a person who suffered from Alzheimer's disease. These include abnormally large numbers of structures called neuritic plaques and neurofibrillary tangles (see Chapter 18). This is clearly an injury to the brain itself. A diagnosis of Alzheimer's disease can be made on the basis of the type of symptoms, the way the symptoms progress over time, the absence of any other cause for the condition and a compatible CAT scan. However, a final diagnosis of Alzheimer's disease rests on the presence of these specific abnormal structures (neuritic plaques and neurofibrillary tangles) in the brain tissue. A brain biopsy is the only way of making this diagnosis. The biopsy is done by removing a piece of skull bone and taking out a small piece of brain tissue. The removal of this small amount of tissue has no effect on mental function. Brain biopsies are not routinely done at present because no treatment is available, even if a diagnosis is made. This may change as research in dementia progresses.

Multi-infarct dementia

In the past, dementing illnesses of old age were thought to be caused by *hardening of the arteries* of the brain. We now know that this is not the case. In multi-infarct dementia, repeated strokes within the brain destroy small areas of the brain. The cumulative effect of this damage leads to a dementia.

Multi-infarct dementias affect several functions, such as memory, coordination or speech, but the symptoms differ somewhat, depending on which areas of the brain are being damaged.

Multi-infarct dementias generally progress in a step-like way. You may be able to look back and recall that the person was worse after a specific time (instead of the gradual, almost imperceptible decline in Alzheimer's disease). Then she may not seem to deteriorate for a period, or she may even appear to improve a little. Some multi-infarct dementias progress as time passes; others may not get any worse for years. Some multi-infarct dementias may be halted by preventing further strokes; in others the progression cannot be stopped.

Sometimes the cause of the repeated strokes can be identified and treated, and further damage prevented. Recent evidence suggests that low doses of aspirin may slow the progression of the disease. Ask your doctor.

Some people may have both Alzheimer's disease and multi-infarct disease.

Depression

Depression is a treatable cause of dementia. In a study of patients seen at the Johns Hopkins Hospital in America, about one-quarter of those who had symptoms of dementia were depressed. Eighty-two per cent of these got better when the patient received treatment for the depression. That depression can cause dementia has been widely accepted only recently and occasionally a doctor may not recognise dementia caused by depression. However, the symptoms of a depression causing dementia are usually easily recognisable.

People with Alzheimer's disease or multi-infarct dementia also often show symptoms of depression, such as tearfulness, hopelessness, poor appetite, restlessness or refusal to pursue activities previously enjoyed. These people are usually forgetful, and have problems with language and motor skills, which suggests that they have both depression and Alzheimer's disease, or multi-infarct dementia.

Whenever a person with a memory problem is depressed, she should be assessed to determine whether the depression is the cause of her dementia or vice versa. *Her depression should be treated whether or not she has an irreversible dementia.* Do not allow a doctor to dismiss depression. However, bear in mind that although the person's depression may improve, her memory problems will not.

Treating a depression, even when the person also has an irreversible dementia, is important. It often relieves her misery, helps her enjoy life, improves her appetite and can reduce annoying behaviours.

Binswanger's disease

Binswanger's disease (sometimes called leukoariosis) is an uncommon vascular (blood vessel-related) dementia. It can be identified on an MRI or CT scan and at post-mortem. It is probably caused by sustained high blood pressure. This entity is controversial. The diagnosis has been made more frequently since MRI scans became available, but experts have not yet developed a standard set of criteria for making the diagnosis. At present, controlling high blood pressure is the only specific treatment available and it is not known whether this slows the progression of the disease.

AIDS

AIDS (acquired immune deficiency syndrome) first appeared in the late 1970s. We now know that it is caused by a virus: the human immunodeficiency virus (HIV). The virus attacks the immune system, making it incapable of fighting off other diseases. It is the other diseases that kill the person. This virus can be spread through sexual contact, through contact with infected blood and through the use of hypodermic needles previously used by someone infected with the virus.

All blood used for transfusions in the United Kingdom is tested for the virus, so transfusions are safe. Those most at risk of contracting the disease are people with multiple sexual partners, intravenous drug users and children born to infected people. Since young adults are more likely to engage in high-risk behaviour, AIDS usually afflicts young and middle-aged people, although cases are now occurring in elderly people.

AIDS often causes dementia. We do not know how frequently this happens, but it is suspected that more than half of the people with AIDS may suffer impairment in thinking at some time during their illness. AIDS dementia occurs when HIV infects the brain. There is some evidence that the AIDS virus specifically attacks certain types of brain cells.

Because of their weakened immune system, AIDS patients may also develop parasitic, fungal, bacterial or other viral infections of the brain. These, too, can cause dementia and delirium (see page 302); the medication used to treat these infections can also cause delirium.

Unfortunately, there is not as yet any cure for AIDS, although treatments have been developed that appear to slow the growth of the virus. There are, however, units in regional hospital centres which supply acute respite and terminal care for AIDS sufferers. Many are also cared for both in the community and by the hospice movement.

Organisations such as the Terence Higgins Trust, London Lighthouse and the Mildmay Mission Hospital in London provide a range of services to help AIDS sufferers live in the community for as long as possible. There are drop-in centres, counselling and support groups, creative therapy sessions, day care and home support teams. All these organisations have residential units which supply respite and terminal care.

Remember that much of the care required by AIDS victims is similar to that required by victims of other dementias. Advice helplines are provided by the organisations mentioned above and can put people in touch with organisations outside London. These are listed in Appendix II.

Other brain disorders

There are several other mental conditions which cannot be classified as dementias.

Delirium

The term *delirium* describes a set of symptoms that can have various causes. Delirium is often confused with dementia. Like the demented patient, the delirious patient may be forgetful or disorientated. Unlike a demented person, *the delirious person shows a changed level of consciousness*. She may have a reduced ability to shift, focus or sustain attention. Other symptoms of delirium may include misinterpretation of reality, false ideas or hallucinations, incoherent speech, either sleepiness in the daytime or wakefulness at night and increased or decreased physical (motor) activity. Symptoms of delirium often develop over a few hours or days. They tend to vary through the day.

Older people who do not have dementing illness may show symptoms – often intermittent – of impaired alertness or confusion, or of an unreliable memory. This may be a delirium caused by some other illness or by medication. Such a delirium should be regarded as a symptom, and the causative disease should be identified and treated, if possible.

People with dementing illnesses are vulnerable to developing a delirium in addition to their dementia. You may observe a sudden worsening in a person who also has other problems, such as constipation, the flu, an infection or even a slight cold. It is important to treat any such problem, because even very minor problems can seriously affect a person with a dementing illness. The complications of conditions like prostate cancer, diabetes, heart failure, chronic lung disease or other serious illnesses also often cause a delirium.

The person with a delirium may become more irritable, seem more confused and drowsy, and be less alert. She may become incontinent, agitated or fearful. She may become apathetic. You may notice an increase or decrease in activity level, a decreased level of alertness, or an increase or decrease in the amount of movement or motor activity.

Visual hallucinations are common in delirium. Such changes are sometimes assumed to be a worsening of the dementia, and the underlying
problem then goes untreated. Always consider the possibility of an illness
and delirium when you observe a sudden change in behaviour. Too
much medication or medication interactions can also cause a delirium,
even weeks after the medication was begun.

Senility, chronic organic brain syndrome, acute or reversible organic brain syndromes

The word *senile* merely means *old*. Thus *senility* does not describe a disease
and is considered by many people to be derogatory or prejudicial.

Chronic organic brain syndrome, and acute or reversible organic brain syndromes
were terms used by some to refer to those dementias that could not be
treated (chronic) and to deliriums that responded to treatment (acute).
These terms are no longer used because they are not specific and because
they include implications of prognosis. We hope that in time there will
be no 'chronic' brain syndromes.

TIA

TIA stands for transient ischemic attack. This is a temporary impairment due to an insufficient supply of blood to part of the brain. The
person may be unable to speak, or may have slurred speech. She may
be weak or paralysed, dizzy or nauseated. These symptoms usually last
only a few minutes or hours before the person recovers. This is in contrast
to a stroke which may have the same symptoms but which cause some
remaining deficit. Very small deficits may not be noticeable. TIAs
should be regarded as warnings of stroke and should be reported to your
GP.

Localised brain injuries

Damage can occur to the brain or head which temporarily or permanently affects either small or greater parts of the brain. Such damage
can be caused by brain tumours, strokes or head injuries.

Unlike dementia, these injuries may not be global, although they may affect more than one mental function. The symptoms can tell a neurologist just where the damage is. This is called a *focal* (localised) *brain lesion* (injury). When the damage is widespread, the symptoms may be those of dementia.

A major *stroke*, which causes such things as sudden paralysis of one side of the body, drooping of one side of the face or speech problems, is an injury to part of the brain. Strokes can be caused by a blood clot blocking vessels in the brain, or by a blood vessel bursting and causing bleeding in the brain. Often the brain cells are injured or impaired by swelling but can recover when the swelling goes down. It may be that other parts of the brain can gradually learn to do the jobs of damaged sections of the brain. People who have had a stroke may recover. Rehabilitation training is important for people who have had a stroke. The chance of having another stroke can be reduced by good medical management.

Head injuries

Head injuries can destroy brain tissue directly or can cause bleeding within the brain. Sometimes blood collects between the skull and the brain, forming a pool of blood. This puts pressure on the brain cells and damages them. It is called a *subdural haematoma*. Even mild falls can cause such bleeding.

People with dementing diseases are vulnerable to falls and may not be able to tell you about them. If you suspect that a person has banged her head, she should be seen promptly by a doctor because treatment can prevent permanent damage. The bleeding beneath the skull may not occur in the same place as the head was hit. Bleeding may be slow, and symptoms may not appear until hours or days after the fall. Bleeding inside the skull may occur on the side opposite the injury.

Anoxia or Hypoxia

When a person suffers a heart attack, the heart may stop pumping blood for a period of time before the person is resuscitated. During that time the brain may not get enough oxygen. This can result in brain damage that looks similar to Alzheimer's disease, except that it does not get progressively worse and usually does not affect language or the ability to carry out actions. People with hypoxic brain damage need much the same care as people with Alzheimer's disease or multi-infarct dementia.

An exciting point as been reached in research into dementia. Not long ago, most people assumed that dementia was the natural result of ageing and only a few pioneers were interested in studying it. In the last ten years that has changed. It is now known that:

1   dementia is not the natural result of ageing;
2   it is caused by specific, identifiable diseases;
3   diagnosis is important in order to identify treatable conditions;
4   a proper assessment is important in the management of contributing diseases that at present are not curable.

Today an increasing amount of research is focusing on the dementing illnesses. With new tools for study, it is possible to have a much clearer look at what goes on in the brain. Because of greater public understanding, there is a growing demand for solutions. These factors acting together have attracted talented men and women to the study of dementia and it is hoped that they will encourage allocation of more research money.

Understanding research

The increased public awareness of Alzheimer's disease has been accompanied by a number of announcements of 'breakthroughs' and 'cures'. Some of these are important building blocks in the search for a cure, but each breakthrough in itself is but one small step in the direction of a cure. Unfortunately, other 'cures' are often hoaxes, aimed at cheating desperate families out of their money.
   Understanding the therapeutic implications of the research can challenge scientists and families alike. Here are some things you need to know about research to help you understand what you read:

● Research scientists need to make their findings public, and the public wants to know what researchers are discovering. The enthusiasm of the press in publicising these findings plays an important role in maintaining public support for research funds, yet families are discouraged when the press makes announcements of 'breakthroughs' that turn out to be disappointing.
● Science must go down some blind alleys. For a while, a development

will look hopeful, and families and scientists will be excited. Then the trail will go cold. This is frustrating, but each time we rule out something, there is one less avenue to investigate. Many clues, like the pieces of a jigsaw puzzle, will eventually fit together to form the answer, but the pieces often do not go where we thought they would.

- Conditions like Alzheimer's disease are different from infectious diseases, such as diphtheria, chicken pox or polio. Each infectious disease has one cause, an infectious agent, leading to one outcome. So far, no single cause for Alzheimer's disease has been identified. Alzheimer's might be a family of diseases, like cancer. This would explain the variability of the disease from one patient to another and the variety of possible causes. It may take a combination of several triggers for a person to develop the disease. If this turns out to be the case, researchers will have to track down several causes and treatments.

- The study of the brain is unlike the study of any other organ. Scientists can study the structure of other organs under a microscope and can often observe a living organ at work. The brain's function cannot be deduced from its appearance and the chemical messengers that do its work quickly dissipate when the brain dies. Until the development of the PET scan (see page 316), scientists had no way of observing the workings of the brain. The brain is extremely complex, it works very quickly and its many parts interact at multiple levels.

- It is essential for studies to eliminate the influence of other factors. Sometimes when a new technique or drug is tried, the patient gets better. Sometimes families who participate in drug studies believe that their family member improved while taking the drug. There are many reasons why this happens, from wishful thinking on the part of clinicians and families, to temporarily cheering up the patient or brightening his thinking. This is called the placebo effect and it is quite common. Good studies of drugs are carefully designed to eliminate the possibility of improvement by other factors.

- Preliminary studies are often carried out on small groups of people. The small size of the sample increases the chances of extraneous factors confusing the outcome. If you hear of exciting results from a small group study, remember that these results may or may not be confirmed by tests on a large group, or by tests done by another researcher.

- The presence of two factors together does not mean that one causes the other. Both A and B might be found in the brains of dementia patients, but this does not mean that A caused B; A and B might both have been caused by an unknown factor, C. It may be years before the relationship between these factors is understood.

- The drugs that may affect the brain of an Alzheimer's victim are likely to cause serious side effects throughout the body. Sometimes research on such drugs must be stopped because their potential damage to other organs outweighs their therapeutic value.

- The Alzheimer's Disease Society releases reports to its local branches on major breakthroughs and on highly publicised claims. These reports are drafted by the Society's Medical Research Advisory Panel and are intended to provide families with accurate information. If you have questions about a particular research project, your branch can telephone the head office of the Society and obtain information from one of the officers there. In addition to the advice sheets, the staff can obtain further information from specialists in the field to help answer your concerns.

Bogus cures

Some unscrupulous individuals promote 'cures' that can be expensive, dangerous or ineffective, or that unfairly raise hopes. The Alzheimer's Disease Society keeps a list of some of the fraudulent products and treatments, and can advise you about which treatments are generally believed by doctors to be of little or no value. If a treatment makes a claim of benefit or cure which exceeds what the Society or the research centres investigating Alzheimer's disease say is possible, we urge you to check it thoroughly before participating.

Research into multi-infarct dementia and stroke

Multiple strokes are the second most common cause of dementia. If ways can be found of preventing stroke or of improving rehabilitation, many thousands of people would benefit.

Scientists are seeking to determine how hypertension, obesity, diet, smoking, heart disease and other factors increase a person's vulnerability to stroke or multi-infarct dementia. They are studying the relationship between larger strokes and the multiple strokes that cause dementia. At present, the best way of preventing stroke is to eliminate the risk factors.

Researchers are also studying which areas of the brain are most likely to be damaged and what changes in brain chemistry take place after a stroke. They are looking at how, when and to what extent rehabilitative training helps a person. They are examining the effectiveness of drugs in preventing stroke, dilating blood vessels, increasing the oxygen supply to the brain and preventing blood clotting. Some studies are evaluating the effects of surgery to remove atherosclerotic plaque from the arteries that deliver blood to the brain.

Scientists are examining the relationship between stroke, depression and the dementia that accompanies depression. They have found that it is important to treat depression when it occurs following a stroke.

Research into Alzheimer's disease

Structural changes in the brain

When Alois Alzheimer looked at tissue taken from the brain of a woman who had the behavioural symptoms of Alzheimer's disease, he saw microscopic changes called neuritic (senile) plaques and neurofibrillary tangles. Similar structures are found in much smaller numbers in the brains of unimpaired older people. Scientists are analysing the structure and chemistry of these plaques and tangles for clues as to their formation and their role in the disease.

Brain cell structure

The brain is made up of billions of nerve cells, which carry out all the tasks of thinking, remembering, feeling emotion and directing body movement, as well as many others. Researchers have learned that a small area deep in the brain loses most of its cells when a person has Alzheimer's disease. The cells in this area look a little like trees with many branches reaching into the front and top of the brain. As the disease progresses, these cells gradually lose their branches and finally die. As the branches are lost, the cells gradually stop communicating with other brain cells, causing problems in thinking.

Neurotransmitters

Researchers have discovered that chemicals in the brain called *neurotransmitters* are necessary for messages to pass from one nerve cell to the next. These neurotransmitters are made, used and broken down within the brain. There are many different neurotransmitters for different types of cells and probably for different kinds of mental tasks. Research indicates that in some diseases there is less than the normal amount of a certain neurotransmitter. For example, a patient with Parkinson's disease can take L-Dopa, which increases the amount of the deficient neurotransmitter dopamine and alleviates the symptoms.

Scientists know that people with Alzheimer's disease suffer from a deficiency in several neurotransmitters, particularly acetylcholine. Somatostatin, noradrenaline, serotonin and corticotrophin-releasing factors may also be deficient.

Researchers have recently learned that a small area of the brain, the Nucleus Basalis of Meynert, shows cell loss in patients with Alzheimer's disease. Moreover, it now appears that this area is the site from which the brain's acetylcholine originates. It may be that the plaques and tangles are remaining fragments of the cells which contained acetylcholine. If a way could be found of increasing the amount of acetylcholine and the other deficient neurotransmitters, then the symptoms of Alzheimer's disease might be relieved.

Abnormal proteins

The cells that make up the human body and the elements inside these cells are made up of proteins. The body takes food, breaks it down into amino acids and then builds the proteins that it needs. Several lines of research are exploring the possibility that Alzheimer's disease results from abnormalities in some of these proteins.

Amyloid protein

Abnormal deposits of a protein called amyloid are found in the brains of patients with Alzheimer's disease. Neuritic plaques (see page 308) have amyloid at the centre and some patients have deposits of amyloid along blood vessels. The production of this protein is controlled by chromosome 21. It is not known how this protein is involved in the disease process.

Protein abnormalities within brain cells

Brain cells contain other proteins, acting like highways, by which chemicals travel within cells. Some patients with Alzheimer's disease appear to have either increased amounts or abnormal forms of these proteins. Among these are tau protein and MAP (microtubule-associated protein). One theory suggests that the systems of people with Alzheimer's disease cannot break down these proteins as they should. This might explain why there are accumulations of abnormal proteins in the brains of people who die from Alzheimer's disease.

Nerve growth factors

Cells within the brain and spinal cord (as well as nerve cells) develop in specific patterns that are directed by chemicals called nerve growth factors. Nerve cells outside the central nervous system (called peripheral nerves) can regrow or regenerate after an injury, but cells within the brain are thought not to have this ability. Scientists are studying whether nerve growth factors might be used to stimulate the replacement or regrowth of damaged nerves in the brains of people with Alzheimer's disease.

Transplants of brain tissue

Much excitement has been generated in recent years about the possibility of replacing damaged brain cells with new ones. Work in animals has shown that certain cells from foetuses or laboratory-grown cell cultures will grow and manufacture neurotransmitters when they are transplanted into animals with brain damage. Cells have been transplanted into the brains of a few people with Parkinson's disease. So far, this has had only limited success. It is not known whether this technique will be applicable for patients with Alzheimer's disease. Because some of the cells for tissue transplants are obtained from tissue taken from human foetuses, this has generated controversy. However, it is most important for research on *animals* to be permitted to continue, to determine whether this procedure has any possibility of helping patients with Alzheimer's disease. It may be possible to grow the needed cells in a laboratory.

Drug studies

Hundreds of drugs have been studied for their effect on Alzheimer's disease. Most of them are quickly found to be ineffective or to have toxic side effects. A few make the news because there is some preliminary evidence that they alleviate symptoms.

In the 1980s, most of the drug research was focused on ways of increasing the amount of the neurotransmitter acetylcholine in the brain. The brain uses chemical raw materials to manufacture acetylcholine within its cells. The acetylcholine then transmits its message to other brain cells. With the message received, these cells break down the used acetylcholine. This gives researchers several possible approaches: to increase the amount of acetylcholine in the brain by giving medication containing it; to encourage increased manufacture of acetylcholine by brain cells; or to prevent the breakdown of the small amount of acetylcholine the brain is producing.

Lethicin and choline, substances occurring in many foods, are known to be used by the body to make acetylcholine. Studies have been carried out in which lethicin has been given to groups of people with dementia, but the results are disappointing. Families often give people lethicin bought from a health food shop, but there is no evidence that this has improved memory, mood or behaviour. Many issues need to be looked at more closely. More needs to be known about why acetylcholine appears to be in short supply in Alzheimer's disease. Newer drugs that have been in the news prevent the breakdown of acetylcholine. A few of these have improved memory for a brief period, but so far none has shown prolonged gains in large numbers of people. One drug which acts in this way (THA or tacrine) was initially shown to help a small group of patients with Alzheimer's disease, but more carefully designed studies have not confirmed these beneficial effects. Acetylcholine is used throughout the body. Therefore, when we alter its level, we can cause serious side effects elsewhere. This factor might limit the use of drugs that affect the acetylcholine system.

Although the drug studies so far might seem discouraging, each one gives researchers more clues about how these drugs react in the body. With enough information, chemists may be able to tailor-make a drug that will alleviate symptoms.

Metals

Aluminium has been found in larger than expected amounts in the brains of some people with Alzheimer's disease. Other metals, such as manganese, are known to be associated with other forms of dementia. It now seems likely that the presence of aluminium is a result of whatever is causing the dementia rather than being a cause of the dementia. People sometimes wonder if they should stop taking antacids, or cooking with aluminium pans, or using deodorants (all sources of aluminium). There is no evidence that their use is a cause of dementia. Studies of people who have been exposed to much larger amounts of aluminium indicate that exposure does not lead to dementia. Treatments that promote the elimination of aluminium from the body have no proven benefit in patients with Alzheimer's disease, and some of these treatments have serious side effects. Some studies of drugs that assist in the elimination of aluminium from the body are being conducted.

Viruses

Some tentative research led scientists to suspect that a viral disease could be causing Alzheimer's disease. You may read about Creutzfeldt-Jacob disease or Kuru. Both of these rare diseases have been studied because they appear to be transmitted by a virus-like agent.

Prions are living particles even smaller than viruses. It has been suggested that these particles might be a cause of Alzheimer's disease. While this has not been totally disproved, it now seems quite unlikely.

There have been many efforts to determine whether Alzheimer's disease is infectious, that is, whether it can be transmitted. At present, there is no evidence to support the hypothesis that Alzheimer's disease is caused by a slow virus, prion or other infectious organism.

Immunological defects

The immune system is the body's defence against infection. Studies of some of the proteins that the body uses to fight infection show abnormal levels in patients with Alzheimer's disease.

Scientists suspect that sometimes the body's defence system, which is designed to attack outside cells such as disease organisms, goes awry and attacks cells within the body. One theory is that this is what happens in Alzheimer's disease. Numerous studies are carried out which approach the problem from this angle.

Other studies are searching for the factor or factors (such as injury, chemical toxin or gene) that might set off an immune response. Some scientists hypothesise that if there is a faulty immune reaction, the body would produce antibodies. Their presence would give a positive tool with which to diagnose the disease.

Head trauma

Several studies report that Alzheimer's patients have suffered more head injuries during their lives than people the same age who do not have Alzheimer's disease. Supporting this theory is the finding that some boxers develop a dementia similar to Alzheimer's disease and have tangles, but not plaques, in the brain. The condition is called *punch drunk*, or *dementia pugilistica, syndrome.* This raises the possibility that subtle brain damage triggered by the head injury eventually leads to a more generalised cell death through immunological or other mechanisms.

One well-designed study has not confirmed the head injury theory. It seems unlikely that head trauma is the cause of Alzheimer's disease in most people.

Epidemiology

Epidemiology is the study of the distribution of diseases in large groups of people. The epidemiology of dementing illnesses may eventually show scientists a link between a dementing illness and something else as yet unknown – for example, a hereditary factor, diet in childhood or the use of medication many years ago. If you have participated in research programmes, you may have been asked many questions that don't seem in any way related to your problem, but these give researchers important epidemiological information.

So far, Alzheimer's disease has been found in all groups of people whose members tend to live long enough to reach late life, when the risk is greater. However, the disease may be less common in Japan than in Europe or North America. Epidemiological research is expensive and can take many years, but studies now under way in the United Kingdom, the United States and other countries may yield valuable clues.

Down's syndrome

People with Down's syndrome (a form of mental retardation) develop plaques and tangles similar to those evident in Alzheimer's patients, as they reach their forties. They do not all develop the symptoms of Alzheimer's disease, although some do experience a further decline in intellectual function. Because Down's syndrome is known to be caused by an extra chromosome 21, or an extra piece of this chromosome, many scientists have been studying the role this chromosome might play in Alzheimer's disease.

Old age

Living into very old age increases the risks of developing Alzheimer's Disease. While an adult's risk of developing the disease is about 1 or 2 in 100 for those over 65, for those over 80 the risk is 1 in 5. Thus, old age itself increases one's risk of developing the disease. But the statistics also mean that 4 out of 5 people over 80 years of age have normal or nearly normal intellectual function.

Heredity

Families often worry that this disease is inherited and that they or their children will develop it. We know that an adult's risk of developing Alzheimer's disease at age 65 is about 1 or 2 in 100, but the odds increase fourfold if a close relative has had the disease, to about 8 in 100. Recently, researchers studying family histories found a few families in which a few members in each generation had the disease. In these rare families the disease is clearly genetic and a family member's risk can be as great as 1 in 2. However, *this is not the case in most families that have one or even more members with the disease*. We do not yet know why this difference between families exists.

If you are worried that you may belong to such a family, consult a genetic counsellor at one of the Regional Genetic Centres or at one of the research centres specialising in Alzheimer's disease. Your GP can make the referral to the Regional Genetic Centre and the Alzheimer's Disease Society also has useful information about genetic counselling. Simply having more than one family member with the disease is *not* evidence of a familial predisposition to Alzheimer's disease. Some individuals have jumped to the conclusion that they are at high risk and have suffered unnecessary anguish because they did not have access to sufficient accurate information. If you find that you *are* at risk, you should make financial plans for yourself and your family as soon as possible.

In 1987, one group of scientists reported finding an extra piece of chromosome 21 in one of the rare families with the genetic form of the disease. Most other people with Alzheimer's disease who have been studied do not have this extra piece of chromosome. It now appears that an abnormality of chromosome 21 is present in some families in which Alzheimer's disease strikes early (the forties or fifties). A different abnormality has been found in chromosome 19 in some families. In these families the disease begins in the sixties, seventies or eighties.

Even if an abnormality on a chromosome is eventually found to be a cause, this will not mean that the disease is always or even usually inherited. A genetic factor may mean only that people inherit a *tendency* to be more vulnerable to the disease, not that they will necessarily develop the disease. Additional triggers may still be necessary for the disease to develop.

To put this in perspective, most of us inherit risk factors for some diseases, such as heart disease or cancer. We know that for these diseases there are additional precipitants, like diet, smoking and exercise, over which we have some control. Researchers are seeking the possible precipitants of Alzheimer's disease.

Gender

Some investigators believe that women are more prone to Alzheimer's disease than men, but that men are more prone to multi-infarct dementia. This may simply be because men are more likely to develop vascular disease, while women tend to live longer and the incidence of Alzheimer's disease increases with age. Researchers are looking for clues as to whether this is so.

Promising clinical and research tools

Neuropsychologists use a combination of questions, simple tasks and observation to evaluate a patient. They can identify the kinds of mental skills a person has lost and those he retains. With this knowledge, clinicians can devise individual plans that help a person use his remaining skills and that place minimal demands on his diminished abilities. Information from a neuropsychological examination helps a family understand why a person cannot do some things but can successfully do others. Neuropsychology can also help to confirm a diagnosis and, potentially, could identify subtypes of Alzheimer's disease.

The PET (positron emission tomography) scan provides a picture of the brain at work. That is, the image it produces shows which areas of the brain are working hardest during a particular kind of mental activity. Like the CT and MRI scan (page 14), the patient lies on an x-ray table and is given a radioactive material that goes through the bloodstream into the brain. (This material is given in a small dose and remains in the body for only a few minutes.) Special equipment measures the amount being used in each area of the brain.

The SPECT (single positron emission computerised tomography) scan is similar to the PET scan but is less expensive and may eventually be used in diagnosis.

These two scans provide scientists with information about how the brain is working and thus hold great potential for research. Because they have not been in use very long, not enough is known about the images a normal brain produces. Therefore, we do not yet know what is abnormal in Alzheimer's disease. We do not yet know whether these scans can identify early Alzheimer's disease.

It has long been known that different parts of the brain carry out different mental tasks (physical activity, talking, feeling emotions, etc.) and that still other parts co-ordinate these mental activities. By identifying the areas of the brain most severely afflicted, neuropsychological evaluations and scans inform researchers about the disease and give clinicians and families information about how to provide good care.

Keeping active

People often wonder if keeping mentally alert and involved, or maintaining physical exercise will prevent a person from developing a dementing illness. As far as is known, neither physical exercise nor keeping mentally active will prevent or alter the course of Alzheimer's disease. However, activity *will* help to maintain general health and improve the quality of life. Some studies that did not differentiate between causes of dementia have produced misleading results about the effect of activity on dementia. Sometimes people seem to develop a dementia after they retire. Upon close examination, however, it usually appears that the early stages of a dementia were developing before the person retired, and that this early, unidentified dementia may have been a factor in the person's decision to retire.

Many people wonder if continuing to exercise after Alzheimer's disease develops will slow the progress of the disease or help people remain active longer. While we know of no good scientific evidence to support this, we believe that common sense supports keeping active within realistic limits (see page 74).

The effect of acute illness on dementia

Sometimes people appear to develop a dementia after a serious illness, hospitalisation or surgery. Again, as far as is known, these things do not affect or alter the course of Alzheimer's disease. Upon close examination, it is often clear that the dementing illness had begun before the person had surgery or developed another disease. The stress of the acute illness and the tendency of people with a dementia to develop a delirium make the dementia worse, so it is noticeable for the first time. Then the person's brain impairment will make it harder for him to adjust after the acute illness, thereby making the dementia more apparent.

Research into the delivery of services

Scientist are now focusing on Alzheimer's disease, multi-infarct disease and stroke. In time we will learn to prevent or treat each disease. But research is not limited to the pursuit of treatments and cures. Also important are studies showing how to help the victims of these diseases live comfortable, satisfying lives despite their illness, and studies that tell us how to assist the families who care for them. No one knows how long it will take to find a cure, but experts suspect that it may take some time. Thus this research is important, to help families and patients *now*.

We already know how to change the quality of life for some people with dementia. We can make changes that help them to function as well as possible, we can reduce their anxiety and fear, and we can make it possible for them to experience enjoyment. Researchers are studying the kinds of living arrangements that are best for those people with dementia who go into care homes, and are seeking ways of helping those who live at home function at their best. This is an exciting and rewarding field. Researchers have watched people who had previously paced, screamed and struck out, become relaxed and begin to participate in enjoyable activities. Even though we cannot cure these diseases, we can treat some symptoms and sometimes reduce suffering.

We know that families need help such as day care, home respite, support groups and other assistance. Researchers are studying how best to reach families, what things families need most, how to encourage families to use respite services and the most cost-effective ways of providing respite. While it may seem that the answers to these questions are obvious, different kinds of families have different needs, and people do not always behave as predicted by researchers. Careful study will prevent money being wasted on unnecessary services or on services families do not know about.

Appendix I: Further reading

There are many good books, magazines and news articles, video-cassettes, and television programmes about dementia and Alzheimer's disease. This list includes only a sample of the available materials. The Alzheimer's Disease Society publishes a Professionals Reading List and Carers Booklist in its information sheets.

It also publishes pamphlets and brochures, information sheets and advice sheets on a variety of topics related to dementia. Some branches also publish materials. You can obtain these through your local branch or by writing to the national office (see Appendix II). Enclose a s.a.e. and ask to see a complete list of the items it publishes, as a local branch may not have all the resources in stock. In addition, booklets, some non-society publications and videotapes are available from the national office.

Suggestions for locating publications primarily intended for professional carers are given at the end of this appendix.

Publications

Personal experience

DOERBERG, M. (1989), *Stolen Mind: The Slow Disappearance of Ray Doernberg*, Chapel Hill, N.C. Algonquin. In paperback; a wife's story.

FORSYTHE, E. (1990), *Alzheimer's Disease: the long bereavement*, London, Faber and Faber.

HONEL, R. W. (1988), *Journey with Grandpa: Our Family's Struggle with Alzheimer's Disease*, Baltimore, John Hopkins University Press. Told by a daughter-in-law; the family included children growing up in the home.

KUSHNER, H. S. (1981), *Bad Things Happen to Good People*, New York, Shocken.

LEWIS, C. S. (1963), *A Grief Observed*, New York, Harper and Row. The books by Kushner and Lewis are drawn from the authors' personal losses and place these experiences in the perspectives of their religions.

General

ADAMS, M. (1986), *A Call to Courage for Caregivers*, Abbey Press (US). Available from Anthony Clarke, 16 Garden Court, Wheathampstead, Hertfordshire AL4 8RF.

COUNSEL AND CARE FOR THE ELDERLY (1986), *What to Look for in a Private or Voluntary Home*. Published by and available from Counsel and Care for the Elderly (see Appendix II).

COHEN, D. AND EISDORFER, C. (1986), *The Loss of Self: A Family Resource for the Care of Alzheimer's Disease and Related Disorders*, New York, Norton.

GILLEARD, C. AND WATT, G. (1983), *Coping with Ageing Parents*, London, MacDonald.

HEALTH EDUCATION AUTHORITY (1986), *Who Cares?: Information and support for the carers of confused elderly people*. Available from Health Education Authority Supplies Department and ADS Central Office (see Appendix II).

HOLDEN, U. P. (1987), *Looking at Confusion: a handbook for those working with the elderly*, Winslow Press, Telford Road, Bicester, Oxon OX6 OTS.

KING'S FUND INFORMAL CARING PROGRAMME (1987), *Taking a Break: a guide for people caring at home*. Published by and available from the King's Fund Centre and ADS Central Office (see Appendix II).

KOHNER, N. (1987), *Caring at Home*. Aimed at all types of carers, covering services available and who to ask. Published by and available from the King's Fund Centre (see Appendix II).

KUBLER ROSS, E. (1970), *On Death and Dying*, New York, Macmillan.

LODGE, B. (1981), *Coping with Caring: A guide to identifying and supporting an elderly person with dementia* (see Appendix II). This booklet spells out the practical steps which can be taken to support and help the elderly confused and their relatives. Published by and available from MIND.

MURPHY, E. (1986), *Dementia and Mental Illness in the Old*, London, Papermac, Macmillan.

NORMAN, A. (1988), *Rights and Risk: a discussion document on civil liberty in old age*. Published by and available from the Centre for Policy on Ageing (see Appendix II).

ORTON, C. (1989), *Care for the Carer*, Make life easier, happier, more fulfilling for you and the elderly person you look after. London, Thorson's Publishing Group Ltd.

RIORDAN, J. AND WHITMORE, B. (1990), *Living with Dementia*, Manchester, Manchester University Press.

STOKES, G. (1987/1988) *Common Problems with the Elderly Confused: Aggression; Incontinence and Inappropriate Urinating; Screaming and Shouting; Wandering*. Bicester, Winslow Press.

WILCOCK, G. K. (1991), *Living with Alzheimer's Disease and Similar Conditions*, London, Penguin Books.

WILSON, J. (1988), *Caring Together: Guidelines for carers self-help and support groups*. Available from ADS Central Office and King's Fund Centre (see Appendix II).

WOODS, R. AND LAY, C. (1989), 2nd Edition. *Caring for the person with dementia: a guide for families and other carers*. Available from ADS Central Office (see Appendix II).

Magazine and news articles

Many of the Alzheimer's Disease Society branches, as well as its central office, publish newsletters. These provide a network for the exchange of information among care-givers. The newsletter also regularly contains reviews of new publications useful for carers. Age Concern England publishes an Information Circular which reviews publications and articles relevant to the elderly. Age Concern Scotland, the Carers National Association and the Health Education Authority also produce useful literature (see Appendix II). The Public Trust Office has a range of free leaflets and booklets on Enduring Powers of Attorney and Court of Protection (see Appendix II).

In foreign languages

The first edition of the 36-Hour Day is available in the following translations. If you cannot obtain these through your local bookshop or the Alzheimer's Disease Society, write to the publisher who will give you details of how to obtain a copy.

DANISH: Hans Reitzels Forlag A.S. Noorre Soogade 35, Postboks 1073, DK-1008, Copenhagen, Denmark.

DUTCH: Wetenschappelijke Uitgeverij Bunge BV, Postbus 13341, 3507 LH Utrecht, The Netherlands.

GERMAN: Hans Huber AG, Medical Publisher and Bookseller, Langgass-Str 76, Postfach, CH-3000, Berne 9, Switzerland.

HEBREW: Melabev, Geriatric Department, P O Box 293, Jerusalem 91002, Israel.

ITALIAN: 11 Pensiero Scientifico Editore SRL, via Panama 48, I-00198 Rome, Italy.

JAPANESE: The Simul Press Inc, Kowa Bldg, no. 9, 1-8-10 Akasaka, Minato-Ku, Tokyo 197, Japan.

NORWEGIAN: Gyldendal Norsk Forlag, Univeristetsgaten 16, P. B. 6860, St Olavs Plass, Oslo 1, Norway.

SPANISH: Editorial pax-Mexico, Libreria Carlos Cesarman, SA, AV. Cuauhtemoc No. 14334, Col. Santa Cruz Atoyac, Mexico 13, DF.

SWEDISH: Bokforlaget Naturoch Kultur Publishers, P O Box 27323, S102 54 Stockholm, Sweden.

For professionals

There is extensive literature on dementia in publications on medicine, psychiatry, psychology, neurology, gerontology, nursing, social work, public policy, long-term care and other related subjects. Professionals will also find the international literature helpful. *Losing a Million Minds*,

Confronting the Tragedy of Alzheimer's Disease and other Dementias, (1987), Washington DC, USA Government Printing Office, is an excellent reference resource (up to 1987), as are the books listed below:

ARIE, T. (ed. 1985), *Recent Advances in Psychogeriatrics: Vol 1*, Edinburgh, Churchill Livingstone.

ASKHAM, J. AND THOMPSON, C. (1990), *Dementia and Home Care: a research report on a home support scheme for dementia sufferers*, London, Age Concern England.

CUMMINGS, J. L., AND BENSON, D. F., (1983), *Dementia: A Clinical Approach*, Boston, Butterworth.

FRASER, M. (1987), *Dementia, Its Nature and Management*, Chichester, Wiley.

HOLDEN, U., AND WOODS, T. (1988), *Reality Orientation: Psychological Approaches to the Confused Elderly*, Edinburgh, Churchill Livingstone.

JACQUES, A. (1988), *Understanding Dementia*, Edinburgh, Churchill Livingstone.

JORM, A. F., et al (1990), *The Epidemiology of Alzheimer's Disease and Related Disorders*, London, Chapman and Hall.

KING'S FUND CENTRE, (1986), *Living well into old age: applying principles of good practice to services for people with dementia*, London, King's Fund Centre.

INEICHAN, B. (1989), *Senile Dementia: policy and services*. London, Chapman and Hall.

LEWIN, E., Sinclair, I. and Gorbach, P. (1989), *Families, services and confusion in old age*, Aldershot, Avebury.

LEVY, R. AND POST, F., (1982), *Psychiatry of Late Life*, Oxford, Blackwell.

LIGHT, E. AND LEBOWITZ, B. D., eds. (1990), *Alzheimer's Disease, Treatment and Family Stress*. London, Hemisphere Publishing Corporation.

LISHMAN, W. A., (1987), *Organic Psychiatry: The psychological consequences of cerebral disorder*, Oxford, Blackwell Scientific Publications.

MACE, N. L. ed. (1990), *Dementia Care: Patient, Family and Community*. Baltimore, John Hopkins University Press, A multidisciplinary book on clinical care.

MARSHALL, M. ed. (1990), *Working with Dementia: guidelines for professionals*, Birmingham, Venture Press.

PITT, B. ed. (1987), *Dementia*, Edinburgh, Churchill Livingstone.

TWINING, C., (1991), *Memory Handbook*, Bicester, Winslow Press.

WILCOCK, G. K. and Muir Gray, J. A. (1981), *Our Elders*, Oxford, Oxford University Press.

ZGOLA, J. M. (1987), *Doing Things: A guide to programming activities for persons with Alzheimer's Disease and related disorders*, Baltimore, John Hopkins University Press.

Journals that carry material on dementia include, but are not limited to, *Annals of Neurology, Archives of Neurology, British Journal of Psychiatry, Community Psychiatry, Current Opinion in Psychiatry, Age and Ageing, Journal of the American Geriatrics Society, Journal of the American Medical Association,*

Journal of Geriatric Psychiatry, Journal of Gerontology, Nature, Neuroscience, New England Journal of Medicine, New Scientist, Science and Journals of social work, nursing, occupational therapy, physiotherapy, policy, public health, genetics, epidemiology and related fields.

The Alzheimer's Disease Society publishes a Professionals Reading List, Information Sheet no. 9. The Dementia Services Development Centre publishes a range of materials for professionals as does Scottish Action on Dementia.

If you are a layperson exploring the professional literature, begin with the references listed in Dementia and Dementia Care (full references shown above). Most public libraries have a computer link to nearby university libraries and can obtain copies of articles from them for you. These libraries will also have access to the British Library Lending Services Division. The literature on dementia has grown enormously in the past ten years; if you use a computer search, you will need to make your request narrow and specific.

For those who wish to search for further literature the following are good sources of reference:

ALZHEIMER DISEASE SOCIETY – monthly newsletter containing articles on research, good practice and book reviews.

CENTRE FOR POLICY ON AGEING – bi-monthly publication – New Literature on Ageing.

NATIONAL INSTITUTE OF SOCIAL WORK – Information Service – Publication monthly – Social Care Update.

BRITISH LIBRARY – medical information service; Document Supply Centre. Publication monthly – current awareness. Topic searches – dementia.

PSYCHIATRY IN OLD AGE – abstracts of current medical literature – neurology section. Published by Sandoz and the Royal Society of Medicine.

(For details of addresses and telephone numbers see Appendix II.)

Videos

For video references and resources for training carers and professionals to manage dementia sufferers, the Alzheimer's Disease Society has an excellent factsheet no. 13, parts 1 and 2.

Appendix II: Organisations

Age Concern England, Astral House, 1268 London Road, London SW16 4ER. Tel: 081–679 8000. Provides advice, information and services for older people, such as day and respite care, through its groups.

Age Concern Northern Ireland, 3 Lower Crescent, Belfast BT7 1NR. Tel. 0232 245729.

Age Concern Scotland, 54A Fountainbridge, Edinburgh EH3 9PT. Tel. 031–228 5656.

Age Concern Cymru, 4th Floor, 1 Cathedral Road, Cardiff CF1 9SD. Tel. 0222 371566.

Alzheimer's Disease Society, Gordon House, 10 Greencoat Place, London SW1P 1PH. Tel. 0171–306 0606 Fax. 0171–306 0808. Supports families, provides information about all forms of dementia, runs local groups for patients and their relatives. Covers England, Wales and Northern Ireland.

Alzheimer Scotland – Action on Dementia, 8 Hill Street, Edinburgh EH2 3JE. Tel. 031–220 4886. (For people caring for someone with dementia who live in Scotland).

Alzheimer's Society of Ireland, St John of God Hospital, Stillorgan, County Dublin, Eire. Tel. 010 353 12881282.

Arthritis Care, 18 Stephenson Way, London NW1 2HD. Tel. 071–916 1500. Also freephone helpline 0800 289170, 1–5pm weekdays. Advice and information, over 150 branches, for people with arthritis and their families.

Association for Continence Advice. Tel. 071–404 6821.

Association of Charity Officers, c/o RICS Benevolent Fund Ltd, 1st Floor, Tavistock House North, Tavistock Square, London WC1H 9RJ. Tel. 071–383 5557. Over 200 member funds including some which run residential and nursing homes for professional, commercial and occupational groups.

BASE (British Association for Service of the Elderly), c/o Mrs C Wyld, Director, 119 Hassell Street, Newcastle Under Lyme, Staffordshire ST5 1AX. Tel. 0782 661033. Provides education and training for those involved in caring for elderly people.

British Association for Continence Care. Tel. 0753 656716.

British Association for Counselling, 1 Regent Place, Rugby, Warwicks CV21 2PJ. Tel. 0788 578328/9. Information about counselling services throughout the UK.

British Association of the Hard of Hearing, 7–11 Armstrong Road, London W3 7JL. Tel. 081–743 1110. Provides information and runs clubs for people who are hard of hearing.

British Federation of Care Home Proprietors, 852 Melton Road, Thurmaston, Leicester LE5 8BN. Tel. 0533 640095. Standards of care in all homes are independently monitored in accordance with national guidelines as a pre-condition of membership. Can provide lists of members in all areas of the country.

British Library, Medical Information Service, Document Supply Centre, Boston Spa, Wetherby, W Yorks LS23 7BQ. Tel. 0937 546039. Provides literature searches.

British Pensioners and Trade Unions Action Association, Norman Dodds

House, 315 Bexley Road, Erith, Kent DA8 3EX. Tel. 0322 335464. Information about its 300 groups throughout the UK.

British Red Cross Society, 9 Grosvenor Crescent, London SW1X 7EJ. Tel. 071–235 5454. Services mainly provided by volunteers and available from local centres. Home nursing, transport, holidays, equipment loan for frail elderly people and those with disabilities. Publications from 9 Grosvenor Crescent, London SW1X 7EJ. Tel. 071–235 5454.

British Telecom, Dial 150, ask for Freephone Telecom Sales and then ask for the Action for Disabled Customers Liaison Officer.

Carers National Association, 20–25 Glasshouse Yard, London EC1A 4JS. Tel. 0171–490 8818 (1–4 pm weekdays). General help and advice for all carers.

Centre for Policy on Ageing, 25–31 Ironmonger Row, London EC1V 3QP. Tel. 071–253 1787. Publishes New Literature on Ageing.

CONCAH, (Continuing Care at Home Association) c/o St Loyes Independent Living Centre, Millbrook House, Millbrook Lane, Topsham Road, Exeter, Devon EX2 6ES. Professional association to improve standards in continuing care.

CONTACT (Helping the Elderly Housebound) 15 Henrietta Street, London WC2E 8QH. Tel. 071–240 0630. Provides young companionship to elderly housebound people.

Councils for Voluntary Service National Association, 3rd Floor, Arundel Court, Arundel Road, Sheffield S1 2NU. Tel. 0742 786636. Provides information about local councils for Voluntary Service.

Counsel and Care, Twyman House, 16 Bonny Street, London NW1 9PG. Tel. 071–485 1566. A charity which provides general advice for older people including information on accommodation and care at home nationwide. Advice can be given on charges and charitable grants available.

Crossroads Care Attendant Schemes, Association of 10 Regent Place, Rugby, Warwickshire CV21 2PN. Tel. 0788 573653. About 190 schemes in the UK which aim to relieve carers. To find out if there is a scheme in your area, contact the national organisation.

Cruse – Bereavement Care, Cruse House, 126 Sheen Road, Richmond, Surrey TW9 1UR. Tel. 081–940 4818. A counselling service for bereaved people throughout the UK.

Dementia Services Development Centre, University of Stirling, Stirling FK9 4LA. Tel. 0786 67740/1. A resource to managers, planners and professionals who are improving or extending services for people with dementia.

DIAL UK, (Disablement Information and Advice Lines), Park Lodge, St Catherine's Hospital, Tickhill Road, Baldy, Doncaster DN4 8QN. Tel 0302–310123. Runs information and advice helplines.

Disability Alliance Education and Research Association, 1st Floor East, Universal House, 88–94 Wentworth Street, London E1 7SA. Tel. 071–247

8776. A federation of over 200 organisations of, and for, people with disabilities who have joined together to press for the introduction of a comprehensive income scheme for all people with disabilities.

Disabled Living Foundation, 380/384 Harrow Road, London W9 2HU. Tel. 071–289 6111. Information about equipment for daily living. Specialist advisory service on clothing. Information about Disabled Living Centres in the UK.

Disablement Income Group, Millmead Business Centre, Millmead Road, London N17 9QU. Tel. 0171–263 8981. Promotes the financial welfare of disabled people through a programme of advice, advocacy and fieldwork, information, publications, research and training.

Elderly Accommodation Counsel, 46A Chiswick High Road, London W4 1SZ. Tel. 0171–995 8320. A registered charity which provides computer print outs from a national database of all forms of private and voluntary accommodation for older people – sheltered housing, residential care, nursing homes and hospices. The charity maintains information about homes which accept people suffering from dementia. With the exception of those on low income, or where a company is supporting the charity, a small payment is requested.

Extend – Exercise Training Ltd (Movement to music for the over sixties and handicapped people of all ages), 22 Maltings Drive, Wheathampstead, Herts AL4 8QJ. Tel/Fax 01582 832760.

Family Welfare Association, 501–505 Kingsland Road, London E8 4AU. Tel. 071–254 6251. Provides counselling and grants to families and individuals in need.

Friends of the Elderly and Gentlefolk's Help, 42 Ebury Street, London SW1W 0LZ. Tel. 071–730 8263. Provides financial assistance to elderly people in need. Runs residential and nursing homes.

Health Education Authority, Distribution Department, Hamilton House, Mabledon Place, London WC1H 9TX. Tel. 071–383 3833. Provides booklet for carers of confused people.

Help the Aged, (Community Alarms Scheme), 16/18 St James's Walk, London EC1R 0BE. Tel. 071–253 0253. Information about personal alarm systems.

Holiday Care Service, 2 Old Bank Chambers, Station Road, Horley, Surrey RH6 9HW. Tel. 0293–774535. Free information and support on holidays for people who are old or disabled, or on a low income. Please enclose a large sae if writing for information.

Hospice Information Service, St Christopher's Hospice, 51–59 Lawrie Park Road, Sydenham, London SE26 6DZ. Tel. 081–778 9252. International resource about hospice services.

Huntington's Disease Association, 108 Battersea High Street, London SW11 3HP. Tel. 071–223 7000. Provides personal support and advice to people with this condition and their families; respite, residential and holiday care.

Jewish Care, Stuart Young House, 221 Golders Green Road, London

NW11 9DQ. Tel. 081–458 3282. Provides services for elderly, mentally ill, disabled people and their families. Runs residential homes.

Kings Fund Centre, 126 Albert Street, London NW1 7NF. Tel. 071–267
6111.

Keep Able Centre, 2 Capital Interchange Way, Brentford, Middlesex
TW8 0EX. Tel. 081–742 2181. Products through a mail order catalogue to assist those living with a disability.

Medic Alert Foundation, 12 Bridge Wharf, 156 Caledonian Road, London
N1 9UU. Tel. 071–833 3034. Produces bracelets and necklaces which
contain medical information about the person.

MENCAP, (Royal Society for Mentally Handicapped Children and
Adults), 123 Golden Lane, London EC1Y 0RT. Tel. 071–454 0454.
Support for mentally handicapped people and their families, through
local branches.

Mildmay Mission Hospital, Hackney Road, London EC2 7NA. Tel. 071–
739 2331.

MIND (National Association for Mental Health), Granta House, 15–19
Broadway, Stratford, London E15 4BQ. Tel. 0181–519 2122. Information Unit offers support for people in mental distress and their
families. Local groups. Publications from 4th floor, 24–32 Stephenson
Way, London NW1 2HD. Tel. 071–387 9126.

National Action on Incontinence. Tel. 091 2130050.

National Association of Citizens Advice Bureaux (NACAB), 115–123 Penton-
ville Road, London N1 9LZ. Tel. 071–833 2181. Provides free advice
through over 1,000 local citizens advice bureaux to anyone on any
subject.

National Association of Widows/Widows Advisory Trust, 54–57 Allison
Street, Digbeth, Birmingham B5 5TH. Tel. 021–643 8348. Offers
specialist information and advice to widows and their families. Local
branches.

National Care Homes Association, 5 Bloomsbury Place, London
WC1A 2QA. Tel. 071–436 1871. More than 70 member associations
of private and voluntary residential care and nursing homes. Will offer
advice on any matters regarding such care.

National Institute for Social Work, Mary Ward House, 5 Tavistock Place,
London WC1H 9SN. Tel. 071–387 9681. Library on social care.

Parkinson's Disease Society of the UK, 22 Upper Woburn Place, London
WC1H 0RA. Tel. 071–383 3513. Information service through
branches across the country. Helps patients and their carers with help
in the home.

Partially Sighted Society, 62 Salusbury Road, London NW6 6NS. Tel. 071–
372 1551. Information service and sight centres round the country.

Patients Association, 18 Victoria Park Square, London E2 9PF. Tel. 081–
981 5676. Advice to patients and carers on patients' rights, complaints
procedures and access to health services or appropriate self-help
groups.

Pensioners' Voice (National Federation of Retirement Pensions Associations), Melling House, 14 St Peter Street, Blackburn, Lancashire BB2 2HD. Tel. 0254 52606. A pressure group formed in 1940 to campaign for improvements in the state pension and other benefits that affect the livelihood of pensioners.

Public Trust Office, Stewart House, 24 Kingsway, London WC2B 6JX. Tel. 071–269 7300/7358.

RADAR (Royal Association for Disability and Rehabilitation), 12 City Forum, 250 City Road, London EC1V 8AF. Tel. 0171–250 3222. Advice and information on access, housing, holidays, mobility and welfare.

Registered Nursing Home Association, Calthorpe House, Hagley Road, Edgbaston, Birmingham B16 8QY. Tel. 021–454 2511. Provides information on registered nursing homes in the United Kingdom and the Republic of Ireland which conform to certain standards and which have been visited by the Association. The Association publishes a book of homes throughout the country.

RELATE (National Marriage Guidance) Herbert Gray College, Little Church Street, Rugby, Warwickshire CV21 3AP. Tel. 0788 573241/560811. Headquarters to about 150 councils. Wide range of publications available concerning marriage and the family.

Royal British Legion, 48 Pall Mall, London SW1Y 5JY. Tel. 071–930 8131. Assistance to people in need, who are, or have been, in the forces and their families. Has sheltered housing and residential homes.

Royal National Institute for the Blind (RNIB), 224 Great Portland Street, London W1N 6AA. Tel. 071–388 1266. Many services for people with visual handicaps.

Royal National Institute for the Deaf, 105 Gower Street, London WC1E 6AH. Tel. 071–387 8033. Advice, information and a wide range of services.

Royal Society of Medicine, 1 Wimpole Street, London W1M 8AE. Tel. 071–290 2900. Publishes abstracts of current medical literature.

St John Ambulance, Medical Department, 1 Grosvenor Crescent, London SW1X 7EF. Tel. 071–235 5231. Local groups loan equipment and provide varying services.

Samaritans, 10 The Grove, Slough, Berks SL1 1QP. Tel. 0753 532713. Support for those feeling suicidal, despairing or in crisis. The number of a twenty four hour helpline is inside the front cover of telephone directories.

Simple Solutions, Marketing Department, Age Concern England, Astral House, 1268 London Road, London SW16 4ER. Tel. 081–679 8000. Catalogue of mail order products for disabled people.

The Stroke Association, CHSA House, 123–127 Whitecross Street, London EC1Y 8JJ. Tel. 071–490 7999. Information and grants for stroke sufferers and their carers. Local volunteer stroke services and stroke clubs.

Soldiers, Sailors and Airmen's Families Association, 19 Queen Elizabeth Street,
   London SE1 2LP. Tel. 071–403 8783. Advice and assistance to all
   service and ex-service men and women and their families.
Terence Higgins Trust, 52–54 Grays Inn Road, London WC1X 8JU. Tel.
   071–242 1010.
United Kingdom Home Care Association, c/o 22 Southway, Carshalton,
   Surrey SM5 4HW. Tel. 081–770 3658. An association of providers of
   care at home, with a code of practice. Lists available of member
   agencies and others in the UK.
Women's Royal Voluntary Service (WRVS), 234–244 Stockwell Road, London
   SW9 9SP. Tel. 071–416 0146. A nationwide network of community
   services.

Appendix III: Monitoring quality in homes

The United Kingdom does not have a 'bill of rights' for people in hospitals, and residential and nursing homes. However, there is a range of
published information about maintaining quality of care in homes.
   The Registered Homes Act 1984 and its associated Regulations control
the registration and inspection of private and voluntary residential care
homes, and of nursing homes. The National Health Services and Community Care Act 1990 created the framework for local authorities to set
up inspection units to inspect *all* residential care homes, including those
run directly by themselves.
   The registration and inspection of nursing homes remains the duty of
district health authorities. In January 1985, the National Association of
Health Authorities (now the National Association of Health Authorities
and Trusts) issued a handbook for health authorities: *Registration and
Inspection of Nursing Homes.* A supplement to this booklet (on terminal
care) was published in 1988. These publications set out guidelines which
are followed by health authorities in carrying out inspection and regu-
lation of nursing homes. They are available from: National Association
of Health Authorities and Trusts, Birmingham Research Park, Vincent
Drive, Birmingham B15 2SQ (tel: 021–471 4444).
   There are many publications giving guidance on maintaining and
monitoring the quality of care in residential homes. In 1984, the Centre
for Policy on Ageing published the report of a working party sponsored
by the then Department of Health and Social Security. *Home Life: A code
of practice for residential care* was intended to provide guidance for home
owners and managers, and for local authority Social Services Departments in their inspection and registration duties for non-statutory residential homes. Many local authorities use *Home Life* as their reference
point for inspection and registration. It is available from: Bailey Distri-

bution, Learoyd Road, Mountfield Industrial Estate, New Romney, TN28 8XU (tel: 0679 66905).

More recently, however, an independent review of residential care was carried out by a working group led by Gillian, Lady Wagner. *Residential Care: a positive choice* was published by the National Institute for Social Work in 1988, and is available from HMSO. It was followed by the development of a number of research projects commissioned by the Department of Health under the title of *Caring in Homes Initiative*. The main work of the projects was completed in 1992. They look at information provision by social services departments; training for care staff; links between care homes and the community; complaints procedures; and quality assurance.

The Social Services Inspectorate (SSI) of the Department of Health publishes a range of documents in their *Caring for Quality* series. These documents include *Guidance on Standards for Residential Homes for Elderly People* (HMSO, 1990), which gives guidance on ways of thinking about standards for homes and their management; clarification of the differences between standards for management, standards for care and a good quality of life; and a summary of the standards developed by SSI in its work.

Homes are for Living In (HMSO, 1989) presents a model for evaluating care in homes. It sets out six basic values under which it groups the many factors which contribute to good quality care. These are:

- privacy
- dignity
- independence
- choice
- rights
- fulfilment (*Homes are for Living In*, p. 7)

The work of local authority inspection units is to be monitored by the Social Services Inspectorate. Policy guidance for local authorities on setting up these units is included in *Community Care: the next decade and beyond. Policy Guidance* (Department of Health, HMSO, 1990). More detailed practice guidance is contained in *Inspecting for Quality. Guidance on practice for inspection units in Social Services Departments and other agencies. Principles, issues and recommendations* (Department of Health, Social Services Inspectorate, HMSO, 1991).

The aim of these initiatives from the Department of Health is to ensure that, as far as possible, residential homes in every part of the country operated by the private, voluntary or statutory sectors, are regulated to similar standards. However, standards which authorities set for homes in their areas are not prescribed by law and they may differ. There is some controversy about the extent to which authorities can control the size and operation of care homes in their area; the Registered Homes

Act sets out only a framework, not specific details about standards to be maintained.

There is also controversy about the distinction between residential care and nursing homes. It is argued by some that the boundaries between residential and nursing care are becoming increasingly blurred. In some areas there are joint arrangements for co-operation in inspection between health and local authorities. There have been calls for the two systems to be brought together.

The inspection processes of care homes by health and local authorities come under the remit of the Commissioner on Local Government and the Commissioner for Health (called the 'Ombudsmen'). Where users of services believe that an authority has not acted properly in carrying out its duties, he or she can apply to the appropriate Ombudsman to make a judgement about whether maladministration has occurred. This also applies to other services provided by health and local authorities. Further information about the work of the Ombudsmen and leaflets about how to complain can be obtained from:

Health

England: The Health Service Commissioner for England
           Church House
           Great Smith Street
           London SW1P 3BW

Scotland: The Health Service Commissioner for Scotland
           Second Floor
           11 Melville Crescent
           Edinburgh EH3 7LU

Wales: The Health Service Commissioner for Wales
         Fourth Floor
         Pearl Assurance House
         Greyfriars Road
         Cardiff CF1 3AG

Local authority

England: Local Government Ombudsman
           21 Queen Anne's Gate
           London SW1H 9BU

(This office should be able to put you in touch with a regional office, if more appropriate.)

Scotland: Local Government Ombudsman
5 Shandwick Place
Edinburgh EH2 4RG

Wales: Local Government Ombudsman
Derwen House
Court Road
Bridgend
Mid-Glamorgan CF31 1BN

Index

Long stay hospital 271
  care 272–3
  sexual problems 293
Losing/hiding things 134
Loving 78
Lumbar puncture 13
Lunch clubs 65, 179

Manganese 312
Masturbation 136
Meal
  not eating 53
  preparation 65–6
Meals-on-Wheels 65, 176
Medic Alert bracelet 126
Medic Alert Foundation 126, 326
Medical help 12–20
Medical problems 100–15
Medical treatment/management 17–20
Medicine(s) (medications) 106–8
  cause of incontinence 86
  easy-to-open pill bottles 108
  forgetting to take 53
  pill dispenser 108
  restlessness induced/reduced by 128
  taking too much 53
Memory
  less in old age 6
    concealed 123
  problems 27–8
Messiness, mealtime 67–8
Misinterpretation 156–7
Mobility Allowance 255
Money, inability to manage 47–8
Mongolism (Down's syndrome) 313
Mouth
  putting things into 62
  sores 84
Movement to music 75
Moving one's bowels 86
Moving to new home 55–8
  adjustment period 57
  inability to adjust 57
Multi-infarct dementia 5, 299
  research 307
Muscle weakness 41
Music 77
  movement to 75
Myoclonus (jerking movements) 115

Naming objects/people, difficulties in 34
National Council for Carers and their
    Elderly Dependants 240
Neighbours
  explanation to 213–14
  help from 176

Nervousness 153–5
Neuritic plaque 299
Neurofibrillary tangle 299, 308
Neuroleptics *see* Tranquillisers
Neurological testing 13
Neurotransmitters 308–9
Nibbling 69
Nonverbal signals 89
Nucleus Basalis of Meynert 309
Nurse 18–19
  community psychiatric 18
  district 18
  private 176
Nursing Agencies, private 18–19
Nursing home
  certificate of registration 275
  choice of 276–8
  organisations recommending 275
  sexual problems 293
Nutrition 65

Occupational therapist
  assessment of motor skills 41, 60
  community 18
    bathroom equipment selection
    85
Occupational therapy, assessment 12
Old friends, visits by 77
Oral hygiene 84
Oral infection 108
Orange Badge scheme 51
Organisation setting-up 244
Outside help 169–79
  friends and neighbours 176
  kinds of services 174
Outside helper 176–8
Overreacting reactions *see* Catastrophic
    reactions
Overstimulation 26

Pain 102
Paint 62
  loose chips, lead-containing 62
Paranoid ideas 54, 156, 158–61
Parkinson's disease
  movement problems 41
Peer support group 245
Pension, state 253
  collection by named person
  265
Personal hygiene 79–80
Personal information wallet 126
Personality changes 7
Petrol 62
PETT (position emission transaxial
    tomography) 316